SpringerWienNewYork

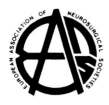

Sponsored by the
European Association of Neurosurgical Societies

Advances
and Technical Standards
in Neurosurgery

Vol. 36

Edited by
J. D. Pickard, Cambridge (Editor-in-Chief),
N. Akalan, Ankara, V. Benes Jr., Prague,
C. Di Rocco, Roma, V. V. Dolenc, Ljubljana,
J. Lobo Antunes, Lisbon, J. Schramm, Bonn,
M. Sindou, Lyon

SpringerWienNewYork

This work is subject to copyright.
All rights are reserved, whether the whole or part of the material is concerned, specifically those of translation, reprinting, re-use of illustrations, broadcasting, reproduction by photocopying machines or similar means, and storage in data banks.

© 2011 Springer-Verlag/Wien
Printed in Austria

SpringerWienNewYork is part of Springer Science Business Media
springer.at

Typesetting: Thomson Press (India) Ltd., Chennai
Printing: Holzhausen Druck GmbH, 1140 Wien, Austria

Product Liability: The publisher can give no guarantee for the information contained in this book.
This does also refers to information about drug dosage and application thereof. In every individual case the respective user must check the accuracy by consulting other pharmaceutical literature.
The use of registered names, trademarks, etc. in this publication does not imply, even in the absence of specific statement, that such names are exempt from the relevant protective laws and regulations and therefore free for general use.

Printed on acid-free and chlorine-free bleached paper
SPIN: 12987481

With 73 (partly coloured) Figures

Library of Congress Control Number: 2010931517

ISSN 0095-4829
ISBN 978-3-7091-0178-0 SpringerWienNewYork

Preface

As an addition to the European postgraduate training system for young neurosurgeons, our predecessors began to publish in 1974 this series of *Advances and Technical Standards in Neurosurgery* which was later sponsored by the European Association of Neurosurgical Societies.

This series was first discussed in 1972 at a combined meeting of the Italian and German Neurosurgical Societies in Taormina, the founding fathers of the series being Jean Brihaye, Bernard Pertuiset, Fritz Loew and Hugo Krayenbühl. Thus were established the principles of European co-operation which have been born from the European spirit, flourished in the European Association, and have been associated throughout with this series.

The fact that the English language is now the international medium for communication at European scientific conferences is a great asset in terms of mutual understanding. Therefore we have decided to publish all contributions in English, regardless of the native language of the authors.

All contributions are submitted to the entire editorial board before publication of any volume for scrutiny and suggestions for revision.

Our series is not intended to compete with the publications of original scientific papers in other neurosurgical journals. Our intention is, rather, to present fields of neurosurgery and related areas in which important recent advances have been made. The contributions are written by specialists in the given fields and constitute the first part of each volume.

In the second part of each volume, we publish detailed descriptions of standard operative procedures and in-depth reviews of established knowledge in all aspects of neurosurgery, furnished by experienced clinicians. This part is intended primarily to assist young neurosurgeons in their postgraduate training. However, we are sure that it will also be useful to experienced, fully trained neurosurgeons.

We hope therefore that surgeons not only in Europe, but also throughout the world, will profit by this series of *Advances and Technical Standards in Neurosurgery*.

The Editors

Contents

List of contributors   XIII

Advances

Detecting residual cognitive function in disorders of consciousness. M. R. COLEMAN[1,2] and J. D. PICKARD[1,2], [1]Cambridge Impaired Consciousness Research Group, Academic Neurosurgery and Wolfson Brain Imaging Centre, Department of Clinical Neurosciences, Addenbrooke's Hospital, Cambridge, UK, [2]Academic Neurosurgery Unit, Addenbrooke's Hospital, University of Cambridge, Cambridge, UK

Abstract   3
Introduction.   4
Positron emission tomography   5
Functional magnetic resonance imaging   6
Using neuroimaging to detect awareness   10
Interpretation of fMRI findings   12
Limitations of neuroimaging   13
Conclusions.   14
References   14

Rationale for hypothalamus-deep brain stimulation in food intake disorders and obesity. N. TORRES[2], S. CHABARDÈS[1,3], and A. L. BENABID[2], [1]Grenoble Institute of Neurosciences, Unite INSERM U836, Grenoble, France, [2]CEA CLINATEC, Grenoble, France, [3]Department of Neurosurgery, University Hospital, Joseph Fourier University, Grenoble, France

Abstract   17
Introduction.   18
Central nervous system control of food intake and weight   19
Deep brain stimulation of the hypothalamus: rationale and putative
hypothalamic targets   21
    Lateral hypothalamus   21
    Ventromedial hypothalamus   22

Experimental studies: Grenoble experience	23
Material and methods	23
Human studies	26
References	28

Gustatory and reward brain circuits in the control of food intake. A. J. OLIVEIRA-MAIA[1,6], C. D. ROBERTS[1], S. A. SIMON[1,3,4], and M. A. L. NICOLELIS[1-5], [1]Department of Neurobiology, Duke University Medical Center, Durham, NC, USA, [2]Department of Psychology and Neurosciences, Duke University Medical Center, Durham, NC, USA, [3]Department of Biomedical Engineering, Duke University Medical Center, Durham, NC, USA, [4]Center for Neuroengineering, Duke University Medical Center, Durham, NC, USA, [5]Edmond and Lily Safra International Institute for Neuroscience of Natal, Natal, Rio Grande do Norte, Brazil, [6]Current addresses: Champalimaud Neuroscience Program, Instituto Gulbenkian de Ciência, Oeiras, Portugal; Department of Psychiatry and Mental Health, Centro Hospitalar de Lisboa Ocidental, Lisbon, Portugal

Abstract	32
Abbreviations	32
Introduction	33
Gustation and gustatory system: definitions	33
Orosensory gustatory input	34
Postingestive sensory processes	38
Central gustatory sensory pathways	41
Amygdala and brain reward pathways	44
Hypothalamus, brainstem and energy homeostasis	45
Novel opportunities in the management of obesity?	48
Conclusions	50
Acknowledgements	50
References	50

SEEG-guided RF-thermocoagulation of epileptic foci: A therapeutic alternative for drug-resistant non-operable partial epilepsies. M. GUÉNOT[1,3-5], J. ISNARD[2-5], H. CATENOIX[2-5], F. MAUGUIÈRE[2-5], and M. SINDOU[1,3,4], [1]Service de Neurochirurgie Fonctionnelle, Hôpital Neurologique Pierre Wertheimer, Hospices Civils de Lyon, Bron, France, [2]Service de Neurologie Fonctionnelle et d'Epileptologie, Hôpital Neurologique Pierre Wertheimer, Hospices Civils de Lyon, Bron, France, [3]Université de Lyon, Université Lyon 1, Lyon, France, [4]Institut Fédératif des Neurosciences de Lyon, Lyon, France, [5]INSERM, U879, Bron, France; Université de Lyon, Université Lyon 1, Lyon, France

Abstract	62
Introduction	63
Technical data	65

Advantages of the technique 65
Patient's selection 66
Placement of the lesion 66
Our experience 68
Patients 68
Targets, follow-up and results 68
Choice of targets 70
Follow-up 70
Results 73
Seizure outcome 73
Safety 74
Discussion 74
Conclusion 76
References 76

Child abuse – some aspects for neurosurgeons. B. MADEA[1], M. NOEKER[2], and I. FRANKE[2], [1]Institute of Legal Medicine, University of Bonn, Bonn, Germany, [2]Department of Pediatrics, University of Bonn, Bonn, Germany

Abstract 80
Introduction 80
Definitions and epidemiology 81
Legal basis 83
Criminology of child abuse 84
Physical examination and taking the history 86
Injuries 86
Blunt force 87
Interpretation of injuries 90
Bone injuries 95
Head injuries, fractures of the skull 99
Non-accidental head injury/shaken-baby-syndrome 104
Shaken-baby-syndrome (SBS) 104
Thermal injuries 109
Injuries of the eyes 114
Differential diagnoses 114
Münchausen syndrome by proxy 116
Lethal child abuse 119
Physical neglect 119
Starvation 120
Taking the case history 121
Structured forensic, investigative interview with the child 122
Documentation 123
General symptoms in cases of child abuse 123
Proceeding in cases of suspected child abuse 124
Child protection team 125

X   Contents

Clinical pathway 126
  Definition of Clinical Pathway 126
Bonn child protection team clinical pathway for suspected child abuse 130
References 130

Technical standards   137

Prophylactic antibiotics and anticonvulsants in neurosurgery. B. RATILAL[1] and C. SAMPAIO[2], [1]Department of Neurosurgery, Hospital de São José, Centro Hospitalar de Lisboa Central, Lisboa, Portugal, [2]Laboratório de Farmacologia Clínica e Terapêutica, Faculdade de Medicina da Universidade de Lisboa, Lisboa, Portugal

Abstract 140
Introduction 140
Antibiotic prophylaxis 142
  Antibiotics for craniotomies 142
  Antibiotics for spinal surgeries 142
  Antibiotics for basilar skull fractures 143
    Background 143
    Clinical material and methods 143
    Results 146
  Non-RCTs that have been systematically reviewed 149
    Discussion 150
    Conclusions 151
  Antibiotics for cerebrospinal fluid shunts 151
    Background 151
    Clinical material and methods 152
    Results 153
    Discussion 166
    Conclusions 167
Anticonvulsant prophylaxis 168
  Anticonvulsants for subarachnoid hemorrhages 168
  Anticonvulsants for acute traumatic brain injuries 168
  Anticonvulsants for chronic subdural hematomas 169
    Background 169
    Clinical material and methods 169
    Results 170
    Discussion 170
    Conclusions 171
  Anticonvulsants for brain tumors 172
    Background 172
    Clinical material and methods 172
    Results 173
    Discussion 177
    Conclusions 178

Commentaries 178
References... 178

The dural sheath of the optic nerve: descriptive anatomy and surgical applications.
P. FRANCOIS[1,2], E. LESCANNE[3], and S. VELUT[1,2], [1]Université François Rabelais de Tours, Laboratoire d'anatomie, Tours, France, [2]CHRU de Tours, Service de Neurochirurgie, Tours, France, [3]CHRU de Tours, Service d'Oto-Rhino-Laryngologie, Tours, France

Abstract 187
Introduction... 188
   Embryology... 188
   The interperiosteodural concept..................................... 190
   Intracranial segment.. 191
   Intracanalicular segment.. 191
      Relations with bony structures 191
      Meningeal relations... 194
   Intraorbital segment 195
Conclusion... 197
References... 198

Surgical indications and techniques for failed coiled aneurysms.
C. RAFTOPOULOS; with the collaboration of G. VAZ, Department of Neurosurgery, University Hospital St-Luc, Université Catholique de Louvain (UCL), Brussels, Belgium

Abstract 199
Introduction... 200
Experience of our group 202
   Our population and illustrative cases................................ 208
   Our classification of FCA and its lessons........................... 213
Experiences of other teams... 217
Conclusions.. 222
References... 222

Author index... 227
Subject index 241

Listed in PubMed

List of contributors

Benabid, A. L., CEA CLINATEC, Grenoble, France

Catenoix, H., Service de Neurologie Fonctionnelle et d'Epileptologie, Hôpital Neurologique Pierre Wertheimer, Hospices Civils de Lyon, Bron, France; Université de Lyon, Université Lyon 1, Lyon, France; Institut Fédératif des Neurosciences de Lyon, Lyon, France; INSERM, U879, Bron, France and Université de Lyon, Université Lyon 1, Lyon, France

Chabardès, S., Grenoble Institute of Neurosciences, Unite INSERM U836 and Department of Neurosurgery, University Hospital, Joseph Fourier University, Grenoble, France

Coleman, M. R., Cambridge Impaired Consciousness Research Group, Academic Surgery and Wolfson Brain Imaging Centre, Department of Clinical Neurosciences, Addenbrooke's Hospital and Academic Neurosurgery Unit, Addenbrooke's Hospital, University of Cambridge, Cambridge, UK

Francois, P., Université François Rabelais de Tours, Laboratoire d'anatomie, Tours, France and CHRU de Tours, Service de Neurochirurgie, Tours, France

Franke, I., Department of Pediatrics, University of Bonn, Bonn, Germany

Guénot, M., Service de Neurochirurgie Fonctionnelle, Hôpital Neurologique Pierre Wertheimer, Hospices Civils de Lyon, Bron, France; Université de Lyon, Université Lyon 1, Lyon, France; Institut Fédératif des Neurosciences de Lyon, Lyon, France; INSERM, U879, Bron, France and Université de Lyon, Université Lyon 1, Lyon, France

Isnard, J., Service de Neurologie Fonctionnelle et d'Epileptologie, Hôpital Neurologique Pierre Wertheimer, Hospices Civils de Lyon, Bron, France; Université de Lyon, Université Lyon 1, Lyon, France; Institut Fédératif des Neurosciences de Lyon, Lyon, France; INSERM, U879, Bron, France and Université de Lyon, Université Lyon 1, Lyon, France

Lescanne, E., CHRU de Tours, Service d'Oto-Rhino-Laryngologie, Tours, France

Madea, B., Institute of Legal Medicine, University of Bonn, Bonn, Germany

Mauguière, F., Service de Neurologie Fonctionnelle et d'Epileptologie, Hôpital Neurologique Pierre Wertheimer, Hospices Civils de Lyon, Bron, France; Université de Lyon, Université Lyon 1, Lyon, France; Institut Fédératif des Neurosciences de Lyon, Lyon, France; INSERM, U879, Bron, Frances and Université de Lyon, Université Lyon 1, Lyon, France

Nicolelis, M. A. L., Department of Neurobiology, Duke University Medical Center; Department of Psychology and Neurosciences, Duke University Medical Center; Department of Biomedical Engineering, Duke University Medical Center; Center for Neuroengineering, Duke University Medical Center, Durham, NC, USA and Edmond and Lily Safra International Institute for Neuroscience of Natal, Natal, Rio Grande do Norte, Brazil

Noeker, M., Department of Pediatrics, University of Bonn, Bonn, Germany

Oliveira-Maia, A. J., Department of Neurobiology, Duke University Medical Center, Durham, NC, USA; Current addresses: Champalimaud Neuroscience Program, Instituto Gulbenkian de Ciência, Oeiras and Department of Psychiatry and Mental Health, Centro Hospitalar de Lisboa Ocidental, Lisbon, Portugal

Pickard, J. D., Cambridge Impaired Consciousness Research Group, Academic Surgery and Wolfson Brain Imaging Centre, Department of Clinical Neurosciences, Addenbrooke's Hospital and Academic Neurosurgery Unit, Addenbrooke's Hospital, University of Cambridge, Cambridge, UK

Raftopoulos, C., Department of Neurosurgery, University Hospital St-Luc, Université Catholique de Louvain (UCL), Brussels, Belgium

Ratilal, B., Department of Neurosurgery, Hospital de São José, Centro Hospitalar de Lisboa Central, Lisboa, Portugal

Roberts, C. D., Department of Neurobiology, Duke University Medical Center, Durham, NC, USA

Sampaio, C., Laboratório de Farmacologia Clínica e Terapêutica, Faculdade de Medicina da Universidade de Lisboa, Lisboa, Portugal

Simon, S. A., Department of Neurobiology, Duke University Medical Center; Department of Biomedical Engineering, Duke University Medical Center and Center for Neuroengineering, Duke University Medical Center, Durham, NC, USA

Sindou, M., Service de Neurochirurgie Fonctionnelle, Hôpital Neurologique Pierre Wertheimer, Hospices Civils de Lyon, Bron, France; Université de Lyon, Université Lyon 1, Lyon, France and Institut Fédératif des Neurosciences de Lyon, Lyon, France

Torres, N., CEA CLINATEC, Grenoble, France

Vaz, G., Department of Neurosurgery, University Hospital St-Luc, Université Catholique de Louvain (UCL), Brussels, Belgium

Velut, S., Université François Rabelais de Tours, Laboratoire d'anatomie and CHRU de Tours, Service de Neurochirurgie, Tours, France

Advances

Detecting residual cognitive function in disorders of consciousness

M. R. COLEMAN[1,2] and J. D. PICKARD[1,2]

[1] Cambridge Impaired Consciousness Research Group, Academic Neurosurgery and Wolfson Brain Imaging Centre, Department of Clinical Neurosciences, Addenbrooke's Hospital, Cambridge, UK
[2] Academic Neurosurgery Unit, Addenbrooke's Hospital, University of Cambridge, Cambridge, UK

With 3 Figures

Contents

Abstract 3
Introduction 4
Positron emission tomography 5
Functional magnetic resonance imaging 6
Using neuroimaging to detect awareness 10
Interpretation of fMRI findings 12
Limitations of neuroimaging 13
Conclusions 14
References 14

Abstract

Clinical audits have suggested up to 40% of patients with disorders of consciousness may be misdiagnosed, in part, due to the highly subjective process of determining, from a patient's behaviour, whether they retain awareness of self or environment. To address this problem, objective neuroimaging methods, such as positron emission tomography and functional magnetic resonance imaging have been explored. Using these techniques, paradigms, which do not require the patient to move or speak, can be used to determine a patient's level of residual cognitive function. Indeed, visual discrimination, speech comprehension and even the ability to respond to command have been demonstrated in some patients who are assumed to be vegetative on the basis of standard behavioural assessments. Functional neuroimaging is now increasingly considered to be a very useful and necessary addition to the clinical assessment process, where there is concern about the accuracy of the diagnosis and the possibility that residual cognitive function has remained undetected. In this essay, the latest neuroimaging findings are reviewed, the limitations and caveats pertaining to interpretation are outlined and the necessary developments, before neuroimaging becomes a standard component of the clinical assessment are discussed.

Keywords: Vegetative state; minimally conscious state; functional magnetic resonance imaging.

Introduction

The management and rehabilitation of severely brain-damaged patients with disorders of consciousness is highly dependent on obtaining an accurate and reliable evaluation of their level of cognitive processing [21]. At present a diagnosis is made predominately on the basis of a patient's clinical history and exhibited behaviour. This assessment, however, is often fraught with difficulties, as many patients are unable to move or vocalise and thus demonstrate awareness of self or environment. The interpretation of exhibited behaviour is therefore highly subjective and attributed as one of the main reasons for the high rate of misdiagnosis found in the vegetative state (VS), minimally conscious state (MCS) and locked-in syndrome [1, 7, 37]. Recent advances in functional neuroimaging, however, have suggested a novel solution to this problem; so-called "activation" studies, which do not require the patient to move or speak, can be used to assess whether a patient retains the ability to comprehend and even respond to speech.

In several recent studies, neuroimaging has been used to detect residual cognitive function and even conscious awareness in patients who behaviourally met the criteria defining the vegetative state [8–10, 26, 28]. These studies are amongst a growing number of examples suggesting neuroimaging may provide important additional information to inform the diagnostic decision making process, inform prognosis and reduce the current rate of misdiagnosis. Crucially, neuroimaging is also enabling scientists and clinicians to glean a greater understanding of the mechanisms underlying conditions of impaired consciousness. In two recent studies this information has been used to guide therapeutic interventions and track recovery [35, 40] and it is anticipated neuroimaging will play an even greater role in guiding therapeutic choices in the future [17, 21].

Positron emission tomography

The first neuroimaging studies in patients with disorders of consciousness used either flurodeoxyglucose (FDG) positron emission tomography (PET) or single photon emission computed tomography (SPECT) to measure resting cerebral blood flow and glucose metabolism [6, 15, 23, 34, 39]. These studies typically found widespread reductions in metabolic activity of up to 50% [2, 36], although in some cases, isolated 'islands' of preserved metabolic activity were identified, suggesting the possibility that some patients may harbour residual function [36]. While these studies undoubtedly provided further impetus to explore residual cognitive function with neuroimaging, metabolic studies were only able to identify functionality at the most general level. Neuroimaging investigations therefore turned to the use of $H_2{}^{15}O$ PET and functional magnetic resonance imaging (fMRI), which are able to link specific changes in blood flow or metabolism to circumscribed cognitive processes [25].

The first activation study using $H_2{}^{15}O$ PET measured regional cerebral blood flow in a post-traumatic vegetative patient during an auditorily presented story told by his mother [14]. Compared to non-word sounds, activation was observed in the anterior cingulate and temporal cortices, possibly reflecting emotional processing of the contents, or tone, of the mother's speech. In another patient diagnosed as vegetative, Menon *et al.* [24], used PET to study covert visual processing in response to familiar faces. When the patient was presented with pictures of the faces of family and close friends, robust activity was observed in the right fusiform gyrus, the so-called human "face area". Importantly, both of these studies involved single, well-documented cases; in group studies of patients meeting the criteria defining the vegetative state, normal brain activity in response to external stimulation has generally been the exception rather than the rule. For example, in one study of fifteen vegetative patients, high intensity noxious electrical stimulation activated midbrain, contralateral thalamus and primary somatosensory cortex in every patient [22]. However, unlike control subjects, the patients did not activate secondary somatosensory, insular, posterior parietal or anterior cingulate cortices.

Early activations studies in patients with disorders of consciousness used $H_2{}^{15}O$ PET, in part because the technique was more widely available and in part because the multiple logistic difficulties of scanning critically ill patients in the strong magnetic field, that is integral to fMRI studies, had yet to be resolved. However, $H_2{}^{15}O$ PET studies are limited by issues of radiation burden which make longitudinal or follow-up studies difficult and prevent a comprehensive examination of multiple cognitive processes within a single session. The power of PET studies to detect statistically significant responses is also low and group studies are often needed to satisfy standard statistical criteria [31]. These limitations thus fall short of clinical demands, which require objective information for each individual in terms of diagnosis, residual function and potential for recovery. fMRI in contrast has no associated radiation burden, offers increased statistical power, improved spatial and temporal resolution and the ability to comprehensively assess the residual function of an individual during a single session.

Functional magnetic resonance imaging

An increasing number of event-related fMRI studies are now being published each year demonstrating various degrees of retained function in patients with disorders of consciousness [4, 8, 9, 16, 38]. fMRI, however, is not without its complexities and challenges when applied to this patient group. Work in a strong magnetic field has well known safety and logistical constraints, but the behaviour of patients with disorders of consciousness also creates challenges. For example, many vegetative patients only have transient periods of eye opening, making the use of visual paradigms difficult. Similarly, scanning a patient who is unable to communicate presents numerous ethical dilemmas, particularly when they are unable to tell you if they are in pain.

Where these difficulties are overcome, the design of fMRI paradigms and their interpretation must also be carefully planned in order to ensure that a specific cognitive process is appropriately assessed and where neural activation is observed this is known to occur in healthy volunteers. Unfortunately, many neuroimaging paradigms are let down by the use of a reverse inference approach, whereby a given cognitive process is inferred based on an observed activation in a particular brain region. For instance, a patient is presented with his/her name spoken by the voice of his/her mother in one condition and the sound of scanner noise in another condition. Using a simple subtraction analysis the experimenters observe greater cortical activation in the primary auditory cortex when the patient hears his mother's voice *versus* the scanner noise. One conclusion could be that the patient recognised his/her name, but the activation observed could equally reflect a low level orienting response to speech in general or an emotional response to the mother's voice. Such a paradigm therefore lacks cognitive specificity and provides limited information about the retained cognitive function of a patient with impaired consciousness. fMRI paradigms require careful planning in order to ensure that they are appropriately counterbalanced and can be directly attributed to a specific cognitive process under study. Using mother voice as an example, a study by Staffen *et al.* [38], compared the response of a patient to hearing their own name *versus* another name. In this case, because identical speech-stimuli were used which differed only with respect to the name itself, activations could be confidently attributed to cognitive processing that is specifically related to the patient's own name. Staffen *et al.* found activation in the medial prefrontal cortex in response to the patient's own, but not in response to other names. This pattern of activation was similar to that observed in three healthy volunteers and corresponds closely to the findings of an electrophysiological study, which reported responses to patients own names (compared to other peoples names) in locked-in, minimally conscious and some vegetative patients [32].

Although knowing that a patient recognises their own name or the voice of a family member is often comforting to their relatives, a response to one's own name is one of the most basic forms of language and may not depend on the higher-level linguistic processes that are assumed to underpin comprehension. We have therefore previously proposed a hierarchical approach to the fMRI assessment of language comprehension in patients with disorders of consciousness; beginning with the simplest form of auditory processing and progressing sequentially through more complex cognitive operations [8, 28, 29].

In a recent study of 22 vegetative and nineteen minimally conscious patients, we assessed each patient's response at three levels of auditory processing to four conditions (sentences containing ambiguous words, sentences containing unambiguous words, signal correlated noise and silence) presented pseudorandomly [10]. At the lowest level we determined whether these patients retained basic primary auditory processing in response to hearing sound (both intelligible speech and unintelligible noise) in contrast to a silent, inter-scan baseline. This level of analysis identifies those brain regions that process the acoustic properties of sound that is common to both speech and non-speech stimuli. In healthy controls this contrast produces activation in primary auditory regions on the superior temporal plane, centred on Heschl's gyrus [33].

The second level of analysis assesses speech-specific perceptual processing by comparing fMRI responses to intelligible speech *versus* acoustically-matched unintelligible noise stimuli. It therefore goes further than our first level of analysis because it specifically isolates the brain's response to intelligible speech, whereas the first level of analysis was designed to identify the brain's response to sound in general (i.e. both intelligible and non-intelligible sounds) when compared to silence.

At the third level of analysis, sentences containing ambiguous words (e.g. bark, or rain/reign) are contrasted with sentences containing no ambiguous words. In healthy volunteers this comparison reveals distributed higher order processing in the left inferior frontal and left temporal cortex reflecting the retrieval of semantic information that is essential in order to process the intended meaning of the ambiguous words. The presence of appropriate activations in this contrast provides strong evidence that some high-level semantic aspects of speech comprehension are preserved.

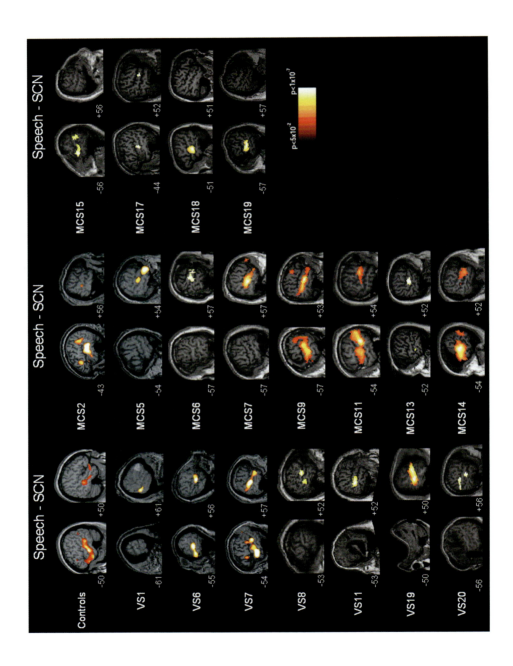

Detecting residual cognitive function 9

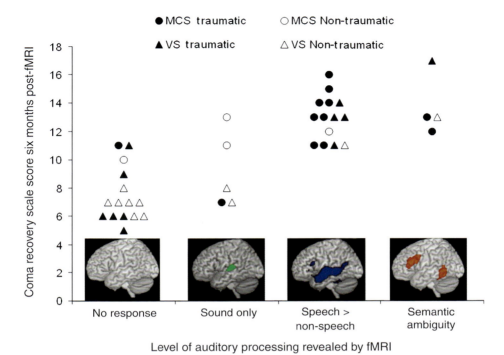

Fig. 2. Level of auditory processing achieved by each patient grouped by diagnosis and aetiology during fMRI, plotted against their six-month highest Coma Recovery Scale (CRS) score. Images at the bottom show left-hemisphere activation for each level of auditory processing from groups of healthy participants in previous control studies. Responses to sound only depicts the contrast of non-speech noise compared to silence from Davis and Johnsrude [13]. Responses to speech *versus* non-speech and high *versus* low ambiguity are reported from Ref. [33]. Reproduced from Ref. [10]

Fig. 1. Residual language function in patients diagnosed as either vegetative or minimally conscious. Seven of the twenty-two patients who had a clinical diagnosis of vegetative state (VS) and twelve of nineteen patients who had a clinical diagnosis of minimally conscious state showed normal responses to sound *versus* silence and intelligible speech *versus* unintelligible noise (shown). Activations are thresholded at $P<0.05$ FDR corrected for multiple comparisons and shown on slices where the peak activation was observed. Numbers represent the x-value of MNI co-ordinates. Reproduced from Ref. [10]

Our fMRI investigation of 22 vegetative and nineteen minimally conscious patients found that seven vegetative patients and twelve minimally conscious patients retained significant temporal-lobe responses in the first and second level of analysis i.e., basic primary auditory cortex responses to sound, but also more elaborate responses to intelligible speech *versus* non-intelligible noise stimuli (Fig. 1; [10]). However, of particular importance, our investigation also found evidence of high level language function (i.e., retrieval of semantic information), in two of the vegetative patients. This striking finding not only showed aspects of normal speech processing in some vegetative patients with negative behavioural markers, but it also revealed a potentially important prognostic tool. When the level of auditory processing achieved by each patient was compared to their subsequent outcome six months post scan, a highly significant correlation (r_s 0.81, $P < 0.001$) was found. Indeed, every patient, who at the time of scanning had shown a behavioural profile consistent with the vegetative state, but a high level of speech processing on brain imaging, subsequently progressed to a minimally conscious state six months post scan (Fig. 2; [10]).

Using neuroimaging to detect awareness

In order for brain imaging to be able to inform the diagnostic decision making process, it needs to be able to provide unequivocal evidence that a patient is aware without requiring him/her to move or speak. Although evidence from a study of healthy sedated volunteers undertaking our speech processing paradigm suggests a person needs to be conscious to demonstrate aspects of speech comprehension [12], a similar pattern of activation in a patient does not necessarily imply they are conscious. Moreover, speech comprehension *per se*, is a subcategory of consciousness; the ability to respond to command and ultimately describe ones feelings, beliefs and experiences being higher examples, which clearly demonstrate a person is aware. In order to address this problem we have recently turned our attention to creating a paradigm that demonstrates that a patient is able to respond to command and answer basic questions without moving or speaking. To do this we instruct patients (who have firstly demonstrated aspects of speech comprehension on our paradigm described above) to perform two mental imagery tasks when cued by the instructions "imagine playing tennis" or "imagine moving around the rooms of your home". In healthy volunteers these tasks elicit robust and reproducible patterns of activation in the supplementary motor cortex and parahippocampal gyrus respectively [5]. Hence, where a patient demonstrates these anatomically distinct patterns of activation, they are not only showing that they understand the instruction (to imagine playing tennis, for example), but also retain the ability to wilfully follow the instruction. This creates the most important benefit of brain imaging to the clinical team, namely a non-verbal means of communication to explore the full extent of retained cognition. Where a patient is able to demonstrate appropriate areas of activation to these commands, they can be further instructed to undertake one of these tasks to indicate "Yes" and the other to indicate "No".

We have recently used this approach to demonstrate that a young woman who fulfilled all internationally agreed criteria for the vegetative state was, in fact, consciously aware and able to make responses using her brain activity, despite her clinical diagnosis [26]. In July 2005, the 23-year-old woman sustained a severe traumatic brain injury as a result of a road traffic accident. During the 5 months between her accident and the fMRI scan, she was assessed by a multidisciplinary team employing repeated standardised assessments consistent with the procedure described by Bates [3] and her condition

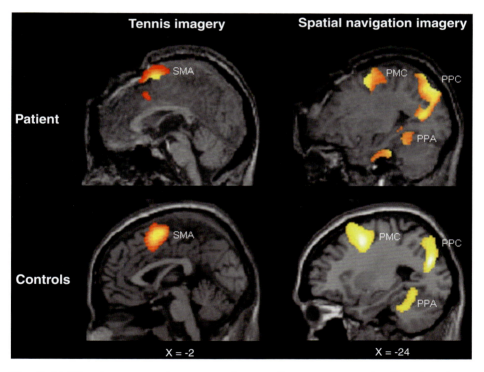

Fig. 3. Volitional responses to command suggesting awareness of self and environment in a patient who fulfilled the clinical criteria defining the vegetative state. In response to the command "imagine playing tennis" the patient showed sustained activity in the supplementary motor area consistent with healthy volunteers. Similarly, in response to the command "imagine moving through the rooms of your home" the patient showed activity in the parahippocampal gyrus, the posterior parietal lobe and the lateral premotor cortex consistent with healthy volunteers. Reproduced from Ref. [26]

was entirely consistent with a diagnosis of vegetative state. During the fMRI scan, the patient was instructed to perform the two mental imagery tasks described above. When she was asked to imagine playing tennis, significant activity was observed in the supplementary motor area (Fig. 3; [26]), that was indistinguishable from that observed in the healthy volunteers scanned by Boly *et al.* [5]. In contrast, when she was asked to imagine moving through the rooms of her home, significant activity was observed in the parahippocampal gyrus, the posterior parietal cortex and the lateral premotor cortex (Fig. 3; [26]), which was again, indistinguishable from those observed in healthy volunteers [5]. We concluded that, despite fulfilling all of the clinical criteria for a diagnosis of vegetative state, this patient retained the ability to understand spoken commands and to respond to them through her brain activity, rather than through speech or movement, confirming beyond any doubt that she was consciously aware of herself and her surroundings. Three years post investigation, this patient has progressed to a severely disabled condition. She retains many physical and cognitive impairment's, but is crucially able to communicate verbally, respond to command and use objects functionally.

The hierarchical fMRI approach described in this essay therefore provides an important additional source of information to the clinical assessment of patients with disorders of consciousness. In patients unable to move, these paradigms are able to reveal evidence of retained cognitive function such as speech comprehension, but they are also able to reveal whether someone is able to willfully respond to command. Crucially, the described hierarchal approach may provide an early communication channel between the patient and clinician, where movement and speech are impaired and provide reliable prognostic information from which to plan therapeutic interventions.

Interpretation of fMRI findings

The interpretation of experimental fMRI data naturally creates scientific debate, especially where the acquired evidence suggests a patient otherwise thought to be in a vegetative state, is in fact, aware of her-self and environment. Indeed, following the publication of the above case, Owen *et al.* [27] responded to several commentaries, which suggested the patient's response to the mental imagery instructions could have been automatic rather than an act of will. It is true that many forms of stimuli, including speech will elicit relatively "automatic" responses, which do not require the patient to participate. However, such responses are transient and occur in the primary sensory cortex. In the mental imagery task described, a participant is asked to imagine playing tennis and importantly to sustain this form of mental imagery for 30 sec, before entering a period of rest for 30 sec on command. This period of mental imagery followed by a period of rest is requested in total five times during the scan. Hence, the participant must wilfully modulate their brain activity in precise sequence with the commands. As both conditions (tennis and rest) are preceded by a verbal instruction, the presence of sustained neural activation to one command and not the other cannot be attributed to merely an automatic response. Indeed, the instruction to imagine playing tennis produced activation in the supplementary motor area (SMA), consistent with motor planning and motor imagery in healthy volunteers [5]. We did not observe any activation in the primary auditory cortex, which would be expected if the response was simply an automatic response to speech. Moreover, the cortical activation seen in the SMA was sustained for a full 30 sec before it ceased on command. We know of no data supporting the inference that such a paradigm can unconsciously elicit sustained hemodynamic responses in these anatomically-specific regions of the brain. Indeed, non-instructive sentences containing the same key words (e.g. "The man enjoyed playing tennis") produce no sustained activity in any of these brain regions in healthy volunteers [27]. Similarly, when the words "tennis" and "house" are presented to uninstructed participants no activity is observed in either the SMA or the PPA.

Limitations of neuroimaging

Although neuroimaging has the potential to inform the clinical assessment of patients with disorders of consciousness, it is not without its own challenges and complexities [17]. Patients with disorders of consciousness have very different behavioural presentations, many creating challenges for functional imaging. For example, some patients demonstrate long periods of eye closure; others demonstrate a bruxism or spontaneous movement of the head. Others intermittently cough and demonstrate flexion/extension through the trunk and limbs. Such spontaneous movement can severely impair the quality of the imaging and limit meaningful interpretation. Similarly, the pathological presentation of patients can also complicate the fitting of functional imaging data to structural imaging data, and the normalisation of these images through reference to a healthy brain. Under these circumstances, statistical assessment of activation patterns is complex and interpretation of activation foci with standard stereotaxic coordinates may be impossible.

As already alluded to, the design of the fMRI task is also critically important. The task must be complex enough that the cognitive process of interest is appropriately studied, but not so complex that the task places too greater demand on a patient who might have fluctuating periods of wakefulness and attention. Moreover, unlike most imaging studies of healthy volunteers, the tasks used must be able to produce robust and reproducible, anatomically specific, patterns of activation in each and every individual, rather than a statistically significant proportion of a healthy cohort.

Whilst the interpretation of positive patterns of activation creates challenges, the absence of appropriate activation requires careful interpretation too. Whilst it may genuinely reflect the severely impaired condition of the patient, it can never be used as evidence of lack of awareness, since 'false negative' results are well documented in healthy volunteers and thus we cannot exclude that at another time that same person may show a response to the task [30]. For example, rather than underlying pathological reasons, the patient may have fallen asleep during the scan or may have even decided not to perform it.

Conclusions

The incidence of misdiagnosis in patients with disorders of consciousness remains alarmingly high [1, 7, 37]. Despite the development of specialist behavioural tools and an acceptance that patient's should be assessed repeatedly over a period of time, behavioural tools continue to require the patient to move or speak in order to demonstrate awareness of self and/or environment [18–20]. The development of objective tools which do not have this handicap is therefore imperative to reducing misdiagnosis and accurately guiding therapeutic choices. One such tool to aid the clinician in addressing this challenge is the use of positron emission tomography and particularly functional magnetic resonance imaging. These techniques are not only able to reveal the pathophysiology underlying these conditions, but are also able to quantify the extent of retained cognitive function, without requiring the patient to move or speak [8]. Indeed, in several neuroimaging studies, patients who have behaviourally met the criteria defining the vegetative state have been found, in fact, to retain evidence of speech comprehension and even ability to respond to command. Whilst the incidence of such retained function is likely to be extremely low, these techniques undoubtedly offer the clinician an additional source of information to aid the challenging diagnostic decision making process. In our opinion there is now sufficient brain imaging evidence to warrant reconvening the Royal College of Physician working party on vegetative state and other International bodies to develop standardised protocols for this purpose [8].

References

1. Andrews K, Murphy L, Munday R, *et al.* (1996) Misdiagnosis of the vegetative state: retrospective study in a rehabilitation unit. BMJ 313: 13–16
2. Agardh CD, Rosen I, Ryding E (1983) Persistent vegetative state with high cerebral blood flow following profound hypoglycemia. Ann Neurol 14(4): 482–86
3. Bates D (2005) The vegetative state and the Royal College of Physicians guidance. Neuropsychol Rehabil 15(3/4): 175–83
4. Bekinschtein T, Leiguarda R, Armony J, *et al.* (2004) Emotion processing in the minimally conscious state. J Neurol Neurosurg Psychiatry 75(5): 788

5. Boly M, Coleman MR, Davis MH, *et al.* (2007) When thoughts become action : an fMRI paradigm to study volitional brain activity in non-communicative brain injured patients. Neuroimage 36: 979–92
6. Beuthien-Baumann B, Handrick W, Schmidt T, *et al.* (2003) Persistent vegetative state: evaluation of brain metabolism and brain perfusion with PET and SPECT. Nucl Med Commun 24(6): 643–49
7. Childs NL, Mercer WN, Childs HW (1993) Accuracy of diagnosis of persistent vegetative state. Neurology 43: 1465–67
8. Coleman MR, Bekinschtein T, Monti M, Owen AM, Pickard JD (2009) A multimodal approach to the assessment of patients with disorders of consciousness. Prog Brain Res 177: 231–47
9. Coleman MR, Rodd JM, Davis MH, *et al.* (2007) Do vegetative patients retain aspects of language comprehension: evidence from fMRI. Brain 130: 2492–507
10. Coleman MR, Davis MH, Rodd JM, *et al.* (2009) Towards the routine use of brain imaging to aid the clinical diagnosis of disorders of consciousness. Brain 132: 2541–52
11. Coleman MR, Menon DK, Fryer TD, *et al.* (2005) Neurometabolic coupling in the vegetative and minimally conscious states: preliminary findings. J Neurol Neurosurg Psychiatry 76: 432–34
12. Davis MH, Coleman MR, Absalom AR, *et al.* (2007) Dissociating speech perception and comprehension and reduced levels of awareness. Proc Nat Acad Sci USA 104: 16032–37
13. Davis MH, Johnsrude IS (2003) Hierarchical processing in spoken language comprehension. J Neurosci 23: 3423–31
14. De Jong B, Willemsen AT, Paans AM (1997) Regional cerebral blood flow changes related to affective speech presentation in persistent vegetative state. Clin Neurol Neurosurg 99(3): 213–16
15. De Volder AG, Goffinet AM, Bol A, *et al.* (1990) Brain glucose metabolism in post-anoxic syndrome. Positron emission tomographic study. Arch Neurol 47(2): 197–204
16. Di HB, Yu SM, Weng XC, *et al.* (2007) Cerebral response to patient's own name in the vegetative and minimally conscious states. Neurology 68: 895–99
17. Giacino J, Hirsch J, Schiff N, *et al.* (2006) Functional neuroimaging applications for assessment and rehabilitation planning in patients with disorders of consciousness. Arch Phys Med Rehabil 87: 67–76
18. Giacino JT, Kalmar K, Whyte J (2004) The JFK coma recovery Scale–Revised: Measurement characteristics and diagnostic utility. Arch Phys Med Rehabil 85: 2020–29
19. Gill-Thwaites H, Munday R (1999) The Sensory Modality Assessment and Rehabilitation Technique (SMART): a comprehensive and integrated assessment and treatment protocol for the vegetative state and minimally responsive patient. Neuropsychol Rehabil 9: 305–20
20. Gill-Thwaites H (2006) Lotteries, loopholes and luck: misdiagnosis in the vegetative state patient. Brain Inj 20(13–14): 1321–28
21. Laureys S, Giacino JT, Schiff ND, *et al.* (2006) How should functional imaging of patients with disorders of consciousness contribute to their clinical rehabilitation needs? Curr Opin Neurol 19(6): 520–27
22. Laureys S, Faymonville ME, Peigneux P, *et al.* (2002) Cortical processing of noxious somatosensory stimuli in the persistent vegetative state. Neuroimage 17(2): 732–41

23. Levy DE, Sidtis JJ, Rottenberg DA, *et al.* (1987) Differences in cerebral blood flow and glucose utilization in vegetative versus locked-in patients. Ann Neurol 22(6): 673–82
24. Menon DK, Owen AM, Williams EJ, *et al.* (1998) Cortical processing in persistent vegetative state. Lancet 352(9123): 200
25. Owen AM, Coleman MR (2008) Neuroscience reviews. Neuroscience 9: 235–43
26. Owen AM, Coleman MR, Boly M, *et al.* (2006) Detecting awareness in the vegetative state. Science 313: 1402
27. Owen AM, Coleman MR, Davis MH, *et al.* (2007) Response to comments on 'Detecting awareness in the vegetative state'. Science 315: 1221c
28. Owen AM, Coleman MR, Menon DK, *et al.* (2005) Using a heirarchical approach to investigate residual auditory cognition in persistent vegetative state. In: Laureys S (ed) The boundaries of consciousness: neurobiology and neuropathology. Progress in Brain Research, Vol. 150. Elsevier, London, pp 461–76
29. Owen AM, Coleman MR, Menon DK, *et al.* (2005) Residual auditory function in persistent vegetative state: A combined PET and fMRI study. Neuropsychol Rehabil 15(3–4): 290–306
30. Owen AM, Coleman MR, Boly M, *et al.* (2007) Using functional magnetic resonance imaging to detect covert awareness in the vegetative state. Arch Neurol 64(8): 1098–102
31. Owen AM, Epstein R, Johnsrude IS (2001) fMRI: applications to cognitive neuroscience. In: Jezzard P, Mathews PM, Smith SM (eds) Functional Magnetic Resonance Imaging. An Introduction to Methods. Oxford University Press, Oxford, UK
32. Perrin F, Schnakers C, Schabus M, *et al.* (2006) Brain response to one's own name in vegetative state, minimally conscious state, and locked-in syndrome. Arch Neurol 63: 562–69
33. Rodd JM, Davis MH, Johnsrude IS (2005) The neural mechanisms of speech comprehension: fMRI studies of semantic ambiguity. Cereb Cortex 15: 1261–69
34. Rudolf J, Ghaemi M, Haupt WF, *et al.* (1999) Cerebral glucose metabolism in acute and persistent vegetative state. J Neurosurg Anesthesiol 11(1): 17–24
35. Schiff ND, Giacino JT, Kalmar K, *et al.* (2007) Behavioural improvements with thalamic stimulation after severe traumatic brain injury. Nature 448(7153): 600–30
36. Schiff ND, Ribary U, Moreno DR, *et al.* (2002) Residual cerebral activity and behavioural fragments can remain in the persistently vegetative brain. Brain 125: 1210–34
37. Schnakers C, Vanhaudenhuyse A, Giacino J, Ventura M, Boly M, Majerus S, Moonen G, Laureys S (2009) Diagnostic accuracy of the vegetative and minimally conscious state: clinical consensus versus standardised neurobehavioural assessment. BMC Neurol 21: 9–35
38. Staffen W, Kronbichler M, Aichhorn M, *et al.* (2006) Selective brain activity in response to one's own name in the persistent vegetative state. J Neurol Neurosurg Psychiatry 77: 1383–84
39. Tommasino C, Grana C, Lucignani G, *et al.* (1995) Regional cerebral metabolism of glucose in comatose and vegetative state patients. J Neurosurg Anesthesiol 7(2): 109–16
40. Voss HU, Uluc AM, Dyke JP, *et al.* (2006) Possible axonal regrowth in late recovery from the minimally conscious state. J Clin Invest 116: 2005–11

Rationale for hypothalamus-deep brain stimulation in food intake disorders and obesity

N. Torres[2], S. Chabardès[1,3], and A. L. Benabid[2]

[1] Grenoble Institute of Neurosciences, Unite INSERM U836, Grenoble, France
[2] CEA CLINATEC, Grenoble, France
[3] Department of Neurosurgery, University Hospital, Joseph Fourier University, Grenoble, France

With 6 Figures

Contents

Abstract 17
Introduction 18
Central nervous system control of food intake and weight 19
Deep brain stimulation of the hypothalamus: rationale
and putative hypothalamic targets 21
    Lateral hypothalamus 21
    Ventromedial hypothalamus 22
Experimental studies: Grenoble experience 23
    Material and methods 23
Human studies 26
References 28

Abstract

Appetite modulation in conjunction with enhancing metabolic rate with hypothalamic lesions has been widely documented in animal and even in humans. It appears these effects can be reproduced by DBS, and the titratability and reversibility of this procedure, in addition to well established safety profile, make DBS an appealing option for obesity treatment. Targeting the hypothalamus with DBS has already been shown to be feasible and potentially effective in managing patients with intractable chronic cluster headache [26]. The surgical risk however must be cautiously taken into account when targeting the hypothalamus, where some mortality cases have been reported when targeting

the posterior part [34]. The development of new surgical approach will probably reduce this surgical risk. Moreover, the role of functional neurosurgery in
obesity is not a new idea. In fact, LH was targeted in obese humans with
electrocoagulation more than 30 years ago, resulting in significant yet transient
appetite suppression and slight weight reduction [36]. All those elements have
made possible the recent regain of interest in DBS for morbid obesity and
open an exciting new area of research in neurosurgery and endocrinology.

Keywords: Eating disorder; obesity; hypothalamus; deep brain stimulation.

Introduction

Obesity is a complex disorder characterized by the accumulation of excess adipose tissue. It is defined in terms of Body Weight Index (BMI), calculated as
weight (kg)/height (m)^2. Although BMI is a continuous variable, epidemiological
studies based on risk of comorbidities have permitted to classify groups of populations. A BMI less than 25 is considered to be normal; 25–29.9 is overweight and
greater or equal to 30, obese [22]. The definition of morbid obese is less consen-
sual, but in general a 45 kg over ideal weight is used in the bariatric surgery
literature [9]. Obesity has reached epidemic proportions globally, with more than
1 billion adults overweight – at least 300 million of them clinically obese. Obesity
accounts for 2–6% of total health care costs in several developed countries; some
estimates put the figure as high as 7%. The true costs are undoubtedly much
greater as not all obesity-related conditions are included in the calculations.

Obesity is associated with diminished quality of life (qol) [37], high risk of
comorbidities [30] and reduced life expectancy by 5 to 20 years [15]. Treatment of
obesity includes non pharmacological measures, pharmacological agents and surgical therapy. Non-pharmacological treatments include behavior therapy, exercise,
and calorie-restricted diets. The main issue remains to overcome barriers to com-
pliance with diet and physical activity. Long-term use of drugs like sibutramine and
orlistat have demonstrated a discreet 4–6% weight loss over a 6 month period in
controlled trials, depending upon the intensity of the diet, exercise, and behavioral
program administered. Other agents (Noradrenergic-releasing agents) induce
more weight loss than placebo in short term studies, but this kind of agents are
only approved for short period using. For the surgery, some patients with morbid
obesity still remain poor candidates for standard Roux en-Y-gastric bypass, in
which a small gastric pouch prevents those patients from eating large quantities
at a single meal. In the longest follow up study of patients after bypass, Pories *et al.*
reported 58%, 55% and 49% loss of excess weight (defined as the patient's weight
minus the patients estimated "ideal" body weight) at 5, 10, and 14 years postoperatively. However, complications occur in 15–55% of bariatric patients, and the
peri-surgical mortality rate is about 1.5% even in experience centers [35]. By
comparison, Deep Brain Stimulation (DBS) Surgery in movement disorders has

a peri-operative morbidity 11.1–19.3% and mortality directly related to the procedure of about 1% [23, 44, 48]. Safer procedures, as laparoscopic adjustable banded gastroplasty are simpler but are not as effective.

While obesity has long been considered as a behavioral disorder, discovery of the hormone "leptin" catalyzed the field of obesity research by demonstrating the existence of an afferent humoral signal from adipose tissue to the central nervous system. Current evidence suggests that once adipose tissue accumulates, a system of overlapping neuroendocrine hormones prevent it from diminishing, making volitional weight loss difficult [49]. As a consequence, modulation of brain circuits emerges as a valuable clinical and research strategy in obesity. Advances in our knowledge of the functional anatomy and electrophysiology of the relevant neural circuitry underlying this condition may unveil novel targets and applications of neuromodulation in obesity. Finally, the possibility to activate or inhibit deep brain structures in a reversible manner with an acceptable range of side effects and morbidity has renewed the interest of modulating the hypothalamus to control food intake disorders and obesity.

In this review, potential neural targets implicated in the pathophysiology of this disease are explored, recent experimental data accumulated in animals are presented and future directions of DBS in this field are discussed.

Central nervous system control of food intake and weight

The brain regulates many aspects of energy homeostasis, adjusting both drive to eat and the expenditure of energy in response to a wide range of nutritional and other signals. This process is highly complex and involves several brain regions ranging from cortex to brainstem, but most interest has focused on the hypothalamus. The understanding of hypothalamic mechanism has increased dramatically in later years. It has become clear that various neural circuits operate to different degrees and probably serve specific functions under particular conditions of altered energy balance.

Central regulation of food intake (FI) and body fat mass is characterized by complex interaction between several brain centers and peripheral signals:

– *A decrease in body fat* is sensed in the arcuate nucleus (ARC) of the hypothalamus by a decrease in Leptin and insulin concentrations. This causes the suppression of anorexigenic signals (melanocyte-stimulating hormones MSH) and the stimulation of orexigenic signals (agouti-related protein ARGP or neuropeptide Y NPY). The net balance of these signals results in an increase in FI and decrease in energy expenditure that ultimately aims to restore fat cell mass.
– *The ingestion of food* generates neural and hormonal satiety signals to the hindbrain: Leptin/insulin-sensitive central effectors pathways interact with hindbrain satiety circuits to regulate the meal size, thereby modulating FI and energy balance [43].

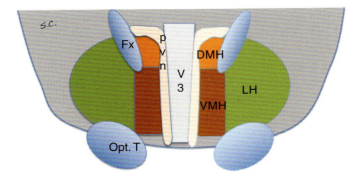

Fig. 1. Schematic representation of the anterior hypothalamus. The ventro-medial region of the hypothalamus, located anteriorly to the mamillary body, contains the dorsomedian, the paraventricular and the ventro-median nuclei. It constitutes the lateral wall of the third ventricle. The fornix crosses the hypothalamus from anterior to posterior in a parasagittal plane and splits the hypothalamus into a ventral and a lateral region. The lateral hypothalamus is a reticular region rather than a nucleus

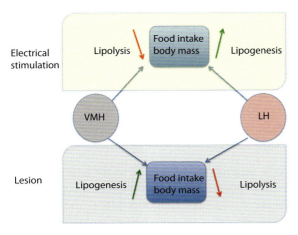

Fig. 2. Schematic representation of the central control of food intake and body mass. The electrical activation of the VMH reduces the food intake and the body mass, and activates the lipolysis. The electrical activation of the LH increases the food intake and the body mass and increases the lipogenesis. In experimental condition, bilateral lesion of the VMH or the LH is known to produce respectively obesity or meagreness (when the animal survives)

Obesity can results from difficulties in sensing changes in metabolic environment. Low leptin and leptin deficiency are all related with low feelings of fullness and ravenous hunger [18]. Leptin receptor resistance produces also morbid obesity and weight loss treatment failures [25]. This is likely to be one way in which FI regulation is adjusted in obese individuals or during weight gaining. In addition, obese subjects failed to display the normal hypothalamic inhibitory responses to glucose infusions, suggesting that there is poor recognition of postprandial satiety signals at the end of the meal [28]. It is a long standing idea that obese people display weak satiety signals, which allow them to consume persistent large meals and gain weight. In general, humans display a system of weight regulation that is asymmetrical – a reduction in body weight is strongly defended but weight gain is not. The body seems to tolerate a positive energy balance. There is no mechanism that can detect a positive energy balance per se and that can induce a behavior which can correct the body weight in an environment that promotes consumption [7].

Deep brain stimulation of the hypothalamus: rationale and putative hypothalamic targets

The imbalance between FI and energy expenditure leads to weight gain in individuals with weak central (hypothalamic) recognition of peripheral signals (Leptin, ghrelin, glucose or insulin) [18]. Activation using Low Frequency Stimulation (LFS) of discreet brain center or inhibition (using High Frequency Stimulation, HFS) of overacting areas may change the body weigh "set point" in intractable morbid obese patient [4, 5].

Lateral hypothalamus

The Lateral Hypothalamus (LH) has long been implicated in feeding behavior and energy expenditure [6]. Its role in appetite regulation is well described in early studies of LH lesions. In 1951, Anand and Brobeck, have shown that bilateral lesions of the lateral hypothalamus provoked weight loss with aphagia [1] and have demonstrated that a diencephalic center that regulates FI in the hypothalamus did exist. This impact on appetite can be partially explained by the presence of orexigenic peptides, expressed predominantly in the LH such as melanin concentrating hormone (MCH) and orexins. Conversely, activation of the LH using electrical stimulation provoked a pronounced bout of eating in previously satiated cats, while electrical stimulation of *The Ventromedial Hypothalamus (VMH)* caused food deprived cats to stop eating [2].

Here also a metabolic effect is suggested by Teitelbaum and Stellar, because theirs rats were able to keep a low weight and regain normal FI after bilateral lesion of LH [46]. Several biochemical and neurophysiological studies have shown activation of LH neurons during fasting period. Recently, Ruffin and

Nicolaidis have confirmed that the metabolic response comes prior to behavioral changes in FI [39].

Given this evidence, it was proposed that chronic bilateral High frequency stimulation (HFS) of LH would mimic the results of lesion studies, just as HFS STN mimics the effects of subthalamotomy. In one study of Sani and colleagues, on post operative day 24, 13% of total body weight reduction was observed in rats that were maintained on 7 day high fat diet undergoing LH-DBS, a difference that was significant compared to controls [41].

Ventromedial hypothalamus

In 1940, Hetherington and Ramson published that the bilateral lesion of the ventro-medial region of the hypothalamus produced hyperphagia followed by obesity with normophagia [19, 21]. Later on, it was confirmed that lesions of the VMH could induce obesity [8]. Like LH, VMH has also been implicated in appetite regulation, as well as maintaining energy homeostasis. VMH lesions results in substantially more lipid and hyperinsulinemia in rats even if pair-fed with sham-lesion controls, suggesting a metabolic bias towards obesity [13].

In contrast to electrolytic lesion, electrical stimulation of VMH at low intensities (20–25 uA) suppresses feeding in rats and increases their metabolic rate [38]. Beltt and Keesey have shown earlier (1975) that VMH low frequency-stimulation was susceptible to inhibit FI [3]. Pauwson in 1987 has also suggested that a metabolic effect is probable during low frequency stimulation of VMH, leading to a chronic decrease in weight without change in FI behavior [32]. This increase in energy expenditure was associated with increased fat oxidation given a concomitant drop in the respiratory quotient (CO_2 produced/O_2 consumed). Thus, heightened metabolism induced by VMH stimulation is sustained by utilization of fat stores via the lipolytic pathway and is most likely due to noradrenergic turnover [40]. Recently, it has been reported that VMH DBS in rats at four different frequencies (25, 50, 75 and 100 Hz) replicated this effect on energy expenditure, demonstrating an increase in metabolism measured by indirect calorimetry [12]. There was a trend towards an indirect relationship between energy expenditure and increase frequencies, confirming that lower frequencies have stimulating effects (Benabid 2006 Personal communication) [29].

In brief, VMH/LH critical involvement in feeding regulation can be summarized as following:

1) suppression and facilitation of feeding regulation can be obtained by electrical stimulation (activation) of the VMH and the LH respectively.
2) hyperphagia and hypophagia are produced by bilateral electrolytic ablations as well as bilateral chemical lesions of the VMH and LH respectively.

3) The presence of neurons in both nuclei that sense the metabolic signals such a glucose, free fatty acid and leptine [14]. It is clear that hypothalamic nuclei play an important role in weight regulation, FI and motivation for feeding.

Attempts have been made to use this knowledge in preclinical settings. In 1984 Brown and collaborators using implantable chronic platinum-tipped electrodes in the ventromedial hypothalamic area (VMH) showed changes in FI in fasted dogs. Dogs that received 1 hour of VMH stimulation every 12 hours for 3 consecutive days maintained an average daily FI of 65% of normal baseline levels [10]. In the light of their results and the availability of this new technology, the authors recommended deep brain stimulation as a potential mean of regulating FI and therefore a possible therapeutic modality for human morbid obesity. Feeding suppression was also elicited by electrical and chemical stimulation in non human primate's hypothalamus. Ventromedial, dorsomedial and ventromedial part of lateral hypothalamus produced prolonged suppression in FI suggesting neuronal inhibitory mechanism of feeding in these centers in awake monkeys [45]. Some concern remains for this target however. Lacan *et al.* assessed the feasibility of ventromedial hypothalamus (VMH) DBS in freely moving vervet monkeys to modulate food intake as a potential treatment of eating disorders, showing interesting results in terms of procedure safety, but failed to reduce weight [24]. Before translating into clinical settings, more work has to be done in preclinical studies, addressing possible collateral sides effects encountered in this area, like changes in blood pressure [11] or changes in memory function [17].

Experimental studies: Grenoble experience

The effect of low and high frequency stimulation of the hypothalamus has been studied in our laboratory on rats and monkeys. We present here data collected after electrical stimulation of the ventro-medial hypothalamus.

Acute and semi-chronic DBS of the VMH in rats.

Material and methods

1) Animals:
Male Whistar rats were used, with at the time of implantation, an average weight of $349 \pm 7\,g$ and $271 \pm 2\,g$ for the acute and chronic stimulation groups respectively. Each rat was fed at libitum with water and food pellets and placed in individual cages, at least 72 hours before any experimentation. The animal house was kept at a constant temperature of $22°C$, with a regular day (8 am to 8 pm)–night (8 pm to 8 am) light cycle.

2) Surgery:
A unilateral electrode implantation in VMH was performed, on a stereotactic Kopf frame under general anaesthesia (chroral hydrate 4%, 1ml/100 g i.p.).

The implantation coordinates were deduced from the Paxinos and Watson Atlas [33]:

- VMH: antero-posterior 2.56 mm behind the bregma, lateral 0.6 mm left from the midline, depth 9.5 mm below the level of the bregma.

3) Implanted electrodes:
Concentric bipolar tungsten electrodes (twisted 200 micron tungsten wires, 400 microns for external diameter), were connected to a socket, in which the stimulation cable could be plugged, and secured on the skull with dental cement.

4) Stimulations:
All stimulations were continuous, bipolar cathode at the tip, anode at the large contac, at 30 Hz for LFS, with a pulse width set at 60 ms.

The applied intensity was determined for each rat during previous preliminary sessions, at about $222 \pm 103\,\mu A$. This value corresponded to the minimal intensity necessary to induce food intake during HFS in VMN.

After surgery, the rats were allowed for 10 days to recover their initial weight and to get accustomed to the new cage as well as holding the connector. The rats were connected to their stimulation cable at least 2 hours before the onset of stimulation. The measures of FI during acute stimulation was repeated for all rats 3 to 5 times, due to important individual variations. Each rat was therefore stimulated at efficient intensity (condition ON) and at zero intensity (condition OFF), 3 to 5 times, each session and each condition being separated by at least 48 hours.

The duration of each stimulation session was 30 minutes for acute stimulation, and 4 hours/day for chronic stimulation.

5) Experimental protocol:
Acute stimulations: The acute effects on food intake of stimulation at high and low frequency were studied in a group of rats ($n = 12$) implanted in VMH. HFS was performed between 11 and 12 am, and LFS between 8 and 9 pm, which correspond to the usual periods during which the animals are fasting or eating respectively. The food intake (FI) was measured at the end of the period of stimulation, and 1 hour later. The sessions of stimulation at high and low frequency were separated by 7 days at least.

The control situation consisted of applying no stimulation, each rat being its own control.

Semi-chronic stimulations: A first group of rats ("chronic" group, $n = 5$) was used to study the long-term effect of HFS on weight and food intake. The chosen intensity (100 µA) was the same for all rats.

Stimulations were continuously applied between 1 and 5 pm, which is the usual period of fasting, for a total of 16 stimulated days (5 days out of 7, during 3 weeks). A second group of rats ("control" group, $n = 10$) were not implanted and used as a control group. The FI, as well as the weight of the animals, were measured during the period of stimulation and 10 days later, every 2 days, the weighing session being done in the morning, between 9 and 10 am. These

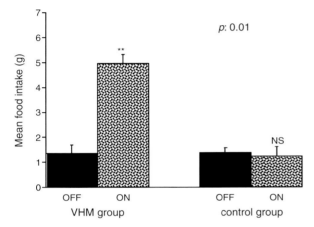

Graph 1. Mean food intake during ON high frequency stimulation compared to sham stimulation in rats implanted in VMH (VMH group) and in rats implanted outside the VMH (control group)

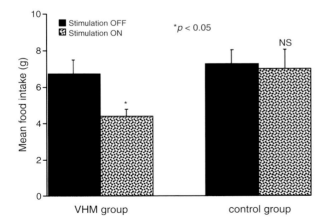

Graph 2. Mean food intake during ON low frequency stimulation compared to sham stimulation in rats implanted in VMH (VMH group) and in rats implanted outside the VMH (control group)

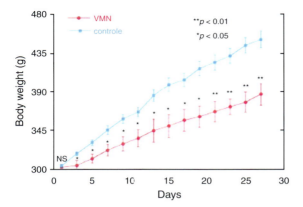

Graph 3. Chronic HFS of the VMH reduces the body weight intake in rats

parameters of stimulation, particularly the duration (4 hours/day) of stimulation, were based on those of the literature.

6) Results:
The main results of this study can be summarized as follows:

1) Acute high frequency stimulation (130 Hz) of the VMH can increase the amount of food intake compared to sham stimulation (Graph 1).
2) Acute low frequency stimulation (30 Hz) of the VMH can reduce the amount of food intake compared to sham stimulation (Graph 2).
3) Chronic electrical stimulation using 130 Hz slows down the body weight intake in juvenile rats compared sham group (Graph 3).

Human studies

In the early 70s, Sano and colleges, explored and selectively destroyed the posteromedial part of the hypothalamus in men in cases of violent, aggressive behavior. This approach also allowed them to stimulate discreet zone and to observe autonomic, somatomotor and other responses. In a series of 51 lesioned patients, a tendency to gain weight after posteromedial hypothalamic destruction was seen. Also during acute electrical stimulation (100 pps, 1 msec, 5–10 V) of the medial hypothalamus, autonomic sympathetic response were obtained, probably related with stress and energy expenditure mechanisms [42]. The first human study specifically centered in treating human obesity using lesion and stimulation of the specific brain centers was carried out by Quaade in 1974. In that study, five patients with morbid obesity were subject to an electro stimulatory exploration of the lateral hypothalamic area. In three cases a convincing transoperatory hunger response was elicited. Two of theses patients received unilateral electro-coagulatory lesion, and in a third a contralateral coagulation was performed. The patients with lesions showed a statistically significant, but transient decrease in caloric intake and a slight and transient decrease of body weight [36]. Although no direct DBS of the hypothalamus has been attempted for weight control, indirect evidence of weight modulation can be found as a secondary effect in the established or experimental indication of DBS in the hypothalamic or near hypothalamic area. For instance, several studies have reported increased body weight and body mass index after high frequency stimulation in the subthalamic nucleus. While the mechanism is still unknown, possible explanations of body weight gain after DBS STN might

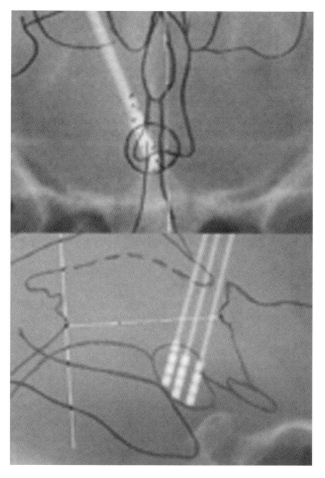

Fig. 3. Hypothalamic hamartoma: Postoperative X-ray of 3 DBS Electrodes implanted in a case of drug resistant gelastic epilepsy. Acute stimulation at a frequency of 130 Hz–100 μs–0.4 mA, reduced Interictal spikes; but chronic high frequency stimulation (130 Hz/90 μs/0.5 V, and then 185 Hz/60 μs/0.1 V) produced 10 kg weight gain, which returned to baseline after turning stimulation off [20]

include reduction of energy output related to elimination of dyskinesias, improved alimentation or direct influence on function of lateral hypothalamus by DBS STN [27, 31, 47].

Chronic unremitting cluster headache refractory to medical treatment is a developing indication of DBS in the posterior hypothalamus. Stimulation in this region in a previous hyperphagic and hypersexual patient has produced pain relief and 25 kg weight reduction [16].

Indirect observations of the effect of DBS applied in the hypothalamic regions, on weight, have been also made in our center. A patient with intractable gelastic epilepsy due to a hypothalamic hamartoma was implanted with 3 DBS quadripolar electrodes in the hamartoma which was attached to the inferolateral part of the floor of the 3rd ventricle (see Fig. 3). While her number and severity of crises were greatly reduced, a 15 kg weight gain associated to menstrual cycle disturbance appeared following high frequency stimulation of the medial hypothalamus [20].

References

1. Anand BK, Brobeck JR (1951) Localization of a "feeding center" in the hypothalamus of the rat. Proc Soc Exp Biol Med 77(2): 323–24
2. Anand BK, Dua S, et al. (1955) Hypothalamic control of food intake in cats and monkeys. J Physiol 127(1): 143–52
3. Beltt BM, Keesey RE (1975) Hypothalamic map of stimulation current thresholds for inhibition of feeding in rats. Am J Physiol 229(4): 1124–33
4. Benabid AL, Wallace B, et al. (2005) Therapeutic electrical stimulation of the central nervous system. C R Biol 328(2): 177–86
5. Benabid AL, Wallace B, et al. (2005) A putative generalized model of the effects and mechanism of action of high frequency electrical stimulation of the central nervous system. Acta Neurol Belg 105(3): 149–57
6. Bernardis LL, Bellinger LL (1996) The lateral hypothalamic area revisited: ingestive behavior. Neurosci Biobehav Rev 20(2): 189–287
7. Blundell JE, Gillett A (2001) Control of food intake in the obese. Obes Res 9 (Suppl. 4): 263S–70S
8. Brobeck JR (1963) Hypothalamus, appetite, and obesity. Physiol Pharmacol Physicians 18: 1–6
9. Brolin, RE (1992) Critical analysis of results: weight loss and quality of data. Am J Clin Nutr 55 (Suppl. 2): 577S–81S
10. Brown FD, Fessler RG, et al. (1984) Changes in food intake with electrical stimulation of the ventromedial hypothalamus in dogs. J Neurosurg 60(6): 1253–57
11. Cortelli P, Guaraldi P, et al. (2007) Effect of deep brain stimulation of the posterior hypothalamic area on the cardiovascular system in chronic cluster headache patients. Eur J Neurol 14(9): 1008–15
12. Covalin A, Feshali A, et al. (2005) Deep Brain Stimulation for Obesity Control: Analyzing Stimulation Parameters to Modulate Energy Expenditure. Neural Engineering, 2005. Conference Proceedings. 2nd International IEEE EMBS Conference, pp 482–85

13. Cox JE, Powley TL (1981) Intragastric pair feeding fails to prevent VMH obesity or hyperinsulinemia. Am J Physiol 240(5): E566–72
14. Dhillon H, Zigman JM, *et al.* (2006) Leptin directly activates SF1 neurons in the VMH, and this action by leptin is required for normal body-weight homeostasis. Neuron 49(2): 191–203
15. Fontaine KR, Redden DT, *et al.* (2003) Years of life lost due to obesity. JAMA 289(2): 187–93
16. Franzini A, Marras C, *et al.* (2007) Chronic high frequency stimulation of the posteromedial hypothalamus in facial pain syndromes and behaviour disorders. Acta Neurochir Suppl 97(Pt 2): 399–406
17. Hamani C, McAndrews MP, *et al.* (2008) Memory enhancement induced by hypothalamic/fornix deep brain stimulation. Ann Neurol 63(1): 119–23
18. Heini AF, Lara-Castro C, *et al.* (1998) Association of leptin and hunger-satiety ratings in obese women. Int J Obes Relat Metab Disord 22(11): 1084–87
19. Hetherington AW (1944) Non-production of hypothalamic obesity in the rat by lesions rostral or dorsal to the ventro-medial hypothalamic nuclei. The Journal of Comparative Neurology 80(1): 33–45
20. Kahane P, Ryvlin P, *et al.* (2003) From hypothalamic hamartoma to cortex: what can be learnt from depth recordings and stimulation? Epileptic Disord 5(4): 205–17
21. Kennedy GC (1950) The hypothalamic control of food intake in rats. Proceedings of the Royal Society of London. Series B, Biological Sciences (1934–1990) 137(889): 535–49
22. Korner J, Aronne LJ (2003) The emerging science of body weight regulation and its impact on obesity treatment. J Clin Invest 111(5): 565–70.
23. Krack P, Batir A, *et al.* (2003) Five-year follow-up of bilateral stimulation of the subthalamic nucleus in advanced Parkinson's disease. N Engl J Med 349(20): 1925–34
24. Lacan G, De Salles AA, *et al.* (2008) Modulation of food intake following deep brain stimulation of the ventromedial hypothalamus in the vervet monkey. Laboratory investigation. J Neurosurg 108(2): 336–42
25. Leitner GC, Roob JM, *et al.* (2000) Leptin deficiency due to lipid apheresis: a possible reason for ravenous hunger and weight gain. Int J Obes Relat Metab Disord 24(2): 259–60
26. Leone M, Franzini A, *et al.* (2003) Hypothalamic deep brain stimulation for intractable chronic cluster headache: a 3-year follow-up. Neurol Sci 24(Suppl 2): S143–45
27. Maschke M, Tuite PJ, *et al.* (2005) The effect of subthalamic nucleus stimulation on kinaesthesia in Parkinson's disease. J Neurol Neurosurg Psychiatry 76(4): 569–71
28. Matsuda M, Liu Y, *et al.* (1999) Altered hypothalamic function in response to glucose ingestion in obese humans. Diabetes 48(9): 1801–06
29. McIntyre CC, Grill WM (2002) Extracellular stimulation of central neurons: influence of stimulus waveform and frequency on neuronal output. J Neurophysiol 88(4): 1592–604
30. Must A, Spadano J, *et al.* (1999) The disease burden associated with overweight and obesity. JAMA 282(16): 1523–29
31. Novakova L, Ruzicka E, *et al.* (2007) Increase in body weight is a non-motor side effect of deep brain stimulation of the subthalamic nucleus in Parkinson's disease. Neuro Endocrinol Lett 28(1): 21–25
32. Pawson PA, Preston E, Haas N, Foster DO (1987) Hypothalamic sites where electrical stimulation increases metabolic rate in the rat. Soc Neurosci Abstr 13: 1163
33. Paxinos G, Watson C (1998) The Rat Brain in Stereotaxic Coordinates. New York: Academic Press

34. Pinsker MO, Bartsch T, *et al.* (2008) Failure of deep brain stimulation of the posterior inferior hypothalamus in chronic cluster headache – report of two cases and review of the literature. Zentralbl Neurochir 69(2): 76–79

35. Pories WJ, MacDonald KG (1993) The surgical treatment of morbid obesity. Curr Opin Gen Surg: 195–205

36. Quaade F (1974) Letter: Stereotaxy for obesity. Lancet 1(7851): 267

37. Roe DA, Eickwort KR (1976) Relationships between obesity and associated health factors with unemployment among low income women. J Am Med Womens Assoc 31(5): 193–94, 198–99, 203–04

38. Ruffin M, Nicolaidis S (1999) Electrical stimulation of the ventromedial hypothalamus enhances both fat utilization and metabolic rate that precede and parallel the inhibition of feeding behavior. Brain Res 846(1): 23–29

39. Ruffin MP, Caulliez R, *et al.* (1995) Parallel metabolic and feeding responses to lateral hypothalamic stimulation. Brain Res 700(1–2): 121–28

40. Saito M, Minokoshi Y, *et al.* (1989) Accelerated norepinephrine turnover in peripheral tissues after ventromedial hypothalamic stimulation in rats. Brain Res 481(2): 298–303

41. Sani S, Jobe K, *et al.* (2007) Deep brain stimulation for treatment of obesity in rats. J Neurosurg 107(4): 809–13

42. Sano K, Mayanagi Y, *et al.* (1970) Results of timulation and destruction of the posterior hypothalamus in man. J Neurosurg 33(6): 689–707

43. Schwartz MW, Woods SC, *et al.* (2000) Central nervous system control of food intake. Nature 404(6778): 661–71

44. Seijo FJ, Alvarez-Vega MA, *et al.* (2007) Complications in subthalamic nucleus stimulation surgery for treatment of Parkinson's disease. Review of 272 procedures. Acta Neurochir (Wien) 149(9): 867–75; discussion 876

45. Takaki A, Aou S, *et al.* (1992) Feeding suppression elicited by electrical and chemical stimulations of monkey hypothalamus. Am J Physiol 262(4 Pt 2): R586–94

46. Teitelbaum P, Epstein AN (1962) The lateral hypothalamic syndrome: recovery of feeding and drinking after lateral hypothalamic lesions. Psychol Rev 69: 74–90

47. Tuite PJ, Maxwell RE, *et al.* (2005) Weight and body mass index in Parkinson's disease patients after deep brain stimulation surgery. Parkinsonism Relat Disord 11(4): 247–52

48. Voges J, Waerzeggers Y, *et al.* (2006) Deep-brain stimulation: long-term analysis of complications caused by hardware and surgery – experiences from a single centre. J Neurol Neurosurg Psychiatry 77(7): 868–72

49. Zhang Y, Proenca R, *et al.* (1994) Positional cloning of the mouse obese gene and its human homologue. Nature 372(6505): 425–32

Gustatory and reward brain circuits in the control of food intake

A. J. Oliveira-Maia[1,6,*], C. D. Roberts[1], S. A. Simon[1,3,4], and M. A. L. Nicolelis[1–5]

[1] Department of Neurobiology, Duke University Medical Center, Durham, NC, USA

[2] Department of Psychology and Neurosciences, Duke University Medical Center, Durham, NC, USA

[3] Department of Biomedical Engineering, Duke University Medical Center, Durham, NC, USA

[4] Center for Neuroengineering, Duke University Medical Center, Durham, NC, USA

[5] Edmond and Lily Safra International Institute for Neuroscience of Natal, Natal, Rio Grande do Norte, Brazil

[6] Current addresses: Champalimaud Neuroscience Program, Instituto Gulbenkian de Ciência, Oeiras, Portugal; Department of Psychiatry and Mental Health, Centro Hospitalar de Lisboa Ocidental, Lisbon, Portugal

[*] To whom correspondence should be addressed at: ajmaia@igc.gulbenkian.pt

With 4 Figures

Contents

Abstract 32
Abbreviations 32
Introduction 33
Gustation and gustatory system: definitions 33
Orosensory gustatory input 34
Postingestive sensory processes 38
Central gustatory sensory pathways 41
Amygdala and brain reward pathways 44
Hypothalamus, brainstem and energy homeostasis 45
Novel opportunities in the management of obesity? 48
Conclusions 50
Acknowledgements 50
References 50

Abstract

Gustation is a multisensory process allowing for the selection of nutrients and the rejection of irritating and/or toxic compounds. Since obesity is a highly prevalent condition that is critically dependent on food intake and energy expenditure, a deeper understanding of gustatory processing is an important objective in biomedical research. Recent findings have provided evidence that central gustatory processes are distributed across several cortical and sub-cortical brain areas. Furthermore, these gustatory sensory circuits are closely related to the circuits that process reward. Here, we present an overview of the activation and connectivity between central gustatory and reward areas. Moreover, and given the limitations in number and effectiveness of treatments currently available for overweight patients, we discuss the possibility of modulating neuronal activity in these circuits as an alternative in the treatment of obesity.

Keywords: Taste; postingestive; feeding; deep brain stimulation.

Abbreviations

AMP	adenosine monophophate
AP	area postrema
ARC	arcuate nucleus of the hypothalamus
ATP	adenosine triphosphate
BLA	basolateral amygdala
CCK	cholecystokinin
CeA	central nucleus of the amygdala
CNS	central nervous system
cNTS	caudal division of the solitary tract nucleus
CoA	coenzyme A
DBS	deep brain stimulation
DMH	dorsomedial nucleus of the hypothalamus
ENaC	epithelial sodium channel
GABA	gamma-aminobutyric acid
GC	gustatory cortex
GIT	gastrointestinal tract
GLP-1	glucagon-like peptide 1
GPCR	G-protein coupled receptors
IC	insular cortex
LH	lateral hypothalamus
MCH	melanin concentrating hormone
MSH	melanocyte stimulating hormone
NAcc	nucleus accumbens
NPY	neuropeptide Y
NTS	solitary tract nucleus

OFC	orbitofrontal cortex
PbN	parabrachial nuclei
PLCβ2	phospholipase C β2
POMC	pro-opiomelanocortin
PP	pancreatic polypeptide
PVH	paraventricular nucleus of the hypothalamus
PYY	peptide YY
rNTS	rostral division of the solitary tract nucleus
SNAP-25	synaptosomal-associated protein of 25 kDa
TRC	taste receptor cell
TRP	transient receptor potential ion channel
VMH	ventromedial nucleus of the hypothalamus
VPpc	parvicellular division of the ventral posterior nucleus of the thalamus
VTA	ventral tegmental area

Introduction

In most societies the prevalence of obesity has risen dramatically to reach epidemic proportions. In the United States alone, a staggering 30% of all adults are obese [158]. Increase in adiposity leads to significant metabolic dysregulation, with important health and economic consequences [158]. Increased availability of palatable and high-calorie food and reduced requirement for energy expenditure through physical activity are usually identified as the main culprits of this obesity epidemic [86]. Nonetheless, the participation of genetic factors in the definition of individual susceptibility for the occurrence of obesity is also widely accepted and has been extensively described [123]. While such factors are commonly assumed to influence metabolic rate or the partitioning of excess calories into fat, current data suggests that a significant part of the genetic influence on human obesity has a direct impact on neural regulation of hunger, satiety and food intake [51]. An important objective in neuroscience research is thus to further understand the central mechanisms of food reward and appetite regulation, which will predictably allow a deeper comprehension of eating disorders such as obesity.

Gustation and the gustatory system: definitions

Gustation has historically been defined as a synonym of taste. Recently, however, this term has been used to define a broader concept, which extends beyond taste [151]. In this broader sense, gustation is considered as the multisensory process that allows for the selection of nutrients and rejection of irritating and/or toxic compounds [151].

Gustatory processing begins when a motivated animal searches for and detects a desired food, usually using visual and/or olfactory cues. Once a desired substance is found, the decision to pursue and maintain consumption usually involves active oral exploration. The unitary sensory perception resulting from taste, odour, texture and temperature of that stimulus, i.e., its flavour, will be a central contributor in the decision of ingestion vs. rejection [153]. Gustatory decision making is also impacted by the organisms' internal state. The central nervous system (CNS) detects a multitude of neural and humoral signals from the periphery, reflecting several aspects of homeostatic balance such as gastrointestinal status, current energy needs and availability, and energy stores [27]. The maintenance of energy homeostasis and stable body weight depends on the integration of these endogenous signals with sensory feedback, and the ability to respond adequately through modulation of both energy expenditure and food intake [145]. Finally, the memories of orosensory, olfactory and postingestive effects of previous encounters with a similar substance also influence food seeking and ingestion [147], as do emotional, cognitive and social factors [178].

The multisensory properties of intra-oral and ingested stimuli are conveyed to the brain through specialized taste, somatosensory, olfactory and visceral sensory neurons that converge on several CNS centres. Thus, once beyond the periphery, many single neurons responding to gustatory stimuli are often found to be broadly tuned to diverse combinations of chemosensory, somatosensory, olfactory and even visual information [140]. Furthermore, the CNS detects humoral signals that cross the blood-brain barrier and transmit information not only about the properties of ingested stimuli, but also about internal physiological states [189], providing additional modulatory influences for central gustatory neurons [115]. Neurons with these multimodal response properties, distributed through several CNS areas, integrate sensory and homeostatic information, participating with neural circuits of affective, cognitive and motor processing to organize ingestive behaviour [87].

Orosensory gustatory input

The peripheral gustatory system extracts multisensory information from substances placed in the mouth, and conveys this information through multiple neural pathways to brainstem structures [84]. Taste receptor cells (TRCs) are responsive to the type and quantity of chemicals dissolved in saliva and allow for the detection of at least five distinctive taste qualities: salt, sweet, bitter, sour (acidic) and umami (savoury taste of amino acids) [157]. Information about less water-soluble compounds, as well as food characteristics such as texture, viscosity and temperature, is primarily transduced by specialized somatosensory neurons with endings distributed throughout the oral epithelium [62].

In vertebrates, TRCs are found in specialized microscopic taste receptor organs – the taste buds. Mammalian taste buds are onion-shaped cell groups embedded at the surface of several intra-oral structures, mainly the palate and tongue, where they cluster into macroscopic structures named gustatory papillae. Each taste bud contains several distinct morphological cell types that can be distinguished by ultrastructural and immunohistochemical features [114]. Type I or dark cells have processes that envelop nerve fibres and other taste cells and, given their expression profile of neurotransmitter-related enzymes and transporters, are thought to have a support function [10]. However, a recent report demonstrated that type I cells have responses that depend on epithelial sodium channels (ENaCs – see below), suggesting a possible role in salt taste transduction [171]. Type II (light or receptor cells) and type III (intermediate or presynaptic cells) are considered the main chemosensing TRCs. Type II receptor cells express G-protein-coupled receptors (GPCRs), phospholipase C $\beta2$ (PLC$\beta2$) and transient receptor potential ion channel M5 (TRPM5). Different type II cell subtypes appear to respond exclusively to sweet, bitter or umami tastants [163]. Given their ultrastructural and molecular characteristics, these cells do not seem to have conventional synapses and, rather, appear to release transmitters via pannexin or connexin hemichannels [77]. Type III presynaptic cells have synaptic contacts with intragemmal nerve fibres and, accordingly, express synapse-related proteins such as SNAP-25 (synaptosomal-associated protein of 25 kDa) [182]. Since they have broadly tuned responses to tastants of multiple qualities, some authors propose that presynaptic cells may receive converging information from receptor cells, presumably via purinergic signaling [163]. Finally, type IV or basal cells, in contrast to the remaining cell types, do not have an elongated shape. They are thought to have a proliferative role to support constant cell turnover in the taste bud [114].

Microvillar processes from taste receptor cells extend towards the bud pore, on the mucosal surface, where contact with sapid chemical stimuli occurs. Taste receptors are transmembrane proteins found on these microvilli and are the basis for many of the chemosensory properties of TRCs. Upon detection of a specific stimulus, they will activate intracellular transduction cascades to initiate the process of gustatory neural signalling [105]. Proteins belonging to the GPCR superfamily have been established as receptors for sweet (T1R2/T1R3 receptors), umami (T1R1/T1R3 receptors), and bitter (T2 R receptors) tastants [113, 188]. The predominant downstream signaling pathways for these receptors require PLC$\beta2$ and TRPM5 [186]. There is also evidence implicating gustducin, a G-protein almost exclusively expressed in TRCs, in bitter and sweet taste transduction [180]. Sour and salt taste qualities rely on a different set of receptors and signaling pathways [186]. Recently, two TRP ion channels from the polycystic kidney disease-like family, co-expressed in a subset of TRCs that are necessary for sour taste transduction [75], were proposed to form a candidate sour receptor [79]. Alternate mechanisms for detection of sour tastants have been described, but it is unclear to what degree these putative pathways for sour taste are specific for different species and/or regions of the tongue [78]. For salt taste, at least two distinct mechanisms exist in rodents: an amiloride-sensitive epithelial sodium channel (ENaC) accounts for part of the responses to sodium and lithium ions [69] while other, amiloride-insensitive mechanisms, serve as receptors for multiple ions including sodium, potassium, ammonium and calcium [42]. A variant of TRPV1, a transient receptor potential vanilloid receptor, has been proposed as an amiloride-insensitive salt taste receptor [104] but the perceptual relevance of this receptor mechanism is still controversial [167].

Perception of a given taste quality seems to reflect the activation of a specific population of TRCs rather than the properties of a specific interaction between a tastant and a taste receptor (such as the kinetics of taste receptor activation). In fact, taste receptors for sweet, bitter, umami and sour are present in largely segregated populations of taste cells that function as narrowly tuned sensors for each of these taste qualities [75, 186]. Additionally, the selective activation of a TRC population expressing a particular taste receptor is, in itself and irrespective of the actual receptor being activated, sufficient to generate approach or rejection behaviours that are specific for that taste quality [113, 188]. It is therefore clear that sweet, bitter, umami and sour taste pathways are segregated at the TRC level. However, this labelled-line model does not seem to be conserved in the CNS, where most authors suggest the occurrence of multisensory and distributed gustatory processing [151].

Adenosine triphosphate (ATP) signaling is necessary for transmission of taste information to the CNS. Tastant evoked ATP release activates $P2X_2/P2X_3$ ionotropic purinoreceptors on primary gustatory afferent nerve terminals [48]. Serotonin and norepinephrine are also released from taste buds upon chemosensory stimulation, but their functional role is not as clear as that of ATP [68, 76]. Other transmitters, peptides and respective receptors, namely acetylcholine, glutamate, cholecystokinin (CCK), vasoactive intestinal peptide, substance P and leptin, have also been identified in taste cells. Many of these compounds are thought to modulate, in an autocrine or paracrine manner, the responses to tastants [68, 76].

The chorda tympani and greater superior petrosal branches of the facial (VIIth) nerve carry sensory axons of cells in the geniculate ganglion and innervate taste buds respectively in the anterior tongue and palate. Sensory axons of the glossopharyngeal (IXth) nerve, with cell bodies in the petrosal ganglion, terminate in taste buds in the posterior tongue (lingual branch) and pharynx (pharyngeal branch). The nodose ganglion of the vagus (Xth) nerve contains primary taste neurons with axons that integrate the pharyngeal, superior laryngeal and internal laryngeal branches to innervate taste buds in the epiglottis, larynx and oesophagus [109]. Primary sensory neurons in these nerves transmit activity generated in TRCs centrally to the solitary tract nucleus (NTS) [151].

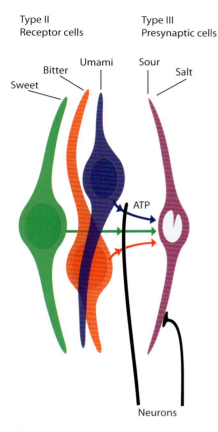

Fig. 1. Peripheral taste mechanisms. Tastants activate two classes of taste bud cells: Type II or receptor cells and Type III or presynaptic cells. Different subclasses of receptor cells (green, red and blue cells), express T1R2/T1R3, T2 R or T1R1/T1R3 G-protein-coupled taste receptors and are activated respectively by sweet, bitter or umami compounds. Downstream signaling pathways in these cells require phospholipase C $\beta2$ and transient receptor potential ion channel M5 (TRPM5). When activated, receptor cells release adenosine triphosphate (ATP), which is then thought to act upon intragemmal taste nerve fibers (black fibres) and/or presynaptic cells. Presypnaptic cells (purple cell) express synapse-related proteins such as synaptosomal-associated protein of 25 kDa and form conventional synapses with intragemmal processes of peripheral taste neurons. In contrast with receptor cells, presynaptic cells are broadly tuned to tastants of multiple qualities – currently, they are thought to be activated directly by sour stimuli, through a different set of receptors and signaling pathways than those used by receptor cells, and indirectly by sweet, bitter and umami compounds, through ATP released from receptor cells. Serotonin (5–HT) is also released from taste buds upon chemosensory stimulation, presumably in synapses between receptor cells and taste neurons. Several taste bud cell types, including receptor cells and type I cells, have been proposed to transduce salt stimuli, but there is still no consensus (see text; adapted from Ref. [163] used with permission)

Peripheral neural taste pathways are functionally and anatomically very close to the somatosensory system, allowing chemical, thermal and tactile detection to act in concert to evaluate substances in the mouth. In fact, the glossopharyngeal and vagal nerves also carry somatosensory nerve fibres from the oral and upper digestive mucosa, as does the lingual branch of the trigeminal (Vth) cranial nerve [107], allowing for the transduction of information relating to the temperature and texture of ingested stimuli [62]. Some intra-oral somatosensory nerve endings are activated by high concentrations of the same chemical stimuli that define some primary tastants, such as NaCl [175], usually producing irritating sensations. Oral mucosa nerve endings may also have other chemosensing properties, as exemplified by the responses to capsaicin, found in chilli peppers and producing a burning sensation [99], and to menthol, producing a cooling sensation [34], mediated by the thermo-sensitive TRPV1 and TRPM8 channels respectively. Furthermore, dietary fats and oils, thought to be sensed mainly by their texture [80] have recently been shown to activate chemosensory mechanisms, such as a fatty acid receptor/transporter, CD36, which is expressed in TRCs and modulates preference for long-chain fatty acid-enriched solutions [97]. On the other hand, physical variables, such as temperature, can affect TRC taste transduction function, as exemplified by thermal modulation of sweet taste intensity [161]. Thus, it becomes clear that, already in the mouth, input to the gustatory system is inherently multisensory.

Postingestive sensory processes

Once a stimulus has been ingested it is not beyond detection by the CNS. In fact, there are multiple and complex humoral and neural postingestive mechanisms that signal not only the presence but also the character of intestinal content. Neural signals depend on the intrinsic and extrinsic enervation of the gastrointestinal tract (GIT). The latter is performed by the autonomic nervous system through both its divisions: parasympathetic (vagal and pelvic nerves) and sympathetic (splanchnic nerves) [189]. These nerves, the vagus in particular, contain afferent neurons that transmit mechanical (i.e., touch, distension, contraction) and chemical sensory information from the GIT to the brain. The neural transmission of chemical information is thought to result from the detection of signaling peptides, such as CCK, produced by enteroendocrine epithelial cells with chemosensing properties [38]. These peptides also reach the circulation, acting on the brain as humoral signals, and are thus called 'gut hormones'. Absorbed nutrients (e.g., glucose) and feeding-related peptides produced in sites other than the gut (e.g., insulin), can also be humoral signals that modulate the activity of central gustatory circuits [189].

With a single exception, discussed below, all known sensory mechanisms originating in the gut are negative feedback signals that lead to decreases in food intake. They are called satiety or satiation signals [38]. Gastric content is detected by vagal afferent fibres in the mucosa, sensitive to touch, while other mechanosensory vagal afferents, in or between muscle layers, report intragastric volume [173]. While gastric satiation processes are predominantly mechanosensory, those originating from the intestine are essentially chemosensory or nutritive [134]. Enteroendocrine cells in the gut lining detect chemical properties of intraluminal content and respond by releasing peptides through their basolateral membrane [38]. Chemosensing activity in enteroendocrine cells is thought to occur through mechanisms and transduction molecules similar to those used in taste, such as T1R3 receptors and gustducin, involved in both orosensory and intestinal responses to sugars [106].

CCK, glucagon-like peptide 1 (GLP-1), oxyntomudulin, peptide YY (PYY) and ghrelin are all examples of gut hormones that have been well established as regulators of food intake [38]. CCK is produced in the duodenal and jejunal mucosa, mainly in response to lipids and proteins, and acts hormonally or via the vagal nerve to reduce food intake [21, 155]. GLP-1, oxyntomudulin and PYY are produced in the more distal segments of the small intestine and the colon, in response to lipids and carbohydrates and, to a lesser extent, proteins [29]. When administered systemically or directly into the CNS, these peptides act as satiation factors [12, 40, 169] and, again, their effects upon peripheral administration involve afferent activity in the vagus nerve [1]. Many other gut peptides have been described but, at this time, the regulation of their secretion and their status as physiologic modulators of feeding is unclear [19].

Ghrelin is the only gut hormone that has been described to act as a positive feed forward stimulus of ingestion [168]. It is secreted from neuroendocrine cells in the gastric mucosa with a temporal pattern of release that is out of phase from all other known gut and pancreatic peptides. Peak circulating levels occur prior to meals and a rapid decrease is observed when nutrients are emptied into the duodenum [39]. Other than ghrelin and palatable oral gustatory stimulation, other ingestion-stimulating mechanisms have been proposed to exist, but remain undefined [147].

Gut peptides are not the only humoral factors that modulate food intake. Free fatty acids, amino acids and glucose, can also convey information about nutritional status to the CNS. In fact, in the first theories for control of energy balance, circulating levels of glucose [108] or of lipids [88] were proposed as the signals of nutritional status. We now know that nutrients in the bloodstream can cross the blood-brain barrier [94] and act directly on the CNS. Oleic acid (a long-chain fatty acid) [125], the amino acid leucine [36] and glucose [22] are examples of nutrients shown to inhibit food intake when administered centrally. Direct CNS nutrient sensing is thought to occur

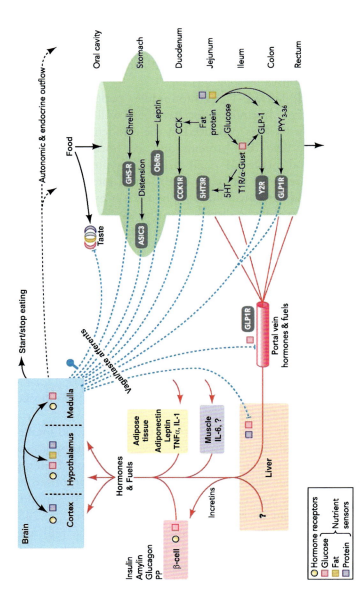

Fig. 2. Gut nutrient signaling pathways. Ingested nutrients elicit mechanosensory and chemosensory responses in the gut, as represented in green on the right. Postingestive responses depend mainly on the production of gut hormones, such as CCK and GLP-1, that signal nutrient presence and quality by activating vagal afferents (blue, dashed lines) and/or entering blood circulation via the portal vein (red, solid lines). Absorbed nutrients (glucose and other 'fuels') and feeding-related peptides produced in sites other than the gut (liver, muscle, adipose tissue and pancreas, on the bottom left), are two other categories of gustatory humoral signals. The postingestive sensory information thus generated, modulates the activity of central neural circuits at several levels of the brain, represented on the top left (from Ref. [189] used with permission)

through key intracellular energy sensors in CNS neurons, found predominantly in the hypothalamus, such as ATP-sensitive potassium channels [124], malonyl-coenzyme A (malonyl-CoA) [100], AMP-activated protein kinase [110], long-chain fatty acyl-CoAs [93] and mTOR (a highly conserved serine-threonine kinase) [36].

Circulating nutrients also activate chemosensors in the pancreas and liver, resulting in the release of hormonal satiation peptides and/or vagal afferent activation [38]. In response to caloric load or vagal efferent activity, the pancreas releases insulin, pancreatic polypeptide (PP) and amylin [83, 103, 146]. With the exception of PP, that acts peripherally [9], these peptides act directly in the CNS to exert an anorectic effect [102, 124]. Portal-hepatic vagal afferents are also sensitive to circulating metabolites such as glucose [117], amino acids [162] and fatty acids [129], and also to gut peptides such as GLP-1 [111]. While the chemosensing mechanisms in the porto-hepatic system are still unclear [95], it is well established that the activity of this system is relevant for the regulation of food intake [164]. Finally, glucose-sensing cells have also been described in the carotid body [132].

Central gustatory sensory pathways

Taste pathways in the CNS are intimately associated with general viscerosensory afferents from the cardiovascular, respiratory and, importantly, gastrointestinal systems [101]. This is the case for all central taste relays, namely the NTS, parabrachial nuclei (PbN) of the pons, parvicellular division of the ventral posterior nucleus of the thalamus (VPpc) and insular or gustatory cortex, through which gustatory taste and visceral projections ascend mostly ipsilaterally [101]. However, in contrast to what happens in rodents, the primate PbN are essentially visceral relays and the NTS projects taste afferents directly to the thalamus [120]. Circulating metabolic signals can also modulate neural responses in relays of the gustatory system, such as the NTS, and in areas that receive direct or indirect gustatory afferents such as the hypothalamic homeostatic centres and reward-related areas in the midbrain [189].

Taste-related information derived from all chemoresponsive cranial nerves, and visceral input, mainly from the vagus nerve, converge in the NTS. The rostral division of the nucleus (rNTS) receives mostly taste afferents while the caudal NTS (cNTS) is the main target for vagal visceral information [4]. Trigeminal somatosensory inputs from oral branches of the fifth nerve also project to the rNTS [165]. Thus, trigeminal stimulants with irritating effects can modulate taste responses in the rNTS [152], as does afferent vagal activity, such as that produced by gastric distension [54]. The NTS has ascending projections to the PbN and local or descending projections to somatic and visceral premotor/motor areas [119]. Local medullary connections with somatic motor or autonomic preganglionic nuclei, either directly or through interneurons in the parvicellular reticular formation, are substrates for reflexes involved in chewing (motor nuclei of the trigeminal and facial nerves), tongue movement (hypoglossal nucleus), salivation (superior and inferior salivatory nuclei), swallowing (nucleus ambiguus) and GI motility and secretion (dorsal motor nucleus of the vagal nerve) [14, 35, 166]. Thus, circuits in the hindbrain are sufficient for decerebrate rats to display both acceptance and rejection behaviours to oral stimulation with tastants [59].

The parabrachial complex is a collection of nuclei located in the dorsolateral aspect of the pons. The PbN nuclei are physically divided into medial and lateral subdivisions by fibres of the superior cerebellar peduncle. In rodents, ascending neural pathways from the NTS synapse in the ipsilateral PbN [121]. The segregation of taste and visceral projections to the rat PbN is not as clear as in the NTS [71]. Nevertheless, visceral afferent projections arising from the cNTS terminate primarily in nuclei of the lateral subdivision while taste responsive neurons are found mainly in the medial PbN [82]. From the rat PbN, third order neurons ascend to form two gustatory projection systems: one projecting dorsally to the thalamus and another projecting ventrally to the forebrain [122].

PbN projections to forebrain centres are mostly reciprocal. In fact, taste-responsive PbN neurons are modulated by electrical stimulation of forebrain sites [44, 98]. The rNTS is also a target of descending forebrain projections from the insular and prefrontal cortices, central nucleus of the amygdala (CeA), lateral hypothalamus (LH), bed nucleus of the stria terminalis and substantia innominata [170]. These descending neural pathways are presumably involved in the modulation of taste activity by physiological and experiential factors [98].

In primates, including humans, rNTS projection fibres have not been shown to terminate in the PbN and synapse directly in the VPpc [15]. Thus, input to the primate PbN is essentially viscerosensory, the bulk of the projections from the PbN are directed towards the ventral forebrain [135] and the VPpc receives most of its gustatory input directly from the NTS [120]. In rodents, the dorsal thalamocortical pathway, originating mainly in the medial PbN, synapses in the VPpc of the thalamus and terminates in the insula. The VPpc is the dorsal thalamic relay for orosensory and visceral information. PbN efferents to this thalamic nucleus are bilateral with an ipsilateral predominance [52]. In fact, while the receptive field for parabrachial gustatory neurons is ipsilateral [67], they can be antidromically driven from the thalamus on either side [126]. However, viscerosensory projections to the thalamus from the external medial parabrachial subnucleus are mainly contralateral [33]. VPpc neurons respond to combinations of chemosensory and/or somatosensory oral stimulation [118] with a medial to lateral arrangement described for taste, thermal and tactile responses [90]. A similar arrangement has also been de-

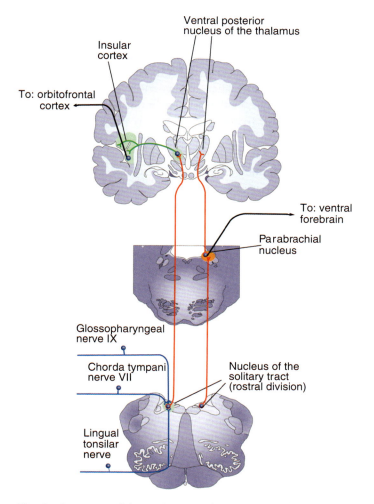

Fig. 3. Anatomy of the main central gustatory pathways. Taste-specific information is conveyed by cranial nerves VII, IX and X (blue lines) to the rostral division of the solitary tract nucleus (rNTS) in the medulla. In primates, fibres (red lines) from second-order taste neurons in the rNTS project ipsilaterally to the parvicellular division of the ventral posterior nucleus of the thalamus (VPpc). Thalamic efferents (green lines) then project to the insula, defining the primary gustatory cortex which, in turn, projects (black lines) to the orbitofrontal cortex, sometimes defined as a secondary cortical taste area. The parabrachial nuclei (PbN) of the pons are shown in orange. In rodents these are a relay for taste afferents from the rNTS. In both primates and rodents, the PbN also receive second order visceral sensory fibres from the caudal division of the solitary tract nucleus (cNTS), transmitted mainly through the vagus nerve (not shown). The PbN has a dorsal thalamocortical projection to the VPMpc and also a ventral projection that terminates in amygdalar and hypothalamic nuclei, among others (adapted from Ref. [151] used with permission)

scribed for taste, GI and cardiovascular/respiratory responses [33]. Neurons in the VPpc projects to the insular cortex and also to the amygdala [131].

The primary taste cortex in macaques is defined as the area receiving afferents from the VPpc, extending posteriorly ~4 mm from its anterior limit at the junction of the orbitofrontal and opercular cortices [148]. Functional neuroimaging studies have shown that, in the human brain, homologous gustatory cortical areas, in the insula and frontal operculum, respond to unimodal taste stimuli [154]. The rodent insula is a cortical region ventral to the oral region of the somatosensory cortex and dorsal to the rhinal sulcus. According to the presence or absence of a granule cell layer, the insular cortex is divided into two histologically distinct subdivisions: the granular and agranular insular cortices. In the dorsal segment of the agranular cortex, adjacent to the granular area, there are scattered granule cells that define a thin strip of dysgranular cortex [101]. It has been noted that insular somatosensory and visceral responses occur in the more dorsal granular insula, whereas taste responses occur ventrally, in the dysgranular area, that is thus proposed to be the primary gustatory cortex (GC) [33, 101]. This stringent definition of the GC as a distinct functional unit, anatomically separated from the more dorsal granular viscerosensory and somatosensory cortex, is challenged by the fact that single neurons in the insula can respond to multiple sensory modalities, namely taste, somatosensory, visceral and nociceptive stimuli [65]. Also, upon stimulation of the entire oral cavity, taste responsive neurons are found not only in the dysgranular but also the granular and, to a lesser extent, the agranular insular cortex [127]. Recent work with optical imaging of the rat insular cortex upon stimulation of the tongue with multiple tastants has equally described responses that include but are not restricted to the dysgranular insula [3].

The different insular regions projects back to their respective thalamic sensory relays and to other cortical areas [150]. The orbitofrontal cortex (OFC), sometimes defined as a secondary taste cortical area [141], receives converging projections from the GC and primary olfactory cortex, proposed as relevant for the perception of flavor [153].

Amygdala and brain reward pathways

The ventral forebrain gustatory projection system includes projections to several structures in the limbic forebrain, such as the hypothalamus [184], amygdala, substantia innominata and bed nucleus of the stria terminalis [52]. The amygdala and the hypothalamus receive other ascending and descending projections from gustatory sensory relays and have important roles in the integration of gustatory input. In the amygdala, the central (CeA) and basolateral (BLA) nuclei are the main sites receiving gustatory projections from the NTS [138], PbN [52, 81], VPpc [131] and insula [130]. The CeA projects back to the NTS and PbN [92] while the BLA has projections to the insula [91]. The two amygdalar areas are also interconnected [130].

The amygdala is reciprocally connected with areas of the midbrain dopaminergic reward system. The latter arises from ventral tegmental area (VTA) dopamine producing neurons that project to the nucleus accumbens (NAcc) and participate in the processing of food reward [179]. The amygdala is connected both with the VTA [133] and the NAcc [89] through the CeA and the BLA. The NAcc also receives afferents directly from other gustatory-related centres, namely the NTS [138], insula [28] and LH [8]. Additionally, circulating pancreatic and gut hormones such as insulin [47], PYY [13] and ghrelin [2] have been shown to directly modulate the activity of midbrain dopamine neurons. The NAcc seems to be a central interface in the integration of sensory, emotional and cognitive controls of food intake [87]. Single accumbens neurons receive convergent inputs from the hippocampus, BLA and prefrontal cortex [49, 50], and dopamine regulates the effect of these afferents on NAcc neurons [55]. NAcc projections to the LH, either direct or through the ventral pallidum, are thought to be its' major effector pathway in the control of feeding behaviours [160].

Food reward, however, is not a unitary concept, and its different conceptual components have been ascribed to different neural substrates. The dissociation between motivational ("wanting" or incentive salience) and hedonic ("liking" or affective salience) components of food reward is one that has been extensively explored [18]. While incentive and affective salience often occur simultaneously and are modulated by neurons found in the same brain areas, such as the NAcc and ventral pallidum, they are behaviourally and neurally distinguishable. "Wanting" reflects the value of a rewarding stimulus in terms of its capacity to elicit an action to obtain that stimulus, and is thought to depend highly on mesolimbic dopamine neurotransmission. "Liking," on the other hand, is the actual pleasurable sensation obtained upon contact with that stimulus, which is often quantified according to stereotypical orofacial responses that can be observed during consumption [17]. While activation of opioid receptors in the NAcc is a potent stimulant of food intake, this effect is specific for palatable foods [181]. Furthermore, opioidergic stimulation of a small subsection of the NAcc ("hedonic hotspot") can specifically modulate orofacial "liking" responses in rats, suggesting a central role for endogenous opioid neurotransmission as a substrate for affective salience [18].

Hypothalamus, brainstem and energy homeostasis

Other than the amygdala, the hypothalamus is the main target of the ventral forebrain gustatory projections system. The NTS projects directly to the median preoptic, paraventricular (PVH), dorsomedial (DMH) and lateral (LH) hypothalamic nuclei [138], while the PbN nuclei project to the median preoptic, PVH, LH, and ventromedial hypothalamus (VMH) [52, 184]. Furthermore, descending projections from the agranular insular cortex target the LH [183]. Lesion studies have established the importance of the hypothalamus for the control of feeding, weight and energy homeostasis. Destruction of the VMH, DMH or PVH induces hyperphagia and obesity [26, 72] while LH lesions induces hypophagia [5]. These findings led to the dual centre model for appetite regulation, with the 'satiety centre' based in the VMH and the 'hunger centre' in the LH [159].

More recently, the VMH has been determined to be the main brain region mediating the effects of leptin [43] – a protein produced and secreted in white adipose tissue that is one of the most important homeostatic mediators of hypophagia [187]. Subsets of LH neurons, on the other hand, contain either orexin (also known as hypocretin) or melanin concentrating hormone (MCH) [45] and both of these peptides are potent stimulators of food intake [136, 143]. The two hypothalamic centres are connected reciprocally to the arcuate nucleus of the hypothalamus (ARC), that is thought to be the master central regulator of energy balance and food intake [74, 185]. Separate subsets of GABAergic ARC neurons have opposed effects on feeding behaviour. Pro-opiomelanocortin (POMC) is a precursor to α- and β-melanocyte stimulating hormones (MSH), two melanocortins that, when released from anorexigenic neurons, act to reduce food intake and body weight while increasing energy expenditure [20]. Orexigenic ARC neurons express neuropeptide Y (NPY) which stimulates feeding and reduces energy expenditure [11]. The same neurons also express agouti gene-related transcript, an antagonist of melanocortin receptors that inhibits the anorectic effects of α-MSH [128]. The ARC is located just above the median eminence, where the blood-brain barrier comprises fenestrated capillaries allowing access to humoral signals that do not reach most other brain areas [53]. Neurons in the ARC are sensitive to glucose [174] and possibly also to intermediates of fatty acid metabolism [100]. Additionally, they express receptors and respond to a variety of other metabolic factors including insulin, leptin and ghrelin [37, 156, 177].

The area postrema (AP), lying immediately dorsal to the NTS, is also a circumventricular organ, that lies outside the blood-brain barrier [25]. Some NTS neurons have dendrites in this zone [70] and AP neurons project to the reticular formation and the PbN in a manner very similar to that of NTS neurons [70, 149]. AP neurons express receptors for, and in some cases have been shown to respond to, amylin [142], CCK [112], GLP-1 [142] and insulin [176]. The AP participates, with the NTS and the dorsal motor nucleus of the vagus, in the control of food intake by the caudal brainstem. In fact, the caudal hindbrain contains glucose-sensitive neurons that are involved in ingestive and

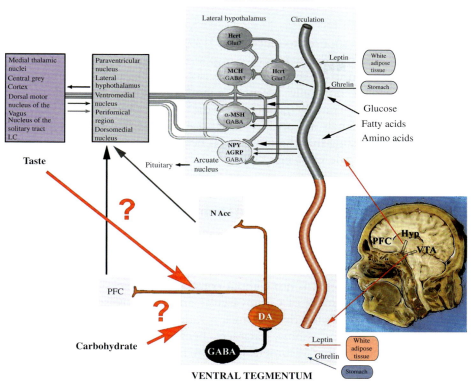

Fig. 4. Hedonic and homeostatic regulation of feeding. Current literature considers the hypothalamus as the main centre for feeding regulation. Lateral hypothalamus neurons that produce orexin (also known as hypocretin – Hcrt) and melanin concentrating hormone (MCH) are potent stimulators of food intake. Neurons in the arcuate nucleus of the hypothalamus synthesize melanocyte stimulating hormone (MSH) or neuropeptide Y (NPY) that have opposed effects in the control of food intake and energy expenditure. The hypothalamic nuclei are traditionally considered a homeostatic centre for feeding regulation since they respond to peripheral metabolic hormones and fuels (such as leptin and ghrelin) that are critical for energy homeostasis [53]. The mesencephalic dopamine system, on the other hand, responds robustly to a diverse array of rewarding stimuli, including food, and plays a critical role in the behavioural responses to these stimuli [179]. Orosensory responses to palatable food are sufficient for the occurrence of dopamine (DA) responses in the mesolimbic system [61], which have generally been considered as a system for 'hedonic' regulation of food intake. However, some of the peripheral hormones that modulate the behavioural components of energy homeostasis also impact the activity in this system (see text). Furthermore, in a recent publication, de Araujo and Oliveira-Maia et al. [41] have shown, using 'taste-blind' mice [186], that the caloric value of sucrose, in the absence of taste transduction, is also sufficient to activate the midbrain reward circuitry. While the physiological details of the signaling mechanisms involved remain to be described, it seems reasonable to suggest that the distinction between hedonic and homeostatic regulation of feeding is redundant. *GABA* gamma-aminobutyric acid; *Glut* glutamate; *Hyp* hypothalamus; *NAcc* nucleus accumbens; *PFC* prefrontal cortex; *VTA* ventral tegmental area (from Ref. [6] used with permission from Elsevier)

sympathoadrenal responses to glucopenia [139] and also neurons that express receptors for, and coordinate ingestive responses to, both leptin [60] and ghrelin [46]. Thus, even when the brainstem is isolated from all forebrain connections, rats exhibit not only acceptance and rejection behaviours to oral stimulation with tastants [59], but also basic satiety-related behaviours [58]. However, these animals are unable to increase meal size in response to food deprivation, suggesting that the forebrain is needed to respond adequately to a long-term homeostatic challenge [57].

Novel opportunities in the management of obesity?

In the introduction to our description of the gustatory system, the dramatic increase in the prevalence of obesity was referred to as the underlying motivation for the study of the central mechanisms of food reward and appetite regulation. In fact, obesity is not without consequence. Excess weight has been linked to the development of cardiovascular and cerebrovascular disease, hypertension, type 2 diabetes, dyslipidemia, a variety of cancers, gallstones, osteoarthritis, sleep apnea, asthma, cataracts, benign prostatic hypertrophy and depression, among other disorders [158]. In fact, obesity is second only to smoking as a leading cause of both preventable mortality and health-related economic burdens. While the health consequences of obesity are important and potentially life-threatening, they are also reversible: even modest reductions in weight lead to improvement in health outcomes such as blood pressure, glucose tolerance and lipid profile [158].

Treating and preventing obesity are thus important objectives in healthcare. However, the treatment options available currently have important limitations. Counselling for dietary modifications, exercise and pharmacologic therapy are the more conservative approaches. Weight loss can be achieved initially but only a small proportion of excess weight is lost and, even so, the maintenance of these losses depends, in most cases, on sustained pharmacologic therapy [24]. In fact, there is extensive evidence that any deviation from a theorized weight "set-point", thought to be based in the hypothalamus, will activate feedback signals, such as leptin and ghrelin, leading to behavioural and metabolic responses that resist and minimize the original weight change [85].

Bariatric surgery is the only effective long-term alternative for the treatment of morbid obesity. In 2005, 140,000 such interventions are estimated to have been performed in the U.S., and reported success rates are high, with up to 80% average excess body weight loss [116]. Furthermore, laparoscopic alternatives, with very low perioperative mortality rates (below 1%), have become available for many bariatric procedures. Nevertheless, bariatric surgery is not devoid of adverse consequences and is not an option for many patients.

Superobese individuals, for example, have higher surgical risks [30], potentially leading to limitations in access to abdominal surgery for those patients that need it most [56]. Moreover, there are important late complications after bariatric surgery, such as metabolic imbalances and nutritional deficiencies [31], and late postoperative mortality rates are thought to be grossly underestimated [30]. In summary, while the effectiveness of bariatric surgery remains unchallenged, it is clear that new alternatives are needed for weight management, especially for extremely obese patients.

The CNS seems to be an important therapeutic target in obesity management. Most of the pharmacological alternatives for obesity treatment act, at least partially, through effects in the brain [23], and modulation of gut hormones constituting the 'gut-brain axis' is thought to be responsible for some of the long-lasting effects of bariatric surgery [7]. The possibility of manipulating food intake and weight by lesions of the hypothalamus was demonstrated in early studies, done in rats, leading to the dual centre model with the VMH as the 'satiety centre' [26, 72] and the LH as the 'hunger centre' [5]. LH lesions have also been performed in a small group of obese patients with significant, albeit temporary, effects in reducing food intake and promoting weight loss [137].The use of electrical stimulation to modify neuronal activity in discrete brain areas has revolutionized functional neurosurgery, with widespread use in the treatment of movement disorders, namely Parkinson's disease [16]. The use of deep brain stimulation (DBS) has also been attempted for several psychiatric disorders, namely Tourette's syndrome, obsessive-compulsive disorder and major depression, with promising results [96]. The consideration of neuropsychiatric factors underlying the pathophysiology of obesity [172] has thus led some to propose the use of DBS in hypothalamic or ventral striatal regions for the treatment of obesity [63]. The feasibility of such an approach is suggested by research in animals, demonstrating inhibition of food consumption [73], or prevention of weight gain [144] by hypothalamic stimulation in rodents. Furthermore, a case of bilateral ventral hypothalamic DBS for treatment of morbid obesity has been reported in the literature, with moderate weight loss and few side effects [64]. While there is still very little information for or against the use of this technique in the treatment of obesity, the possibility of conducting DBS surgery under local anaesthesia [16] may prove to be an advantage for those patients where abdominal surgery poses a significant risk.

Neural stimulation outside of the brain might also prove to be a valid alternative for obese patients. Several experimental treatments, such as gastric electrical stimulation [66] and intra-abdominal vagal blocking therapy [32] are currently being pursued with this purpose. It is critical to validate these approaches to weight control and accurately understand the mechanisms by which they act.

Conclusions

Gustatory, homeostatic and reward circuits in the mammalian brain are part of a complex and distributed neural system that coordinates feeding and other aspects of energy homeostasis. Therapeutic or experimental manipulation of neuronal activity in this system can reduce food consumption and promote weight control, in some cases with dramatic and/or long-lasting effects. Furthermore, with an ever-growing arsenal of neurobiological approaches to understanding brain function, knowledge on the physiology and pathophysiology of feeding behaviour, especially as it relates to hyperphagia and obesity, is already substantial. There are, however, still many unanswered questions. Treatments for obesity that reduce food intake are thought to modulate CNS activity mostly indirectly, through mechanisms that are still poorly understood but presumed to involve changes in neural and/or humoral input to the brain. On the other hand, experimental interventions that directly modify anatomical and/or functional properties of the brain and result in weight loss are yet to be applied clinically. In years to come, new approaches for the management of obesity are critically necessary. Research on the central neural mechanisms of gustation could contribute significantly towards uncovering novel avenues for the treatment of obesity and even related metabolic disorders such as diabetes.

Acknowledgements

We thank Susan Halkiotis for assistance in reviewing our original manuscript. This work was supported by Grant Number R01DC001065 to Sidney Simon from the National Institute on Deafness and Other Communication Disorders (NIDCD). The content is solely the responsibility of the authors and does not necessarily represent the official views of the NIDCD or the National Institutes of Health.

References

1. Abbott CR, Monteiro M, *et al.* (2005) The inhibitory effects of peripheral administration of peptide YY(3–36) and glucagon-like peptide-1 on food intake are attenuated by ablation of the vagal-brainstem-hypothalamic pathway. Brain Res 1044(1): 127–31
2. Abizaid A, Liu ZW, *et al.* (2006) Ghrelin modulates the activity and synaptic input organization of midbrain dopamine neurons while promoting appetite. J Clin Invest 116(12): 3229–39
3. Accolla R, Bathellier B, *et al.* (2007) Differential spatial representation of taste modalities in the rat gustatory cortex. J Neurosci 27(6): 1396–404
4. Altschuler SM, Bao XM, *et al.* (1989) Viscerotopic representation of the upper alimentary tract in the rat: sensory ganglia and nuclei of the solitary and spinal trigeminal tracts. J Comp Neurol 283(2): 248–68

5. Anand BK, Brobeck JR (1951) Localization of a "feeding center in the hypothalamus of the rat. Proc Soc Exp Biol Med 77(2): 323–24
6. Andrews ZB, Horvath TL (2008) Tasteless food reward. Neuron 57(6): 806–08
7. Ashrafian H, le Roux CW (2009) Metabolic surgery and gut hormones – a review of bariatric entero-humoral modulation. Physiol Behav 97(5): 620–31
8. Baldo BA, Daniel RA, *et al.* (2003) Overlapping distributions of orexin/hypocretin- and dopamine-beta-hydroxylase immunoreactive fibers in rat brain regions mediating arousal, motivation, and stress. J Comp Neurol 464(2): 220–37
9. Banks WA, Kastin AJ, *et al.* (1995) Regional variation in transport of pancreatic polypeptide across the blood-brain barrier of mice. Pharmacol Biochem Behav 51(1): 139–47
10. Bartel DL, Sullivan SL, *et al.* (2006) Nucleoside triphosphate diphosphohydrolase-2 is the ecto-ATPase of type I cells in taste buds. J Comp Neurol 497(1): 1–12
11. Baskin DG, Breininger JF, *et al.* (1999) Leptin receptor mRNA identifies a subpopulation of neuropeptide Y neurons activated by fasting in rat hypothalamus. Diabetes 48(4): 828–33
12. Batterham RL, Cowley MA, *et al.* (2002) Gut hormone PYY(3–36) physiologically inhibits food intake. Nature 418(6898): 650–04
13. Batterham RL, ffytche DH, *et al.* (2007) PYY modulation of cortical and hypothalamic brain areas predicts feeding behaviour in humans. Nature 450(7166): 106–09
14. Beckman ME, Whitehead MC (1991) Intramedullary connections of the rostral nucleus of the solitary tract in the hamster. Brain Res 557(1–2): 265–79
15. Beckstead RM, Morse JR, *et al.* (1980) The nucleus of the solitary tract in the monkey: projections to the thalamus and brain stem nuclei. J Comp Neurol 190(2): 259–82
16. Benabid AL, Chabardes S, *et al.* (2009) Deep brain stimulation of the subthalamic nucleus for the treatment of Parkinson's disease. Lancet Neurol 8(1): 67–81
17. Berridge KC (1996) Food reward: brain substrates of wanting and liking. Neurosci Biobehav Rev 20(1): 1–25
18. Berridge KC (2009) 'Liking' and 'wanting' food rewards: brain substrates and roles in eating disorders. Physiol Behav 97(5): 537–50
19. Berthoud HR (2008) Vagal and hormonal gut-brain communication: from satiation to satisfaction. Neurogastroenterol Motil 20(Suppl 1): 64–72
20. Biebermann H, Castaneda TR, *et al.* (2006) A role for beta-melanocyte-stimulating hormone in human body-weight regulation. Cell Metab 3(2): 141–46
21. Blevins JE, Stanley BG, *et al.* (2000) Brain regions where cholecystokinin suppresses feeding in rats. Brain Res 860(1–2): 1–10
22. Booth DA (1968) Effects of intrahypothalamic glucose injection on eating and drinking elicited by insulin. J Comp Physiol Psychol 65(1): 13–16
23. Bray GA, Greenway FL (2007) Pharmacological treatment of the overweight patient. Pharmacol Rev 59(2): 151–84
24. Bray GA, Wilson JF (2008) In the clinic. Obesity. Ann Intern Med 149(7): ITC4-1-15; quiz ITC4-16
25. Broadwell RD, Brightman MW (1976) Entry of peroxidase into neurons of the central and peripheral nervous systems from extracerebral and cerebral blood. J Comp Neurol 166(3): 257–83
26. Brobeck JR, Tepperman J, *et al.* (1943) Experimental hypothalamic hyperphagia in the albino rat. Yale J Biol Med 15: 831–53

27. Broberger C (2005) Brain regulation of food intake and appetite: molecules and networks. J Intern Med 258(4): 301–27
28. Brog JS, Salyapongse A, *et al.* (1993) The patterns of afferent innervation of the core and shell in the "accumbens" part of the rat ventral striatum: immunohistochemical detection of retrogradely transported fluoro-gold. J Comp Neurol 338(2): 255–78
29. Brubaker PL, Anini Y (2003) Direct and indirect mechanisms regulating secretion of glucagon-like peptide-1 and glucagon-like peptide-2. Can J Physiol Pharmacol 81(11): 1005–12
30. Buchwald H, Estok R, *et al.* (2007) Trends in mortality in bariatric surgery: a systematic review and meta-analysis. Surgery 142(4): 621–32; discussion 632–35
31. Bult MJ, van Dalen T, *et al.* (2008) Surgical treatment of obesity. Eur J Endocrinol 158(2): 135–45
32. Camilleri M, Toouli J, *et al.* (2008) Intra-abdominal vagal blocking (VBLOC therapy): clinical results with a new implantable medical device. Surgery 143(6): 723–31
33. Cechetto DF, Saper CB (1987) Evidence for a viscerotopic sensory representation in the cortex and thalamus in the rat. J Comp Neurol 262(1): 27–45
34. Chuang HH, Neuhausser WM, *et al.* (2004) The super-cooling agent icilin reveals a mechanism of coincidence detection by a temperature-sensitive TRP channel. Neuron 43(6): 859–69
35. Contreras RJ, Gomez MM, *et al.* (1980) Central origins of cranial nerve parasympathetic neurons in the rat. J Comp Neurol 190(2): 373–94
36. Cota D, Proulx K, *et al.* (2006) Hypothalamic mTOR signaling regulates food intake. Science 312(5775): 927–30
37. Cowley MA, Smart JL, *et al.* (2001) Leptin activates anorexigenic POMC neurons through a neural network in the arcuate nucleus. Nature 411(6836): 480–84
38. Cummings DE, Overduin J (2007) Gastrointestinal regulation of food intake. J Clin Invest 117(1): 13–23
39. Cummings DE, Purnell JQ, *et al.* (2001) A preprandial rise in plasma ghrelin levels suggests a role in meal initiation in humans. Diabetes 50(8): 1714–19
40. Dakin CL, Gunn I, *et al.* (2001) Oxyntomodulin inhibits food intake in the rat. Endocrinology 142(10): 4244–50
41. de Araujo IE, Oliveira-Maia AJ, *et al.* (2008) Food reward in the absence of taste receptor signaling. Neuron 57(6): 930–41
42. DeSimone JA, Lyall V, *et al.* (2001) A novel pharmacological probe links the amiloride-insensitive NaCl, KCl, and NH(4)Cl chorda tympani taste responses. J Neurophysiol 86(5): 2638–41
43. Dhillon H, Zigman JM, *et al.* (2006) Leptin directly activates SF1 neurons in the VMH, and this action by leptin is required for normal body-weight homeostasis. Neuron 49(2): 191–203
44. Di Lorenzo PM (1990) Corticofugal influence on taste responses in the parabrachial pons of the rat. Brain Res 530(1): 73–84
45. Elias CF, Saper CB, *et al.* (1998) Chemically defined projections linking the mediobasal hypothalamus and the lateral hypothalamic area. J Comp Neurol 402(4): 442–59
46. Faulconbridge LF, Cummings DE, *et al.* (2003) Hyperphagic effects of brainstem ghrelin administration. Diabetes 52(9): 2260–65
47. Figlewicz DP (2003) Adiposity signals and food reward: expanding the CNS roles of insulin and leptin. Am J Physiol Regul Integr Comp Physiol 284(4): R882–92

48. Finger TE, Danilova V, *et al.* (2005) ATP signaling is crucial for communication from taste buds to gustatory nerves. Science 310(5753): 1495–99
49. French SJ, Totterdell S (2002) Hippocampal and prefrontal cortical inputs monosynaptically converge with individual projection neurons of the nucleus accumbens. J Comp Neurol 446(2): 151–65
50. French SJ, Totterdell S (2003) Individual nucleus accumbens-projection neurons receive both basolateral amygdala and ventral subicular afferents in rats. Neuroscience 119(1): 19–31
51. Friedman JM (2009) Obesity: causes and control of excess body fat. Nature 459(7245): 340–42
52. Fulwiler CE, Saper CB (1984) Subnuclear organization of the efferent connections of the parabrachial nucleus in the rat. Brain Res 319(3): 229–59
53. Gao Q, Horvath TL (2007) Neurobiology of feeding and energy expenditure. Annu Rev Neurosci 30: 367–98
54. Glenn JF, Erickson RP (1976) Gastric modulation of gustatory afferent activity. Physiol Behav (16): 561–68
55. Goto Y, Grace AA (2005) Dopaminergic modulation of limbic and cortical drive of nucleus accumbens in goal-directed behavior. Nat Neurosci 8(6): 805–12
56. Gottig S, Daskalakis M, *et al.* (2009) Analysis of safety and efficacy of intragastric balloon in extremely obese patients. Obes Surg 19(6): 677–83
57. Grill HJ, Kaplan JM (2001) Interoceptive and integrative contributions of forebrain and brainstem to energy balance control. Int J Obes Relat Metab Disord 25(Suppl 5): S73–77
58. Grill HJ, Norgren R (1978) Chronically decerebrate rats demonstrate satiation but not bait shyness. Science 201(4352): 267–69
59. Grill HJ, Norgren R (1978) The taste reactivity test. II. Mimetic responses to gustatory stimuli in chronic thalamic and chronic decerebrate rats. Brain Res 143(2): 281–97
60. Grill HJ, Schwartz MW, *et al.* (2002) Evidence that the caudal brainstem is a target for the inhibitory effect of leptin on food intake. Endocrinology 143(1): 239–46
61. Hajnal A, Smith GP, *et al.* (2004) Oral sucrose stimulation increases accumbens dopamine in the rat. Am J Physiol Regul Integr Comp Physiol 286(1): R31–37
62. Halata Z, Munger BL (1983) The sensory innervation of primate facial skin. II. Vermilion border and mucosa of lip. Brain Res 286(1): 81–107
63. Halpern CH, Wolf JA, *et al.* (2008) Deep brain stimulation in the treatment of obesity. J Neurosurg 109(4): 625–34
64. Hamani C, McAndrews MP, *et al.* (2008) Memory enhancement induced by hypothalamic/fornix deep brain stimulation. Ann Neurol 63(1): 119–23
65. Hanamori T, Kunitake T, *et al.* (1998) Responses of neurons in the insular cortex to gustatory, visceral, and nociceptive stimuli in rats. J Neurophysiol 79(5): 2535–45
66. Hasler WL (2009) Methods of gastric electrical stimulation and pacing: a review of their benefits and mechanisms of action in gastroparesis and obesity. Neurogastroenterol Motil 21(3): 229–43
67. Hayama T, Ito S, *et al.* (1987) Receptive field properties of the parabrachiothalamic taste and mechanoreceptive neurons in rats. Exp Brain Res 68(3): 458–65
68. Heath TP, Melichar JK, *et al.* (2006) Human taste thresholds are modulated by serotonin and noradrenaline. J Neurosci 26(49): 12664–71

69. Heck GL, Mierson S, *et al.* (1984) Salt taste transduction occurs through an amiloride-sensitive sodium transport pathway. Science 223(4634): 403–05

70. Herbert H, Moga MM, *et al.* (1990) Connections of the parabrachial nucleus with the nucleus of the solitary tract and the medullary reticular formation in the rat. J Comp Neurol 293(4): 540–80

71. Hermann GE, Kohlerman NJ, *et al.* (1983) Hepatic-vagal and gustatory afferent interactions in the brainstem of the rat. J Auton Nerv Syst 9(2–3): 477–95

72. Hetherington AW, Ranson SW (1940) Hypothalamic lesions and adipocity in the rat. Anat Record 78: 149

73. Hoebel BG, Teitelbaum P (1962) Hypothalamic control of feeding and self-stimulation. Science 135: 375–77

74. Horvath TL, Diano S, *et al.* (1999) Synaptic interaction between hypocretin (orexin) and neuropeptide Y cells in the rodent and primate hypothalamus: a novel circuit implicated in metabolic and endocrine regulations. J Neurosci 19(3): 1072–87

75. Huang AL, Chen X, *et al.* (2006) The cells and logic for mammalian sour taste detection. Nature 442(7105): 934–38

76. Huang YA, Maruyama Y, *et al.* (2008) Norepinephrine is coreleased with serotonin in mouse taste buds. J Neurosci 28(49): 13088–93

77. Huang YJ, Maruyama Y, *et al.* (2007) The role of pannexin 1 hemichannels in ATP release and cell-cell communication in mouse taste buds. Proc Natl Acad Sci USA 104(15): 6436–41

78. Huque T, Cowart BJ, *et al.* (2009) Sour ageusia in two individuals implicates ion channels of the ASIC and PKD families in human sour taste perception at the anterior tongue. PLoS One 4(10): e7347

79. Ishimaru Y, Inada H, *et al.* (2006) Transient receptor potential family members PKD1L3 and PKD2L1 form a candidate sour taste receptor. Proc Natl Acad Sci USA 103(33): 12569–74

80. Kadohisa M, Verhagen JV, *et al.* (2005) The primate amygdala: Neuronal representations of the viscosity, fat texture, temperature, grittiness and taste of foods. Neuroscience 132(1): 33–48

81. Karimnamazi H, Travers JB (1998) Differential projections from gustatory responsive regions of the parabrachial nucleus to the medulla and forebrain. Brain Res 813(2): 283–302

82. Karimnamazi H, Travers SP, *et al.* (2002) Oral and gastric input to the parabrachial nucleus of the rat. Brain Res 957(2): 193–206

83. Katsuura G, Asakawa A, *et al.* (2002) Roles of pancreatic polypeptide in regulation of food intake. Peptides 23(2): 323–29

84. Kawamura Y, Okamoto J, *et al.* (1968) A role of oral afferents in aversion to taste solutions. Physiol Behav 3: 537–42

85. Keesey RE, Powley TL (2008) Body energy homeostasis. Appetite 51(3): 442–45

86. Keith SW, Redden DT, *et al.* (2006) Putative contributors to the secular increase in obesity: exploring the roads less traveled. Int J Obes (Lond) 30(11): 1585–94

87. Kelley AE, Baldo BA, *et al.* (2005) Corticostriatal-hypothalamic circuitry and food motivation: integration of energy, action and reward. Physiol Behav 86(5): 773–95

88. Kennedy GC (1953) The role of depot fat in the hypothalamic control of food intake in the rat. Proc R Soc Lond B Biol Sci 140(901): 578–96

89. Kirouac GJ, Ganguly PK, (1995) Topographical organization in the nucleus accumbens of afferents from the basolateral amygdala and efferents to the lateral hypothalamus. Neuroscience 67(3): 625–30

90. Kosar E, Grill HJ, *et al.* (1986) Gustatory cortex in the rat. II. Thalamocortical projections. Brain Res 379(2): 342–52

91. Krettek JE, Price JL (1977) Projections from the amygdaloid complex to the cerebral cortex and thalamus in the rat and cat. J Comp Neurol 172(4): 687–722

92. Krettek JE, Price JL (1978) Amygdaloid projections to subcortical structures within the basal forebrain and brainstem in the rat and cat. J Comp Neurol 178(2): 225–54

93. Lam TK, Pocai A, *et al.* (2005) Hypothalamic sensing of circulating fatty acids is required for glucose homeostasis. Nat Med 11(3): 320–7

94. Lam TK, Schwartz GJ, *et al.* (2005) "Hypothalamic sensing of fatty acids. Nat Neurosci 8(5): 579–84

95. Langhans W (1996) Role of the liver in the metabolic control of eating: what we know – and what we do not know. Neurosci Biobehav Rev 20(1): 145–53

96. Larson PS (2008) Deep brain stimulation for psychiatric disorders. Neurotherapeutics 5(1): 50–8

97. Laugerette F, Passilly-Degrace P, *et al.* (2005) CD36 involvement in orosensory detection of dietary lipids, spontaneous fat preference, and digestive secretions. J Clin Invest 115(11): 3177–84

98. Li CS, Cho YK, *et al.* (2005) Modulation of parabrachial taste neurons by electrical and chemical stimulation of the lateral hypothalamus and amygdala. J Neurophysiol 93(3): 1183–96

99. Liu L, Simon SA (1996) Capsaicin-induced currents with distinct desensitization and Ca^{2+} dependence in rat trigeminal ganglion cells. J Neurophysiol 75(4): 1503–14

100. Loftus TM, Jaworsky DE, *et al.* (2000) Reduced food intake and body weight in mice treated with fatty acid synthase inhibitors. Science 288(5475): 2379–81

101. Lundy RF Jr, Norgren R (2004) Gustatory system. In: Paxinos G (ed) The Rat Nervous System. Academic Press, San Diego, CA and London, Elsevier, pp 891–921

102. Lutz TA, Del Prete E, *et al.* (1995) Subdiaphragmatic vagotomy does not influence the anorectic effect of amylin. Peptides 16(3): 457–62

103. Lutz TA, Geary N, *et al.* (1995) Amylin decreases meal size in rats. Physiol Behav 58(6): 1197–202

104. Lyall V, Heck GL, *et al.* (2004) The mammalian amiloride-insensitive non-specific salt taste receptor is a vanilloid receptor-1 variant. J Physiol 558(Pt 1): 147–59

105. Margolskee RF (2002) Molecular mechanisms of bitter and sweet taste transduction. J Biol Chem 277(1): 1–4

106. Margolskee RF, Dyer J, *et al.* (2007) T1R3 and gustducin in gut sense sugars to regulate expression of Na+-glucose cotransporter 1. Proc Natl Acad Sci U S A 104(38): 15075–80

107. Matsumoto I, Emori Y, *et al.* (2001) A comparative study of three cranial sensory ganglia projecting into the oral cavity: in situ hybridization analyses of neurotrophin receptors and thermosensitive cation channels. Brain Res Mol Brain Res 93(2): 105–12

108. Mayer J (1953) Glucostatic mechanism of regulation of food intake. N Engl J Med 249(1): 13–16

109. Miller IJ Jr (1995) Anatomy of the peripheral taste system. In: Doty RL (ed) Handbook of Olfaction and Gustation. Marcel Dekker Inc., New York, pp 521–47

110. Minokoshi Y, Alquier T, *et al.* (2004) AMP-kinase regulates food intake by responding to hormonal and nutrient signals in the hypothalamus. Nature 428(6982): 569–74

111. Mithieux G, Misery P, *et al.* (2005) Portal sensing of intestinal gluconeogenesis is a mechanistic link in the diminution of food intake induced by diet protein. Cell Metab 2(5): 321–29

112. Moran TH, Robinson PH, *et al.* (1986) Two brain cholecystokinin receptors: implications for behavioral actions. Brain Res 362(1): 175–79

113. Mueller KL, Hoon MA, *et al.* (2005) The receptors and coding logic for bitter taste. Nature 434(7030): 225–29

114. Murray RG (1971) Ultrastructure of taste receptors. In: Beidler LM (ed) Handbook of Sensory Physiology. Volume IV. Chemical Senses Part 2: Taste. Springer-Verlag, Berlin, pp 31–50

115. Nakano Y, Oomura Y, *et al.* (1986) Feeding-related activity of glucose- and morphine-sensitive neurons in the monkey amygdala. Brain Res 399(1): 167–72

116. Nguyen NT, Wilson SE (2007) Complications of antiobesity surgery. Nat Clin Pract Gastroenterol Hepatol 4(3): 138–47

117. Niijima A (1969) Afferent impulse discharges from glucoreceptors in the liver of the guinea pig. Ann NY Acad Sci 157(2): 690–700

118. Nomura T, Ogawa H (1985) The taste and mechanical response properties of neurons in the parvicellular part of the thalamic posteromedial ventral nucleus of the rat. Neurosci Res 3(2): 91–105

119. Norgren R (1978) Projections from the nucleus of the solitary tract in the rat. Neuroscience 3(2): 207–18

120. Norgren R (1984) Central neural mechanisms of taste. In: Darien-Smith I (ed) Handbook of Physiology – The Nervous System III. Sensory Processes 1. American Physiological Society, Washington, DC, pp 1087–128

121. Norgren R, Leonard CM (1971) Taste pathways in rat brainstem. Science 173(2): 1136–39

122. Norgren R, Leonard CM (1973) Ascending central gustatory pathways. J Comp Neurol 150(2): 217–37

123. O'Rahilly S, Farooqi IS (2006) Genetics of obesity. Philos Trans R Soc Lond B Biol Sci 361(1471): 1095–105

124. Obici S, Feng Z, *et al.* (2002) Decreasing hypothalamic insulin receptors causes hyperphagia and insulin resistance in rats. Nat Neurosci 5(6): 566–72

125. Obici S, Feng Z, *et al.* (2002) Central administration of oleic acid inhibits glucose production and food intake. Diabetes 51(2): 271–75

126. Ogawa H, Hayama T, *et al.* (1984) Location and taste responses of parabrachio-thalamic relay neurons in rats. Exp Neurol 83(3): 507–17

127. Ogawa H, Ito S, *et al.* (1990) Taste area in granular and dysgranular insular cortices in the rat identified by stimulation of the entire oral cavity. Neurosci Res 9(3): 196–201

128. Ollmann MM, Wilson BD, *et al.* (1997) Antagonism of central melanocortin receptors in vitro and in vivo by agouti-related protein. Science 278(5335): 135–38

129. Orbach J, Andrews WH (1973) Stimulation of afferent nerve terminals in the perfused rabbit liver by sodium salts of some long-chain fatty acids. Q J Exp Physiol Cogn Med Sci 58(3): 267–74

130. Ottersen OP (1982) Connections of the amygdala of the rat. IV: Corticoamygdaloid and intraamygdaloid connections as studied with axonal transport of horseradish peroxidase. J Comp Neurol 205(1): 30–48

131. Ottersen OP, Ben-Ari Y (1979) Afferent connections to the amygdaloid complex of the rat and cat. I. Projections from the thalamus. J Comp Neurol 187(2): 401–24

132. Pardal R, Lopez-Barneo J (2002) Low glucose-sensing cells in the carotid body. Nat Neurosci 5(3): 197–98

133. Phillipson OT (1979) Afferent projections to the ventral tegmental area of Tsai and interfascicular nucleus: a horseradish peroxidase study in the rat. J Comp Neurol 187(1): 117–43

134. Powley TL, Phillips RJ (2004) Gastric satiation is volumetric, intestinal satiation is nutritive. Physiol Behav 82(1): 69–74

135. Pritchard TC, Hamilton RB, *et al.* (2000) Projections of the parabrachial nucleus in the old world monkey. Exp Neurol 165(1): 101–17

136. Qu D, Ludwig DS, *et al.* (1996) A role for melanin-concentrating hormone in the central regulation of feeding behaviour. Nature 380(6571): 243–47

137. Quaade F, Vaernet K, *et al.* (1974) Stereotaxic stimulation and electrocoagulation of the lateral hypothalamus in obese humans. Acta Neurochir (Wien) 30(1–2): 111–17

138. Ricardo JA, Koh ET (1978) Anatomical evidence of direct projections from the nucleus of the solitary tract to the hypothalamus, amygdala, and other forebrain structures in the rat. Brain Res 153(1): 1–26

139. Ritter RC, Slusser PG, *et al.* (1981) Glucoreceptors controlling feeding and blood glucose: location in the hindbrain. Science 213(4506): 451–52

140. Rolls ET, Baylis LL (1994) Gustatory, olfactory, and visual convergence within the primate orbitofrontal cortex. J Neurosci 14: 5437–52

141. Rolls ET, Yaxley S, *et al.* (1990) Gustatory responses of single neurons in the caudolateral orbitofrontal cortex of the macaque monkey. J Neurophysiol 64(4): 1055–66

142. Rowland NE, Crews EC, *et al.* (1997) Comparison of Fos induced in rat brain by GLP-1 and amylin. Regul Pept 71(3): 171–74

143. Sakurai T, Amemiya A, *et al.* (1998) Orexins and orexin receptors: a family of hypothalamic neuropeptides and G protein-coupled receptors that regulate feeding behavior. Cell 92(4): 573–85

144. Sani S, Jobe K, *et al.* (2007) Deep brain stimulation for treatment of obesity in rats. J Neurosurg 107(4): 809–13

145. Schwartz MW, Porte D Jr (2005) Diabetes, obesity, and the brain. Science 307(5708): 375–79

146. Schwartz MW, Woods SC, *et al.* (2000) Central nervous system control of food intake. Nature 404(6778): 661–71

147. Sclafani A (2004) Oral and postoral determinants of food reward. Physiol Behav 81(5): 773–79

148. Scott TR, Plata-Salaman CR (1999) Taste in the monkey cortex. Physiol Behav 67(4): 489–511

149. Shapiro RE, Miselis RR (1985) The central neural connections of the area postrema of the rat. J Comp Neurol 234(3): 344–64

150. Shi CJ, Cassell MD (1998) Cortical, thalamic, and amygdaloid connections of the anterior and posterior insular cortices. J Comp Neurol 399(4): 440–68

151. Simon SA, de Araujo IE, *et al.* (2006) The neural mechanisms of gustation: a distributed processing code. Nat Rev Neurosci 7(11): 890–901
152. Simons CT, Boucher Y, *et al.* (2003) Suppression of central taste transmission by oral capsaicin. J Neurosci 23(3): 978–85
153. Small DM, Prescott J (2005) Odor/taste integration and the perception of flavor. Exp Brain Res 166(3–4): 345–57
154. Small DM, Zald DH, *et al.* (1999) Human cortical gustatory areas: a review of functional neuroimaging data. NeuroReport 10(1): 7–14
155. Smith GP, Jerome C, *et al.* (1981) Abdominal vagotomy blocks the satiety effect of cholecystokinin in the rat. Science 213(4511): 1036–37
156. Spanswick D, Smith MA, *et al.* (2000) Insulin activates ATP-sensitive K+ channels in hypothalamic neurons of lean, but not obese rats. Nat Neurosci 3(8): 757–58
157. Spector AC, Travers SP (2005) The representation of taste quality in the mammalian nervous system. Behav Cogn Neurosci Rev 4(3): 143–91
158. Stein CJ, Colditz GA (2004) The epidemic of obesity. J Clin Endocrinol Metab 89(6): 2522–25
159. Stellar E (1954) The physiology of motivation. Psychol Rev 61(1): 5–22
160. Stratford TR, Kelley AE (1999) Evidence of a functional relationship between the nucleus accumbens shell and lateral hypothalamus subserving the control of feeding behavior. J Neurosci 19(24): 11040–48
161. Talavera K, Yasumatsu K, *et al.* (2005) Heat activation of TRPM5 underlies thermal sensitivity of sweet taste. Nature 438(7070): 1022–25
162. Tanaka K, Inoue S, *et al.* (1990) Amino acid sensors sensitive to alanine and leucine exist in the hepato-portal system in the rat. J Auton Nerv Syst 31(1): 41–46
163. Tomchik SM, Berg S, *et al.* (2007) Breadth of tuning and taste coding in mammalian taste buds. J Neurosci 27(40): 10840–48
164. Tordoff MG, Friedman MI (1986) Hepatic portal glucose infusions decrease food intake and increase food preference. Am J Physiol 251(1 Pt 2): R192–96
165. Torvik A (1956) Afferent connections to the sensory trigeminal nuclei, the nucleus of the solitary tract and adjacent structures; an experimental study in the rat. J Comp Neurol 106(1): 51–141
166. Travers JB, Norgren R (1983) Afferent projections to the oral motor nuclei in the rat. J Comp Neurol 220(3): 280–98
167. Treesukosol Y, Lyall V, *et al.* (2007) A psychophysical and electrophysiological analysis of salt taste in Trpv1 null mice. Am J Physiol Regul Integr Comp Physiol 292(5): R1799–809
168. Tschop M, Smiley DL, *et al.* (2000) Ghrelin induces adiposity in rodents. Nature 407(6806): 908–13
169. Turton MD, O'Shea D, *et al.* (1996) A role for glucagon-like peptide-1 in the central regulation of feeding. Nature 379(6560): 69–72
170. van der Kooy D, Koda LY, *et al.* (1984) The organization of projections from the cortex, amygdala, and hypothalamus to the nucleus of the solitary tract in rat. J Comp Neurol 224(1): 1–24
171. Vandenbeuch A, Clapp TR, *et al.* (2008) Amiloride-sensitive channels in type I fungiform taste cells in mouse. BMC Neurosci 9: 1
172. Volkow ND, O'Brien CP (2007) Issues for DSM-V: should obesity be included as a brain disorder? Am J Psychiatry 164(5): 708–10

173. Wang FB, Powley TL (2000) Topographic inventories of vagal afferents in gastrointestinal muscle. J Comp Neurol 421(3): 302–24

174. Wang R, Liu X, *et al.* (2004) The regulation of glucose-excited neurons in the hypothalamic arcuate nucleus by glucose and feeding-relevant peptides. Diabetes 53(8): 1959–65

175. Wang Y, Erickson RP, *et al.* (1993) Selectivity of lingual nerve fibers to chemical stimuli. J Gen Physiol 101(6): 843–66

176. Werther GA, Hogg A, *et al.* (1987) Localization and characterization of insulin receptors in rat brain and pituitary gland using in vitro autoradiography and computerized densitometry. Endocrinology 121(4): 1562–70

177. Willesen MG, Kristensen P, *et al.* (1999) Co-localization of growth hormone secretagogue receptor and NPY mRNA in the arcuate nucleus of the rat. Neuroendocrinology 70(5): 306–16

178. Wilson CS (2002) Reasons for eating: personal experiences in nutrition and anthropology. Appetite 38(1): 63–7

179. Wise RA (2006) Role of brain dopamine in food reward and reinforcement. Philos Trans R Soc Lond B Biol Sci 361(1471): 1149–58

180. Wong GT, Gannon KS, *et al.* (1996) Transduction of bitter and sweet taste by gustducin. Nature 381(6585): 796–800

181. Woolley JD, Lee BS, *et al.* (2006) Nucleus accumbens opioids regulate flavor-based preferences in food consumption. Neuroscience 143(1): 309–17

182. Yang R, Crowley HH, *et al.* (2000) Taste cells with synapses in rat circumvallate papillae display SNAP-25-like immunoreactivity. J Comp Neurol 424(2): 205–15

183. Yasui Y, Breder CD, *et al.* (1991) Autonomic responses and efferent pathways from the insular cortex in the rat. J Comp Neurol 303(3): 355–74

184. Zaborszky L, Beinfeld MC, *et al.* (1984) Brainstem projection to the hypothalamic ventromedial nucleus in the rat: a CCK-containing long ascending pathway. Brain Res 303(2): 225–31

185. Zaborszky L, Makara GB (1979) Intrahypothalamic connections: an electron microscopic study in the rat. Exp Brain Res 34(2): 201–15

186. Zhang Y, Hoon MA, *et al.* (2003) Coding of sweet, bitter, and umami tastes: different receptor cells sharing similar signaling pathways. Cell 112(3): 293–301

187. Zhang Y, Proenca R, *et al.* (1994) Positional cloning of the mouse obese gene and its human homologue. Nature 372(6505): 425–32

188. Zhao GQ, Zhang Y, *et al.* (2003) The receptors for mammalian sweet and umami taste. Cell 115(3): 255–66

189. Zheng H, Berthoud HR (2008) Neural systems controlling the drive to eat: mind versus metabolism. Physiology (Bethesda) 23: 75–83

SEEG-guided RF-thermocoagulation of epileptic foci: A therapeutic alternative for drug-resistant non-operable partial epilepsies

M. Guénot[1,3–5], J. Isnard[2–5], H. Catenoix[2–5], F. Mauguière[2–5], and M. Sindou[1,3,4]

[1] Service de Neurochirurgie Fonctionnelle, Hôpital Neurologique Pierre Wertheimer, Hospices Civils de Lyon, Bron, France
[2] Service de Neurologie Fonctionnelle et d'Epileptologie, Hôpital Neurologique Pierre Wertheimer, Hospices Civils de Lyon, Bron, France
[3] Université de Lyon, Université Lyon 1, Lyon, France
[4] Institut Fédératif des Neurosciences de Lyon, Lyon, France
[5] INSERM, U879, Bron, France; Université de Lyon, Université Lyon 1, Lyon, France

With 5 Figures and 2 Tables

Contents

Abstract 62
Introduction 63
Technical data 65
   Advantages of the technique 65
   Patient's selection 66
   Placement of the lesion 66
Our experience 68
   Patients 68
   Targets, follow-up and results 68
      Choice of targets 70
      Follow-up 70
   Results 73
      Seizure outcome 73
      Safety 74
Discussion 74
Conclusion 76
References 76

Abstract

Background: Previous literature includes numerous reports of acute stereotactic ablation for epilepsy. Most reports focus on amygdalotomies or amygdalohippocampotomies, some others focus on various extra-limbic targets. These stereotactic techniques proved to have a less favourable outcome than that of standard surgery, so that their rather disappointing benefit/risk ratio explains why they have been largely abandoned.

However, depth electrode recordings may be required in some cases of epilepsy surgery to delineate the best region of cortical resection. We usually implant depth electrodes according to Talairach's stereo electroencephalography (SEEG) methodology. Using these chronically implanted depth electrodes, we are able to perform radiofrequency (RF)-thermolesions of the epileptic foci. This paper reports the technical data required to perform such multiple cortical thermolesions, as well as the results in terms of seizure outcome in a group of 41 patients.

Technical data: Lesions are placed in the cortex areas showing either a low amplitude fast pattern or spike-wave discharges at the onset of the seizures. Interictal paroxysmal activities are not considered for planning thermocoagulation sites. All targets are first functionally evaluated using electrical stimulation. Only those showing no clinical response to stimulation are selected for thermolesion, including sites located inside or near primary functional area.

Lesions are performed using 120 mA bipolar current (50 V), applied for 10–30 sec. Each thermocoagulation produces a 5–7 mm diameter cortical lesion. A total of 2–31 lesions were performed in each of the 41 patients. Lesions are placed without anaesthesia.

Results: 20 patients (48.7%) experienced a seizure frequency decrease of at least 50% that was more than 80% in eight of them. One patient was seizure free after RF thermocoagulation. In 21 patients, no significant reduction of the seizure frequency was observed. Amongst the characteristics of the disease (age and sex of the patient, lobar localization of the EZ) and the characteristics of the thermocoagulations (topography, lateralization, number, morphology of the lesions on MRI) no factor was significantly linked to the outcome. However, the best results were clearly observed in epilepsies symptomatic of a cortical development malformation (CDM), with 67% of responders in this group of 20 patients ($p = 0.052$). Three transient post-procedure side-effects, consisting of paraesthetic sensations in the mouth (2 cases), and mild apraxia of the hand, were observed.

Conclusion: SEEG-guided-RF-thermolesioning is a safe technique. Our results indicate that such lesions can lead to a significant reduction of seizure frequency. Our experience suggests that SEEG-guided RF thermocoagulation should be dedicated to drug-resistant epileptic patients for whom conventional resection surgery is risky or contra-indicated on the basis of invasive pre-surgical evaluation, particularly those suffering from epilepsy symptomatic of cortical development malformation.

Keywords: Radio frequency thermocoagulations; epilepsy; SEEG; epilepsy surgery.

Introduction

Performing *stereotactic lesions* of the brain in order to relieve, or even cure, epilepsy is not a new idea.

Prior literature comprises numerous reports of acute stereotactic ablation for epilepsy. Most reports focus on amygdalotomies or amygdalohippocampotomies [1, 2, 6–8, 10, 16, 17, 21–23, 26, 27, 29, 31, 34, 40, 42, 44, 46], some others focus on various extra-limbic targets [9, 12, 14, 24, 30, 32, 36, 37, 39], Others deal with stereotactic ablation of epileptogenic lesions, especially hamartomas of the hypothalamus [33].

Between 1965 and 1987, twenty-one studies were found to have been carried out to assess the efficiency of stereotactic lesioning of various cerebral targets for the control of intractable seizures. These studies involved from 5 to 107 patients, and 15 of them consisted of stereotactic lesioning of the amygdalo-hippocampal structures solely. The rate of improvement, in terms of seizure frequency, was reported to vary from 50 to 85%. However, many of these studies were initially performed to assess the effect of stereotactic amygdalotomy for the control of unmanageable behaviour, and it was secondarily found that some of the patients had a bonus relief from seizures. This explains why, in those early studies, literature pertaining to stereotactic amygdalotomy, hippocampotomy or fornicotomy displays results, which are difficult to interpret given the surgical techniques and outcome assessment used. Pre-surgical assessment was less rigid, it was rare to be able to verify the site and size of the lesion and follow-up data were poor being short and inaccurate. Finally, the relationship of outcome to the surgery was often indeterminate.

In 1999, Parrent and Blume [34] carried out a single study to assess the safety and efficacy of stereotactic ablation of the amygdala and hippocampus for the treatment of medial temporal lobe epilepsy. Twenty-two stereotactic amygdalohippocampotomies were performed in 19 patients with unilateral temporal lobe seizures. Two lesion groups were defined. In group I, discrete lesions were made, encompassing the amygdala and anterior hippocampus. In group II, a large number of confluent lesions were made encompassing the amygdala and a larger part of the hippocampus. In five group I patients, one (20%) experienced a favourable seizure outcome. Of 15 group II patients, nine (60%) experienced a favourable seizure outcome, with two seizure free. They conclude that extensive amygdalohippocampal ablation improved seizure outcome compared with more limited ablation, but that these results were not so good as those from temporal lobectomy in a similar patient group.

Two different review articles dealing with stereotactic ablation for refractory epilepsy were then published in 2000 by Parrent and Lozano [35], and by Polkey [38]. Both concluded that these techniques, although being well tolerated with fewer adverse effects than observed with conventional surgical procedures, and although current image-guided technology offers the opportunity to revisit some of these techniques, have a definitively less favourable outcome than that of standard surgery [4, 43, 47].

This might be related with several causes, such as the variability of the reported targets and indications (which often mixed behavioural disorders and epilepsy), or the small size of the lesions. Moreover, despite the recent use of image-guided technology, the risk of intra-cerebral bleeding due to the stereotactic positioning of the lesioning probe is a real risk.

Finally, the rather disappointing benefit/risk ratio of previously published stereotactic lesioning for epilepsy does explain that this technique, popular in the 60s and 70s, has been largely abandoned, and was not widely performed up to now.

Irrespective to this matter of fact, *invasive pre-surgical EEG recordings of seizures* may be required in many patients suffering from drug-resistant partial epilepsy to define the optimal cortical resection [3, 5, 13, 18, 28]. In many epilepsy surgery centres, as in ours, such invasive explorations are carried out using stereo electroencephalography (SEEG), according to the method first developed in the 60s by Talairach and Bancaud [45]. Principles and methodology of SEEG have been reported in detail in previous publications [13, 18]. Briefly, SEEG consists of stereotactic implantation of depth electrodes in the brain, in order to identify the exact location(s) of the epileptogenic area(s), as well as the pathways of discharge propagation. The sites of implantation depend, for each particular patient, upon the outcome of prior non-invasive pre-surgical investigations. Because MRI is coupled with angiography, each electrode can reach its implantation site without injuring cerebral vessels. Each electrode is made of stainless steel, and has 5–18 contacts. The dimensions of each contact are 2 mm in length, and 0.8 mm in diameter. From 5 to 16 electrodes are implanted per patient (mean of 11). On the average, 150 contacts per patient reflect local EEG activity in the depth of the sulci, as well as the medial aspects of the hemispheres (Fig. 1). This electrode coverage allows a very accurate tridimensional exploration of the epileptiform network, and in our hands provides a map superior to that given by subdural grid electrodes recordings, particularly, if the epileptogenic area is deeply situated. The electrodes are left in place for up to 21 days, or until sufficient information is obtained on localization of seizure onset and propagation.

Most often, the video-SEEG recording of spontaneous seizures leads to "a tailored resection" of the epileptogenic zone (EZ). Some patients, however, are not eligible for surgery after this invasive procedure because the EZ are

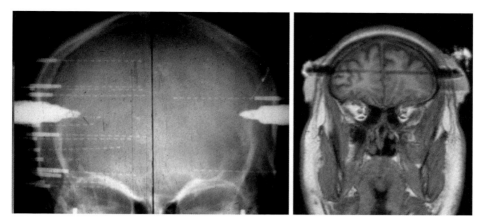

Fig. 1. Example of a post-implantation control antero–posterior X-ray (left) and MRI scan, T1 weighted, frontal slice (right). The depth electrodes are implanted orthogonally, according to the Talairach's SEEG methodology. sixteen depth electrodes are implanted in this particular case, each of them having from 5 to 15 contacts

multiple and/or located close to or inside highly eloquent cortical areas (primary language, motor or visual zones).

In this context, in addition to passive recording, *the use of these SEEG electrodes to generate focal lesions of the epileptogenic zone* and of seizures propagation pathways seemed to us worth to be investigated. Such lesions can be produced by thermocoagulation, using a radiofrequency (RF) generator connected to the electrode contacts. This is named SEEG-guided RF-thermocoagulation of the epileptogenic foci.

Based on a personal experience of this method in a 41 patients series, this paper aims:

1. at presenting the feasibility and safety of multiple cortical RF-thermolesions made by means of chronically implanted SEEG electrodes;
2. at reporting the results obtained in 41 consecutive patients who, amongst those referred to our department for surgical treatment of drug-resistant partial epilepsy between 2003 and 2007, have accepted this procedure as a first therapeutic step before surgery, or as a palliative treatment when surgery was not possible.

Technical data

Advantages of the technique

The advantages of using SEEG electrodes for performing multiple RF-thermolesions are supported by several lines of evidence [19, 20]:

1. The high number of implanted electrodes offers the possibility for producing several thermolesions;
2. Confluent lesions can be generated by contiguous placement of multiple thermolesions;
3. The clinical and electrophysiological status of the patient can be monitored in real-time before, during and after the lesion is performed. Such monitoring allows interruption of the procedure as soon as a sensation of heat is reported. Heat perception can be due to proximity of the lesion site and pericerebral cisternea, and can be a warning against unintentional injury to the optic tract or brainstem;
4. As electrical stimulations are systematically performed during video-SEEG recording sessions, the possible side-effects of a lesion can be anticipated in detail. Consequently, there is no need for supplementary stimulation or a temporary lesion to test for adverse effects during the SEEG-guided-RF-thermolesion procedure;
5. The SEEG-guided-RF-thermolesion procedure does not require anaesthesia;
6. Placement of thermolesions does not preclude subsequent conventional surgery in case of failure;
7. The bleeding risk is nil, as the electrodes are already in place, for recording purpose;
8. As revealed by our experience, these lesions are well-tolerated by the patient.

Patient's selection

Obviously, not all the patients having benefited from a SEEG during the same period ($n = 132$), underwent a SEEG-guided RF thermocoagulation procedure. RF thermocoagulation is only considered as soon as one or more of the implanted electrodes fulfils the following conditions:

1. To be located in the cortex areas showing either a low amplitude fast pattern or spike-wave discharges at the onset of the seizures. Interictal paroxysmal activities were not considered for planning thermocoagulation sites.
2. All targets are first functionally evaluated using electrical stimulation. Only those showing no clinical response to stimulation are selected for thermolesion, including sites located inside or near primary functional area.

The SEEG-guided RF thermocoagulation procedure is always performed at the very end of the video-SEEG recording session, which usually lasts between 2 and 3 weeks.

Placement of the lesion [20]

All SEEG-guided-RF-thermolesion procedures are performed without anaesthesia. Lesions are made using a radiofrequency lesion generator system model

RFG-5 manufactured by Radionics (Radionics Medical Products Inc., 22 Terry Av., Burlington, MA 01803, USA). The SEEG electrodes are manufactured by Dixi (Dixi Medical, 4, chemin de Palente, BP 889, 25025 Besançon, France). The lesions are produced between two contiguous contacts of the selected electrodes. Temperature cannot be monitored *in vivo* at electrode contacts, so the lesions are made using a 50 V, 120 mA current, which was found *in vitro* to increase the local temperature to 78–82°C within a few seconds, thus producing a lesion around the electrode contact in 10–30 sec (Fig. 2). A depth EEG recording is performed during the procedure at the relevant contacts after each coagulation, which shows the absence of focal epileptiform activity at the lesion site after thermolesion. For each patient, several (2–31, median: 12 in our

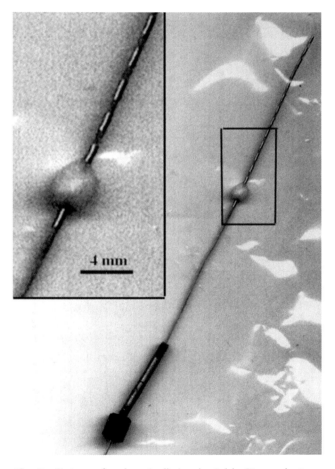

Fig. 2. Picture of a chronically implantable Stereoelectroencephalography (SEEG) electrode. *In vitro* thermocoagulation in egg white. The coagulated zone, 5 mm in diameter, is visible between the two selected contacts of the electrode

experience) bipolar lesions can be performed in one or more anatomical targets. The electrical activity recorded at the contact pairs used for RF thermocoagulation immediately after the procedure shows either a voltage reduction or a frequency slowing consistently associated to a decrease or a disappearance of interictal spikes.

The SEEG electrodes are removed at the end of the SEEG-guided-RF-thermolesion procedure, and the patient is discharged 24 h after its completion.

Post-operative MRI scans, with T1 and T2 sequences in horizontal, frontal and sagittal planes are performed three months after placement of the lesions, in order to assess the anatomical extent of the lesions.

Our experience [11, 19]

Patients (Table 1)

Forty-one patients (16 female, 25 male; mean age, 28 ± 8.6 years, range: 8–46), investigated by SEEG in the department of Functional Neurosurgery of Lyon, France, underwent multiple SEEG-guided RF thermocoagulation between 2003 and 2007.

All patients benefited from pre-surgical non-invasive investigation, including continuous video-EEG recordings, high-resolution Magnetic Resonance Imaging (MRI), [18]Fluorodeoxyglucose Positron Emission Tomography (PET) scan and sometimes ictal and interictal Single Photon Emission Computerized Tomography (SPECT). In all these patients, data obtained from the non-invasive pre-surgical investigations were not sufficiently congruent for localizing reliably the EZ. Intracerebral recording of spontaneous seizures (i.e. video-SEEG recording) was thus undertaken before any surgical decision. All electrodes were implanted according to pre-surgical diagnostic necessities, so that the RF thermocoagulation procedure had no influence on the number of electrodes and did not increase the risk of the stereotactic implantation. All patients gave their consent. They were all informed that the RF thermocoagulation procedure may be an opportunity to obtain, at the price of a minimal invasive procedure (as the electrodes are already in place) a significant chance of improvement of the epilepsy. The very low probability of being seizure free was clearly explained. They were also informed that, whenever possible, they will be offered conventional EZ surgical resection if they estimated RF thermocoagulation results as insufficient.

Targets, follow-up and results

The data obtained from this unique clinical series may be exposed as follows:

Table 1. *Patient data, location of the RF thermolesions and epileptological outcome*

No.	Sex, age	Etiology	Side	Anatomical targets	Outcome (% improvement)	Engel's class
1	F, 24	Cryptogenic	R	Parietal cortex	0	IV
2	M, 31	Cryptogenic	L	T5	0	IV
3	M, 40	Cryptogenic	R	Hipp, insula, T4, T pole	0	IV
4	M, 43	Cryptogenic	L	supplementary motor area	0	IV
5	F, 23	Cryptogenic	L	Amygdala, hipp, T pole	0	IV
6	F, 34	Cryptogenic	L	Entorhinal cortex, T3, T5	0	IV
7	M, 15	Cryptogenic	R	Insula	0	IV
8	M, 13	Cryptogenic	R	Insula, T and F operculum	0	IV
9	M, 34	Cryptogenic	L	Hipp, T operculum, insula	30	III
10	M, 26	Cryptogenic	L	Amygdala, hipp	60	III
11	M, 24	Cryptogenic	L	SMA, cingulate gyrus	80	II
12	F, 23	Cryptogenic	L	T pole, T2, T3, T4	95	II
13	F, 33	Cryptogenic	L	Amygdala, hipp	95	II
14	M, 46	Hipp sclerosis	R	Amygdala, hipp	0	IV
15	M, 24	Hipp sclerosis	L	Hipp, T1, T2, T. pole	0	IV
16	M, 32	Hipp sclerosis	R	Amygdala, hipp	0	IV
17	F, 26	Hipp sclerosis	R	Amygdala, hipp, T4, T pole	0	IV
18	M, 28	Hipp sclerosis	L	Amygdala, hipp, T5	80	III
19	F, 30	Hipp sclerosis	R	Amygdala, hipp	80	III
20	F, 21	Cort dyspl	R	T1, T2, T3, T pole	0	IV
21	F, 35	Cort dyspl	R	Occipital cortex	0	IV
22	M, 23	Cort dyspl	L	Hipp, temporal cortex	0	IV
23	M, 26	Cort dyspl	R	F cortex, F operculum	0	IV
24	F, 33	Cort dyspl	L	Orbitofrontal cortex, F3	0	IV
25	F, 20	Cort dyspl	R	Post-cing gyrus, O pole	0	IV
26	M, 32	Cort dyspl	R	Post-central gyrus	0	IV
27	M, 21	Cort dyspl	R	T1	50	III
28	F, 16	Cort dyspl	R	Frontal cortex	50	III
29	F, 8	Cort dyspl	L	Occipital cortex	50	III
30	F, 27	Cort dyspl	L	Frontal cortex	50	III
31	M, 28	Cort dyspl	L	Post-cing gyrus, O pole	50	III
32	M, 25	Cort dyspl	L	Insula	70	III
33	M, 36	Cort dyspl	L	T2	70	III
34	M, 33	Cort dyspl	R	F operculum, insula	70	III
35	M, 43	Cort dyspl	L	Amygdala, hipp, T pole	80	II
36	M, 36	Cort dyspl	R	Insula, F operculum	80	II
37	F, 33	Cort dyspl	L	Hipp, entorhinal cortex	95	II
38	M, 17	Cort dyspl	L	Occipital cortex	100	I
39	M, 42	Post-trauma	R	T1, T3, T pole	0	IV
40	F, 22	Heterotopia	L	T and O cortex	50	III

(*continued*)

Table 1. (*continued*)

No.	Sex, age	Etiology	Side	Anatomical targets	Outcome (% improvement)	Engel's class
40	F, 22	Heterotopia	L	T and O cortex	50	III
41	M, 23	Heterotopia	L	O peri-ventr heterotopia	50	III

M Male, *F* female, *R* right side, *L* left side, *Cort dyspl* cortical dysplasia, *Hipp* hippocampus, *T1* superior temporal gyrus, *T2* middle temporal gyrus, *T3* inferior temporal gyrus, *T4* temporo-occipital gyrus, *T5* parahippocampal gyrus, *T* temporal, *F* frontal, *SMA* supplementary motor area, *F3* inferior frontal gyrus, *O* occipital, *post-cing gyrus* posterior cingular gyrus, *peri-ventr* peri-ventricular

Choice of targets

The choice of targets has been explained in the previous chapter (patient's selection). It depended upon data from video-SEEG recordings regarding the localization of the epileptogenic focus. All targets were located in the cortex areas showing either a low amplitude fast pattern or spike-wave discharges at the onset of the seizures. Interictal paroxysmal activities were not considered for planning thermocoagulation sites. Only those showing no clinical response to stimulation were selected for thermolesion. This often implied that a partial damage only could be caused to the epileptogenic zone, as the electrode contacts being located in cortex areas showing paroxysmal ictal activities, but also clinical effects to stimulation could not be used for RF thermocoagulation.

Follow-up

The frequency of seizures and the possible adverse effects of RF thermocoagulation procedure were collected during consultations made at one month, three months, six months and then once a year after RF thermocoagulation.

The median follow-up after the RF thermocoagulation procedure, until the last consultation or the surgery, was 19 months (mean: 25 ± 21; range: 8–60). 21 of the 28 patients who were eligible for surgical resection have been operated a few months (mean: 8.9 ± 5; range: 4–28) after the RF thermocoagulation procedure. In the 13 patients who were not eligible for surgery, the mean follow-up duration was 43 months ± 18 (range: 15–72) between RF thermocoagulation and the last consultation.

The anatomic localization and extent of the thermolesions were assessed in every patient by a brain MRI scan performed 3 months after RF thermocoagulation. MRIs depicted isolated or multiple areas of coagulation necrosis, which were clearly visible along the electrode trajectories. The diameter of lesions ranged from 5 to 7 mm. The total length of lesioned area, made of

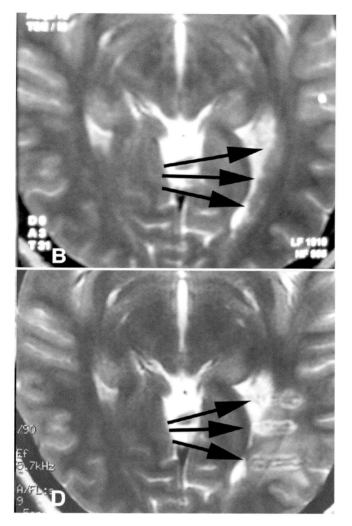

Fig. 3. Example of pre- (above) and post- (below) SEEG-guided thermolesions MRI (horizontal slices, T2 sequences). The lesions (arrows, lower picture) were placed in a left periventricular heterotopia (arrows, upper picture)

confluent discrete lesions along the electrode path, varied according to the number of electrode contacts used for bipolar coagulations (Figs. 3–5).

Anti-epileptic drugs treatment was left unchanged during the six months following RF thermocoagulation. In some patients, the antiepileptic drug regimen was modified after the first six months of follow-up, but in no patient these changes modified the seizure outcome.

Patients were classified as responders if the decrease in seizures frequency was of 50% or more, and non-responders if not. The results were also expressed in

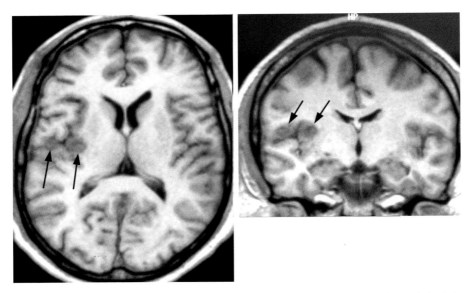

Fig. 4. Example of a post RF-thermolesion MRI. Horizontal (left) and frontal (right) T1 slices. Arrows: RF-thermolesions in the right insula and frontal operculum

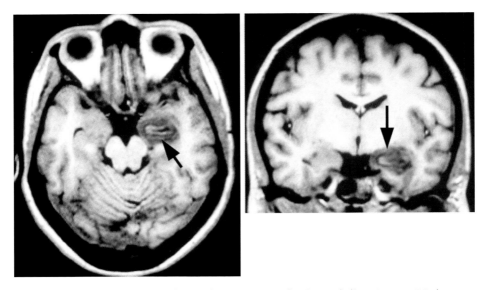

Fig. 5. Example of a post RF-thermolesion MRI. T2 horizontal slice. Arrow: RF-thermolesion of the left amygdala

Engel's classification, based on the facts that this is a palliative technique where the combined results of Engel I, Engel II and Engel III are considered worthwhile results. Groups were compared with the non-parametric Mann–Whitney test for

SEEG-guided thermocoagulation in epilepsy

continuous data (age, number of RF thermocoagulation, follow-up) because of small sample sizes. For categorical data (etiology, epileptogenic focus and RF thermocoagulation localization), Chi-squared or Fisher's exact test was applied. A p-value less than 0.05 was considered as statistically significant.

Results

Seizure outcome (Tables 1 and 2)

- 20 patients (48.7%) experienced a seizure frequency decrease of at least 50% that was more than 80% in eight of them. One patient was seizure free after RF thermocoagulation.
- In 21 patients, no significant reduction of the seizure frequency was observed.
- No patient showed any increase of seizure frequency.

The results are similar when expressed in Engel's classification: 21 patients (51.2%) were in Engel's class I–III (one is Engel Ia), whereas 20 patients (48.8%) did not experience any improvement after RF thermocoagulation (Engel's class IV).

Improvement of the epilepsy was observed at the first evaluation one month after RF thermocoagulation in 32 patients (78%). In 11 of them, this initial clinical benefit disappeared rapidly i.e. 3.8 ± 3 months after RF thermocoagulation and in one at 12 months. Beyond this lapse of time, the effect remained stable.

Table 2. *Seizure outcome according to the etiology of the epilepsy and the localization of the epileptogenic focus*

	Responders (>50% seizure reduction)	Non-responders (<50% seizure reduction)
Etiologies		
Cortical dysplasia	12 (1 seizure free)	7
Heterotopia	2	0
Cryptogenic	5	8
Hippocampal sclerosis	2	4
Post-traumatic	0	1
Localization		
Temporal	12	11
Frontal	3	3
Occipital	3	2
Parietal	1	2
Insula	2	2

Amongst the characteristics of the disease (age and sex of the patient, lobar localization of the EZ) and the characteristics of the thermocoagulations (topography, lateralization, number, morphology of the lesions on MRI) no factor was significantly linked to the outcome. However, the best results were clearly observed in epilepsies symptomatic of a cortical development malformation (CDM), with 67% of responders in this group of 20 patients ($p = 0.052$).

In the group of non-eligible patients for resective surgery ($n = 13$), due either to the insular topography of the epileptogenic focus, or to the high probability of a post-surgical visual deficit, or to bilateral epileptic foci, or to an EZ localization inside primary motor zone or language areas, 9 presented with CDM, and 6 of them were responders to SEEG-guided RFTC. One of them was seizure free.

Safety

No permanent neurological or cognitive impairment occurred after any of the procedures. Three patients showed transient adverse effects: mouth dysaesthesia during a few days and two months after intra-insular RF thermocoagulation in two patients, motor apraxia in the left hand after RF thermocoagulation within the right supplementary motor area that completely disappeared after six months. In one case, one of the coagulations was interrupted because it produced a slightly painful heat sensation in the ipsilateral side of the head. This sensation disappeared immediately after cessation of the radiofrequency current. In this particular case, the coagulation site was located in the temporo-mesial area, very close to the choroidal fissure.

Discussion

Multiple SEEG-guided RF thermocoagulation finally provides a therapeutic capability to a technique (i.e. SEEG) previously devoted to a diagnostic purpose only.

As a matter of fact, the use of SEEG electrodes for performing multiple RF-thermolesions appears to provide a unique opportunity to have large access to the epileptogenic network without additional risk from the implantation of lesioning electrodes.

Whenever it is feasible, lobectomy, cortectomy or hemispherotomy, based on precise localization of the EZ remains the most efficient treatment of partial drug-refractory epilepsies [15, 25, 41]. Some palliative procedures, such as multiple subpial trans-sections, callosotomy or vagus nerve stimulation, can be efficient to decrease, sometimes strongly, seizure frequency. Based on this principle, SEEG-guided RF thermocoagulation is a technique, which aims at causing a partial damage of the EZ, as tailored in each individual patient by the SEEG exploration.

Complications are minor, rare and reversible in all cases. No long-term side effects, particularly on cognitive function, are observed. The fact that RF thermocoagulation is guided by SEEG recordings and carried out only in cortical sites where focal stimulation did not elicit any clinical response probably accounts for the small number, and complete reversibility, of post RF thermocoagulation focal deficits. Thus it is possible to treat targets located very near to cortical areas with high functional value (language or primary visual zone), or poorly accessible to conventional surgical procedure (insular cortex).

The benefit-risk ratio of the SEEG-guided RF thermocoagulation procedure proves particularly favourable for the patients in whom surgery is not feasible or risky. Such was the case for 13 of our 41 patients, of whom seven benefited from RF thermocoagulation with a reduction of 50% or more in seizure frequency in six cases and a complete seizures control in one. In these cases, SEEG-guided RF thermocoagulation proved to be a safe therapeutic option, the results of which compare favourably to those of other palliative therapeutic procedures such as vagus nerve stimulation, multiple subpial transection, callosotomy or deep intracerebral stimulations [15]. These favourable results however, will require further long-term reevaluation, as the average follow-up, of less than 2 years, of our series, may bring reservation for the very long-term efficacy of the technique.

Conversely RF thermocoagulation results in patients eligible for cortectomy proves inferior to those of surgery. Indeed, 21 of our 28 patients went through conventional surgery in a second step, of whom 19 are in Engel's class I and four are awaiting surgery. These results show that the SEEG-guided RF thermocoagulation procedure is not an alternative to resection surgery and incited us to stop proposing RF thermocoagulation to patients eligible to conventional surgery, and especially to patients eligible for temporo-mesial resection, which bears the best surgical prognosis [43, 47]. This can partially be explained by the relatively small size of the thermocoagulation lesions, as compared to the extent of the epileptogenic area.

The best results of RF thermocoagulation are observed in epilepsies symptomatic of cortical development malformations that are not accessible to surgery. Indeed, a seizure frequency reduction more than 50% is noted in 67% of patients suffering from epilepsy symptomatic of dysplasia or heterotopia, of whom one remains seizure free with a follow-up of 40 months. Thus, the favourable outcomes that we observe cannot be explained by a complete lesion of the epileptogenic area, as assumed after surgical cortectomy. SEEG-guided RF-thermocoagulations, when efficient, may instead cause a partial volume reduction of the epileptogenic cortex and disturb its synaptic circuitry and electrophysiological organization, sufficiently to stop, or to reduce, the occurrence of seizures.

Conclusion

Despite its limits, the SEEG-guided RF-thermolesion procedure we describe here appears to be feasable, reliable, well-tolerated and safe. Its risk-benefit ratio remains favourable, so that we advocate it as a first step, even if a standard curative surgery is needed in a second step. Our experience suggests that SEEG-guided RF thermocoagulation should be dedicated to drug-resistant epileptic patients for whom conventional resection surgery is risky or contra-indicated on the basis of invasive pre-surgical evaluation, particularly those suffering from epilepsy symptomatic of cortical development malformation. Knowing the excellent congruence between the completeness of the lesion resection and the favourable evolution of the epileptic disease in cortical development malformations, we now tend, for such patients, to increase the number of electrodes implanted in the lesion itself in order to produce the greatest possible number of thermolesions inside the malformation.

References

1. Anderson R (1970) Psychological differences after amygdalotomy. Acta Neurol Scand 46(Suppl 43): 94
2. Balasubramanian V, Kanaka TS (1976) Stereo tactic surgery of the limbic system in epilepsy. Acta Neurochir (Wien) 23: 225–34
3. Behrens E, Zentner J, Van Roost D, Hufnagel A, Elger CE, Schramm J (1994) Subdural and depth electrodes in the presurgical evaluation of epilepsy. Acta Neurochir (Wien) 128: 84–87
4. Bien CG, Kurthen M, Baron K, Lux S, Helmstaedter C, Schramm J, Elger CE (2001) Long-term seizure outcome and antiepileptic drug treatment in surgically treated temporal lobe epilepsy patients: a controlled study. Epilepsia 42: 1416–21
5. Binnie CD, Elwes RDC, Polkey CE, Volans A (1994) Utility of stereoelectroencephalography in preoperative assessment of temporal lobe epilepsy. J Neurol Neurosurg Psychiatry 57: 58–65
6. Blume WT, Parrent AG, Kaibara M (1997) Stereo tactic amygdalohippocampotomy and medial temporal spikes. Epilepsia 38: 930–36
7. Bohbot VD, Allen JJ, Nadel L (2000) Memory deficits characterized by patterns of lesions to the hippocampus and parahippocampal cortex. Ann NY Acad Sci 911: 355–68
8. Bohbot VD, Kalina M, Stepankova K, Spackova N, Petrides M, Nadel L (1998) Spatial memory deficits in patients with lesions to the right hippocampus and to the right parahippocampal cortex. Neuropsychologia 36(11): 1217–38.
9. Bouchard G. Basic targets and the different epilepsies (1976) Acta Neurochir 23: 193–99.
10. Bouvier G, Saint-Hilaire JM, Maltais R, Belique R, Desrochers P (1980) Stereo tactic lesions in primary epilepsy of the limbic system. Acta Neurochir (Wien) 30: 151–59

11. Catenoix H, Mauguiere F, Guenot M, Ryvlin P, Bissery Y, Sindou M, Isnard J (2008) SEEG-guided thermocoagulations: a palliative treatment of nonoperable partial epilepsies. Neurology 71(21): 1719–26
12. Ciganek L, Sramka S, Nadvornik P, Fritz G (1976) Effects of stereotactic operations in the treatment of epilepsies, neurological aspects. Acta Neurochir (Wien) 23: 201–04
13. Cossu M, Cardinale F, Castana L, Citterio A, Francione S, Tassi L, Benabid AL, Lo Russo G (2005) Stereoelectroencephalography in the presurgical evaluation of focal epilepsy: a retrospective analysis of 215 procedures. Neurosurgery 57: 706–18
14. Crow HJ, Cooper R (1972) Stimulation, polarization and coagulation using intracerebral implanted electrodes during the investigation and treatment of psychiatric and other disorders. Med Prog Technol 1(2): 92–102
15. Clusmann H, Schramm J, Kral T, Hemstaedter C, Ostertun B, Fimner R, Haun D, Elger CE (2002) Prognostic factors and outcome after different types of resection for temporal lobe epilepsy. J Neurosurg 97: 1131–41
16. Exley KA, Parsonage MJ, Wall AL (1967) Electrocoagulation of the amygdalae in an epileptic patient. Electrencephalogr Clin Neurophysiol 43(Suppl 31): 172
17. Flanigin HF, Nashold BS (1976) Stereo tactic lesions of the amygdala and hippocampus in epilepsy. Acta Neurochir (Wien) 23: 235–39
18. Guenot M, Isnard J, Ryvlin P, Fischer C, Ostrowsky K, Mauguiere F, Sindou M (2002) Neurophysiological monitoring for epilepsy surgery: the Talairach SEEG method. Stereotact Funct Neurosurg 73: 84–87
19. Guenot M, Isnard J (2008) Multiple SEEG-guided RF-thermocoagulations of epileptic foci. Neurochirurgie 54(3): 441–47
20. Guenot M, Isnard J, Ryvlin P, Fischer C, Mauguiere F, SindouM (2004) SEEG-guided RF-thermocoagulation of epileptic foci: feasibility, safety, and preliminary results. Epilepsia 45(11): 1368–74
21. Heimburger RF,Whitlock CC, Kalsbeck JE (1966) Stereo tactic amygdalotomy for epilepsy with aggressive behavior. JAMA 198: 741–45
22. Heimburger RF, Small IF, Milstein V, Moore D (1978) Stereo tactic amygdalotomy for convulsive and behavioral disorders. Appl Neurophysiol 41: 43–51
23. Hood TW, Siegfried J, Wieser HG (1983) The role of stereotactic amygdalotomy in the treatment of temporal lobe epilepsy associated with behavioral disorders. Appl Neurophysiol 46: 19–25
24. Hullay J, Gombi R, Velok G (1976) Surgical and stereotactic attempts in intractable epilepsy. Acta Med Acad Sci Hung 33(2): 119–24
25. Kumlien E, Doss RC, Gates JR (2002) Treatment outcome in patients with mesial temporal sclerosis. Seizure 11: 413–17
26. Marossero F, Ravagnati L, Sironi VA, Miserocchi G, Franzini A, Entorre G, Cabrini GP (1980) Late results of stereotactic radiofrequency lesions in epilepsy. Acta Neurochir (Wien) 30: 145–49
27. Mempel E, Witkiewicz B, Stadnicki R (1980) The effect of medial amygdalotomy and anterior hippocampotomy on behavior and seizures in epileptic patients. Acta Neurochir (Wien) 30: 161–67
28. Munari C, Hoffman D, Francione S, Kahane P, Tassi L, Lo Russo G, Benabid AL (1994) Stereo-electroencephalography methodology: advantages and limits. Acta Neurol Scand (Suppl 152): 56–67

29. Nadvornik P, Sramka M (1975) Anatomical considerations for the stereotaxic longitudinal hippocampectomy. Confin Neurol 36: 177–81
30. Nadvornik P, Sramka M, Gajdosova D (1974) Critical remarks on the stereotaxic treatment of epilepsy. J Neurosurg Sci 18: 133–35
31. Narabayashi H (1980) From experiences of medial amygdalotomy on epileptics. Acta Neurochir Suppl (Wien) 30: 75–81
32. Ojeman GA, Ward AA (1975) Stereo tactic and other procedures for epilepsy. Adv Neurol 8: 241–63
33. Parrent AG (1999) Stereo tactic radiofrequency ablation for the treatment of gelastic seizures associated with hypothalamic hamartoma. Case report. J Neurosurg 91(1): 881–84
34. Parrent AG, Blume WT (1999) Stereo tactic amygdalohippocampotomy for the treatment of medial temporal lobe epilepsy. Epilepsia 40(10): 1408–16
35. Parrent AG, Lozano AM (2000) Stereo tactic surgery for temporal lobe epilepsy. Can J Neurol Sci 27(1): 79–84
36. Patil AA, Andrews R, Torkelson R (1995) Stereo tactic volumetric radiofrequency lesioning of intracranial structures for control of intractable seizures. Stereotact Funct Neurosurg 64(3): 123–33
37. Patil AA, Andrews R, Torkelson R (1995) Minimally invasive surgical approach for intractable seizures. Stereotact Funct Neurosurg 65: 86–89
38. Polkey CE (2003) Alternative surgical procedures to help drug-resistant epilepsy, a review. Epileptic Disord 5: 63–75
39. Schaltenbrand G, Spuler H, Nadjmi M, Hopf HC, Wahren W (1966) The stereotactic treatment of symptomatic epilepsy. Munch Med Wochenschr 108(35): 1707–11
40. Schwab RS, Sweet WH, Mark VH, Kjellberg RN, Ervin FR (1965) Treatment of intractable temporal lobe epilepsy by stereotactic amygdala lesions. Trans Am Neurol Assoc 90: 12–19
41. Schramm J, Kral T, Kurthen M, Blumcke I (2002) Surgery to treat focal frontal lobe epilepsy in adults. Neurosurgery 51: 644–54
42. Schumann G, Nadvornik P, Schroder T (1987) Results of stereotactic treatment of drug-resistant epilepsy. Psychiatr Neurol Med Psychol 39: 38–43
43. Sindou M, Guenot M, Isnard J, Ryvlin P, Fischer C, Mauguiere F (2006) Temporo-mesial epilepsy surgery: outcome and complications in 100 consecutive adult patients. Acta Neurochir (Wien) 148(1): 39–45
44. Small IF, Heimburger RF, Small JG, Milstein V, Moore DF (1977) Follow-up of stereotaxic amygdalotomy for seizure and behavior disorders. Biol Psychiatry 12(3): 401–11
45. Talairach J, Bancaud J (1973) Stereo tactic approach to epilepsy. Methodology of anatomo-functional stereotactic investigations. Prog Neurol Surg 5: 297–354
46. Vaernet K (1972) Stereo tactic amygdalotomy in temporal lobe epilepsy. Confin Neurol 34: 176–80
47. Wiebe S, Blume WT, Girvin JP, Eliasziw M (2001) A randomized, controlled trial of surgery for temporal lobe epilepsy. N Eng J Med 345: 311–18

Child abuse – some aspects for neurosurgeons

B. Madea[1], M. Noeker[2], and I. Franke[2]

[1] Institute of Legal Medicine, University of Bonn, Bonn, Germany
[2] Department of Pediatrics, University of Bonn, Bonn, Germany

With 24 Figures and 22 Tables

Contents

Abstract	80
Introduction	80
Definitions and epidemiology	81
Legal basis	83
Criminology of child abuse	84
Physical examination and taking the history	86
Injuries	86
Blunt force	87
Interpretation of injuries	90
Bone injuries	95
Head injuries, fractures of the skull	99
Non-accidental head injury/shaken-baby-syndrome	104
Shaken-baby-syndrome (SBS)	104
Thermal injuries	109
Injuries of the eyes	114
Differential diagnoses	114
Münchausen syndrome by proxy	116
Lethal child abuse	119
Physical neglect	119
Starvation	120
Taking the case history	121
Structured forensic, investigative interview with the child	122
Documentation	123
General symptoms in cases of child abuse	123

Proceeding in cases of suspected child abuse 124
Child protection team 125
Clinical pathway 126
    Definition of Clinical Pathway.. 126
Bonn child protection team clinical pathway for suspected
child abuse 130
References... 130

Abstract

Neurosurgeons are mainly concerned with child abuse in cases of severe cranio-cerebral trauma. Aim of the present paper is to highlight the clinical picture and symptoms in cases of child abuse and our multidisciplinary approach to reveal a solid diagnosis. The detection of child abuse requires a high index of suspicion, especially in cases of subtle injuries. Besides reporting to the appropriate agencies primary goals are to terminate suspected abuse and to prevent further harm to the child. All this requires a confirmed diagnosis.

Keywords: Child abuse; epidemiology; case history; head injury; fall from height; bruises.

Introduction

Many medical disciplines have to deal with the diagnosis and therapy of child abuse, predominantly pediatricians and – in fatal cases – forensic pathologists. The diagnosis of child abuse is often not just a simple diagnosis but requires knowledge from different medical disciplines (pediatrics, neurology, ophthalmology, dermatology, surgery, forensic medicine, toxicology) to reveal a solid diagnosis taking all differential diagnoses of accidental trauma or confounding diseases into account [43].

The diagnosis of child abuse may have several legal consequences (e.g. child is withdrawn from the family). To avoid legal consequences against the treating physicians – in cases of unreported suspected child abuse as well as in reported but not proven child abuse – the diagnosis has to be validated. Although the classical features of child abuse have already been described by Ambroise Tardieu, a French forensic pathologist, in 1860 [40, 91], the modern recognition of the syndrome dates back about less than five decades (Kempe 1962) [29, 30, 32]. Since then many excellent monographs [2, 3, 7, 9, 12, 29, 30, 33–36, 38, 39, 45, 46, 56, 61, 68, 72, 76, 78, 83, 87, 94] and a huge literature (clinical, experimental, legal, psychological) have been published. Programs to protect children have been developed, however, the national approaches differ widely as well as the legal background.

Definitions and epidemiology

A standardized definition of child abuse is still missing; it is even said that a definition itself is controversial as what is unacceptable now may have been considered as valid and desirable at other times [6, 33, 35, 36, 78, 83]. A definition should comprise:

— physical abuse
— neglect/deprivation/failure to thrive (FTT)
— mental or emotional abuse/neglect
— sexual abuse
— Munchausen by proxy syndrome (Mbps)

A definition is also depending on general conditions of the respective society. Thus, the German Bundestag (Drucksache 10/4560, dated 13.06.1986) issued the following definition [7]:

Abuse is an intentional conscious or unconscious physical or mental harm which is occurring in families or in institutions, thus, in systems of cohabitation, and which is causing damages and/or arrested developments or even death and, thus, derogates or menaces the welfare and the rights of a child.

Similar definitions are accepted in most European countries [83, 98]. In the UK, child abuse was formally defined in the 1999 Department of Health guidelines and redefined in 2000 (Department of Health 2000):

— Physical abuse involves hitting, shaking, throwing, poisoning, burning or scalding, drowning, suffocating or otherwise causing physical harm to the child which is actual or likely.
— Fictitious (or factitious) illness by proxy is also included under physical abuse.
— From a clinical perspective, the severity of the injury, the number of injuries, the age of the child and any previous injuries and other abuses (neglect, child sexual abuse, emotional abuse) are all part of the jigsaw which leads to a diagnosis of physical abuse.

In the US, child abuse is defined by the Child Abuse Prevention and Treatment Act (CAPTA) of 1974 as "Any recent act or failure to act on the part of a parent or caretaker which results in death, serious physical or emotional harm, sexual abuse or exploitation, or an act or failure to act which represents an imminent risk of serious harm" to a child under the age of 18 [83]. Child abuse is not only an intentional act but might also be the result of carelessness by the parent or the caretaker.

While gross forms of abuse are self evidently abuse in lesser degrees of trauma it may be questionable whether injuries resulted from deliberate battering, inexpert rough handling or accident.

The pathognomonic symptom of physical abuse are signs of repeated impact of violence that become manifest in injuries of different age or can not be caused by a single act of violence, respectively (multi-temporal).

The American paediatrician Henry Kempe (1922–1984) formed the term "battered-child-syndrome" in 1962 when he first identified injuries and/or patterns of injuries as a result of parental violence [29, 30, 36]. For a long time signs of external violence were interpreted as accidental. For instance in 1946

Table 1. *Number of child maltreatment deaths (Innocenti Report Card)*

	Children under 15 years	of which under 1 year
Australia	156	39
Austria	66	16
Belgium	98	26
Canada	284	91
Czech Republic	105	23
Denmark	40	8
Finland	41	12
France	765	161
Germany	523	148
Greece	16	3
Hungary	113	51
Iceland	1	1
Ireland	12	4
Italy	104	13
Japan	916	257
Korea	414	55
Luxembourg	2	1
Mexico	4974	1006
Netherlands	84	26
New Zealand	55	19
Norway	14	1
Poland	363	131
Portugal	320	29
Slovak Republic	51	16
Spain	44	9
Sweden	53	8
Switzerland	56	11
UK	502	143
USA	7081	1889
Total	17253	4197

The table shows the total number of maltreatment deaths among children under the age of 15 and under the age of one year. The totals are over a five-year period and include deaths that have been classified as "of undetermined intent".

Caffey [13] described the combination of chronic subdural haematomas and (multiple) fractures of the long bones in children. He was convinced of the traumatic origin of these injuries, however, the mechanism by which they occurred was obscure. It seems that at this time nobody could imagine that those injuries were the result of physical child abuse caused by carers.

According to crime statistics physical child abuse is an apparently rare type of crime. Nevertheless the estimated number of unreported cases is high and there is – at least in Germany and in contrast to other countries – no obligation to report suspected cases to the police. According to a UNICEF study (Innocenti Report 2003) [95] 523 children died due to non accidental external violence in Germany in the last five years (among them 148 children younger than one year) (Table 1, including data of several other countries). Almost 3500 children under the age of 15 die from maltreatment (physical abuse and neglect) every year in the industrialized world. Every week 2 children die from abuse and neglect in Germany and the United Kingdom, 3 children in France, 4 in Japan and 27 a week in the United States. The risk of death by maltreatment is approximately 3 times greater for the under-ones than for those aged 1–4, who in turn face double the risk of those aged 5–14 (UNICEF, Innocenti Report 2003). Based on these data 157,000 cases of child abuse are expected per year in Germany [35, 95]. From these children who are treated in hospital 12–15% die. According to a WHO-study 2.2 boys and 1.8 girls younger than 5 years per 100,000 children die due to child non accidental trauma [41]. The number of deaths per 100,000 children in the age group 0–16 years is given with 80 for Germany, 370 for Portugal, 300 for Mexico, 240 for the USA and 10 for Spain. According to the official police statistics 1700–2100 cases of child abuse are reported to the authorities in Germany per year, however, the number of unreported cases is with 95% very high [35]. In the US 16.5 children per 1000 were found to be victims of abuse in 2005. Child neglect was the most frequent form of abuse followed by physical abuse in 16.6% of all reported cases. In Canada the rate of substantiated child maltreatment was 21.71 per 1000 in 2003, of which 10% involved physical harm. In England in 2001 24 children in every 10,000 were abused, of which 7300 were victims of physical harm [83, 98].

Legal basis

The German criminal code (StGB, Strafgesetzbuch) like the criminal codes of other European countries provides different forms of penalty for physical abuse, dependent on the severity of the criminal act (assault or aggravated assault – also with fatal consequences, (attempted) murder, (attempted) man-slaughter). Of special importance are § 171 StGB – breach of duty of care and upbringing (includes e.g. the substantial damage of physical and psychical devel-opment) and § 225 StGB – abuse of wards (comprises torment, cruel abuse, malicious neglect; higher penalty in cases of possible death and substantial damage of physical and psychic development) [6].

Legal definitions are for instance:

Torment: Causation of continuing and repeating substantial (physical or psychic) pain or suffering (also by omission).

Cruel abuse: Causation of substantial pain or suffering while being of insensible attitude disregarding third parties suffering (not as a consistent characteristic); criminal act by omission: malicious neglect of duty of care (omission of averting the abuse). The application of these criteria is a purely juridical decision.

The amendment of the § 1631 of the German Civil Code (BGB, Bürgerliches Gesetzbuch) dated 2.11.2000 restricts the principals of upbringing:

Children have a right to be brought up without violence. Physical punishment, psychical injuries and other degrading methods are prohibited.

The crime statistic of 1999 included 2257 complaints subject to § 225 StGB (abuse of wards). According to this statistic appr. 60% of the offenders and victims are male. The estimated number of unreported cases is much higher – according to estimations about 20,000–100,000 cases per year [6, 35]. Thus, the problem is rather under – than overestimated in practice.

Reasons for the high number of unreported cases are [34, 83, 98]:

– Child abuse is an intra-familiar incident with no independent witnesses
– Lacking awareness of witnesses and treating physicians
– Misjudging of injuries as result of accidents
– Childrens' dependence on their parents
– Abused children are usually too young to report what happened

Criminology of child abuse

– Infants (2–4-year-old) are notably at risk. About 75% of all cases affect children <7 years. Often one child of several siblings is concerned; if this child is taken out of the family it should be thought of protective methods for the siblings (risk of recurrence).
– Endangerment of unwanted, handicapped children.
– Offenders are parents of younger age or companions of the mother; all kinds of social background are involved. Men are thought to be more often "active" abusers, women more often "passive" abusers.
– Most cases take place at home with mothers more hitting than fathers, but men causing more damage.
– The act is mostly impulsive and takes place in stressful situations (lacking frustration tolerance); alcohol abuse is considered as a supporting factor.

- The persons having the care and custody of the child give no or only insufficient explanations for the injuries, the explanations differ partly or are adapted to the diagnostic findings. In some cases siblings are made responsible for the injuries or an akwardness of the child itself is said to be the reason for the injuries.
- A doctor is consulted with temporal delay although the injuries are obviously severe. Older and non treated injuries do exist.
- When pre-treating physicians are contacted it becomes obvious that there had been no continuous treatment but several different doctors had been consulted (so-called "doctor-hopping").

Several influencing factors in physical abuse have been identified (Table 2).

Table 2. *Summary of influencing factors in physical abuse. From Hobbs, Hanks, Wynne (1999)*

Socio-cultural:	attitudes towards punishment, values placed on children as individuals versus chattels, property, ownership.
Socio-economic:	poverty is a mayor stress which promotes violence, deprivation and child abuse. Not all poor families abuse.
Unemployment:	a special kind of social stress, linked with poverty.
Family breakdown:	unstable martial relationships, spouse violence, separation and divorce. Loss of extended family supports from increased social mobility.
Health:	poor health in parents, especially mother, reduces coping and tolerance levels. Psychiatric illness or poor psychological health including symptoms of stress. Alcohol and drug usage including prescribed psychotropic drugs.
Handicap:	one child factor that is important. Difficult children to care for – e.g. screamers, poor feeders – are other examples.
Education:	lack of education and the personal resources this brings results in fewer ways of coping. Low intelligence is another factor.
Poor parenting:	either from poor childhood experiences, or lack of opportunity to learn.
Individual:	youth, immaturity, isolation, criminality are all adverse factors.
Generational:	the tendency to repeat the cycle of abuse from generation to generation.
Environmental:	effects of cold, damp, overcrowded housing, nowhere for the children to play, enforced proximity.
Services:	lack of appropriate, accessible services – e.g. day care, nurseries, maternal and child health services.

Physical examination and taking the history

There are many different types of physical child abuse and it is the task of any physician to give the right interpretation of the injury, its nature and origin and not to over-interpret lesions. In cases of an injury which is detected during an examination of a child or if a child is brought to a doctor because of an injury an examination of the whole body of the child is indispensable.

In cases of infantile injuries physical abuse has to be considered as differential diagnosis. A thorough physical examination with clear documentation of findings is the basis for the further management of the case [17, 31, 48, 49, 76].

Injuries

There is a large variety of injuries in cases of child abuse from superficial wounds to severe life-threatening conditions. Most injuries in child abuse are due to blunt force and caused manually by hitting or beating with the hands, shaking, throwing or dropping [6, 34, 78, 98]. Often instruments like sticks or belts are used. Burning, scalding and suffocation are seen less often. Suffocation and poisoning play an important role in MbpS [37, 65–67]. Shooting, strangulation and stabbing are seen in classical childhood homicides [6, 80].

Injuries due to child abuse can be classified as follows [6, 34, 78, 98]:

— Superficial (dermatological): bruises, abrasions, lacerations, scratches, bites, stab wounds, pin pricks, pinch marks, ligature marks, broken or avulsed hair or nails, burns or scalds, chemical injury.
— Deeper lesions: haematoma, cephalhaematoma, mouth injury (tear of lip frenulum), strangulation.
— Fractures, dislocations, wrenched limbs, periosteal injury.
— Thoraco-lumbar internal injury – stomach, gut, solid viscera, lung.
— Intracranial (including eyes) and spinal injury: whiplash, shaken, subdural haematoma, epidural haematoma, cerebral haemorrhage, contusion or oedema, spinal cord injury.
— Asphyxia, drowing and poisoning.
— Fabricated disorders (Munchausen by proxy).

While all types of violence can occur in cases of child abuse, injuries due to blunt force are seen most frequently. Mostly it are skin and bone lesions which raise suspicion of child abuse and a classic aphorism by forensic pathologists says: "The skin and bones tell a story which the child is either too young or to frightened to tell" [14].

Blunt force

Typical types of infliction and consequences are summarized in Table 3 and shown in Fig. 1.

Inflicted bruises show a number of different patterns:

— Hand marks (on arms, trunk, cheeks) (Fig. 2). While accidental injuries often involve unprotected parts of the body like shin bone, knee or elbow, injuries of "protected" areas (backside, thighs and chest) should raise suspicion whether physical abuse did happen (Figs. 3 and 4) [34, 98].

Table 3. *Consequences of different forms of blunt violence. According to Ref. [49]*

Violence	Injury
Ear pulling	Pulling the earlap
Hair pulling	Pulling the hair, bald areas
Beating the head	Haematomas, lacerations, scars
Biting	Dental impression, oval or semilunar haematomas
Forceful gripping	Traces of grips, haematomas measuring 0.5–2.5 cm, possibly grouped, trace of the thumb at the opposite side
Pinching	Uncharacteristic haematomas, possibly abrasions from fingernails
Traces of grips	Haematomas at arms or at the sides of the thorax
Captivation	Erythema, abrasions, haematomas at joints
Violent feeding	Injuries of oral mucosa including frenulum of upper and/or lower lip (by opening with spoon or bottle), broken teeth
Beating with flat hand	Formed haematomas of the cheek, retroauricular haematomas (ENT-examination), myringorupture
Beating with fist	Eyeglass haemorrhage (injuries of the eye), haematomas of the oral mucosa including break off of tooth, rupture of inner organs (liver, spleen, gastrointestinal organs) in front of the spine (without external signs of injuries!)
Beating with knuckles	Roundish haematomas arranged side by side
Beating with stick or similar item	Double striae design (fine striped haematomae with central fading)
Beating with other items (e.g. belt, coat-hanger, leg of a chair...)	Extensive haematomas; typical localization on the back of the body (bottom, back of the legs), possibly defending injuries on the arms
Kicks	Possibly impression of shoe profile, cave: kicks into the abdomen could cause severe injuries without external signs (see beats with fist)
Dropping, throwing against a wall	Extensive haematomas, skull fractures, ...

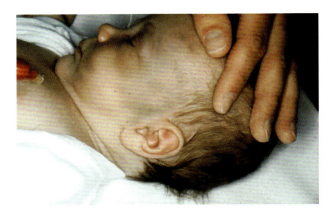

Fig. 1. Four-month-old child, haematoma of the left cheek and forehead, brought to hospital by parents after "fall from table" immediately prior to hospitalization, died four weeks later due to hypoxic brain damage. Bruises on cheek and forehead not fresh, typical handmark on the left cheek caused by hitting with the right hand

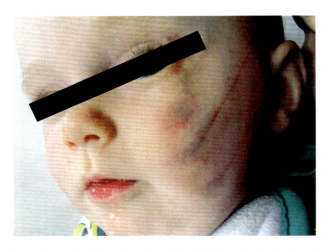

Fig. 2. Typical handmark on the left cheek with a handprint

- Marks of implements – e.g. straps, sticks, buckles (patterned intradermal bruises, tram-line bruising) (Fig. 5) [78].
- Bruises from throwing, swinging or pushing the child onto a hard object (Fig. 6).
- Bites with a 3–3.5 cm in diameter ring or arc bruises (Fig. 7).
- Bizarre marks (Fig. 8).
- Kicks with footwear with patterned shoe sole (Fig. 9).

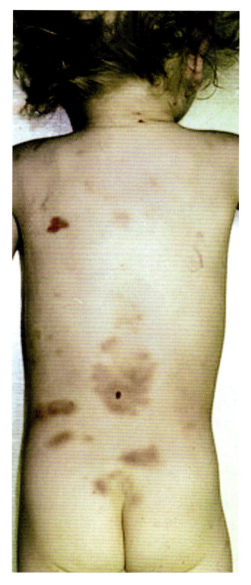

Fig. 3. Bruises on the back, typical fingertip bruises

Hand marks may be seen as grab mark or fingertip bruises, for example on limbs, face, chest wall. Another form is a hand print or linear finger mark, e.g. on the cheek. Slap marks – often vaguely two or three finger-sized linear marks – are seen with stripe effect [78]. Rings may leave a tell-tale mark. Bruising around the limbs (wrist, forearm, upper arm, thigh) are due to grip-

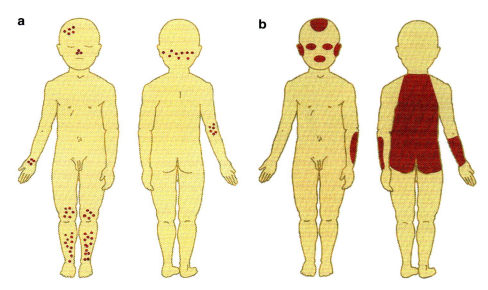

Fig. 4. Accidental injuries in unprotected areas like chin, knee, elbow, forehead (a); inflicted injuries in "protected" areas like back, buttocks, chest, furthermore cheek and top of the scalp (b) [7]

ping the child. Bruising on the backside and back are due to beating with the hand or a strap. Bruising of the face is due to beating with the hand. Besides cheek, mouth [44], ear and forehead are concerned. The upper lips may be swollen, the inner lips be lacerated, the upper lip frenulum damaged [6, 34, 78, 98]. Bruises on the chest and back are usually from finger pressure. Deep visceral injuries with liver laceration or rupture of pancreas and duodenum may occur without external visible signs of violence of the abdomen [8, 20, 46, 77].

Of special importance is the aging of bruises [49, 56, 82]. The observed age may be contradictory to history given by the parents or bruises of different age indicate injuries at different times. Table 4 and Fig. 10 give some hints. There is of course a great interindividual variability of colour changes and it is impossible to give an exact age of the bruises from their colour [6, 78, 98]. Therefore it is of utmost importance to document the colour and the demarcation of bruises instead of giving a too precise estimation of the age.

Interpretation of injuries

Injuries caused by accidents and injuries caused by abuse can be differentiated by location of the injury. Injuries due to falls are seen at prominent

Child abuse – some aspects for neurosurgeons

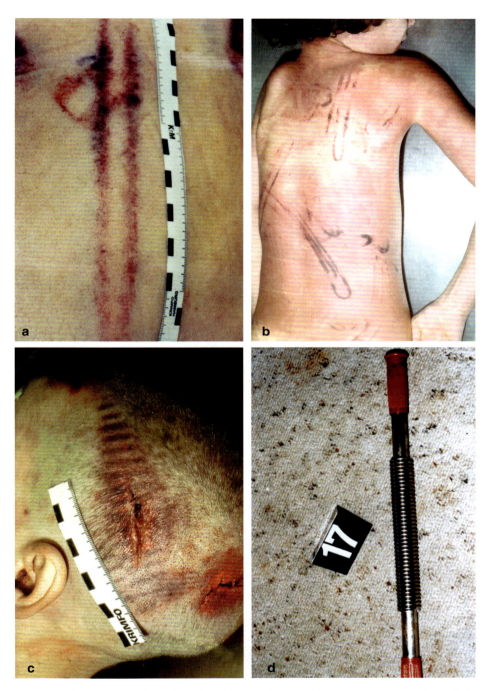

Fig. 5. Patterned intradermal bruise. (a) Tramline bruising after hitting with a stick, (b) bruising after beating with a strap, (c) patterned bruising of the scalp with a laceration using a patterned instrument (d)

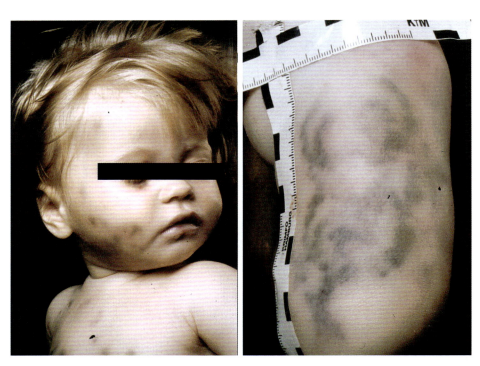

Fig. 6. Fingertip bruising of the cheek and chest, patterned bruising of the left thigh due to throwing the child on a patterned object

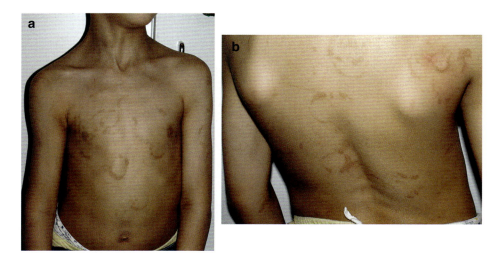

Fig. 7. Several bit marks of the chest

Child abuse – some aspects for neurosurgeons

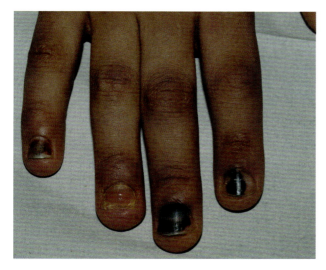

Fig. 8. Subunugal bruises due to hitting on the fingers

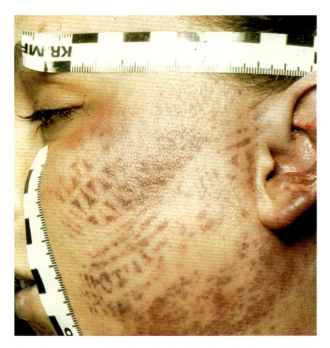

Fig. 9. Patterned bruise of the left cheek due to kicking with a shoe sole

areas of the head, e.g. the forehead, the chin or the zygomatic bone [6, 16, 31, 51, 58, 70] while injuries due to abuse are seen above the top of the head, the cheeks and the mouth (Fig. 4).

Table 4. Aging of bruises. From Hobbs, Hanks, Wynne 1999

	Age	Colour
One scheme (Schmitt 1987):	0–2 days	swollen, tender
	0–5 days	red, blue, purple
	5–7 days	green
	7–10 days	yellow
	10–14 days (or more)	brown
	2–4 weeks	cleared
other scheme:	Recent (24–48 hours)	reddish, purple, swollen, tender
	2–3 days	brownish purple
	4–7 days	brownish green
	7 days+	yellow

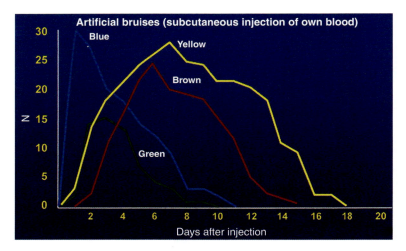

Fig. 10. Aging of bruises after subcutaneous injection of own blood. Fresh bruises are reddish-purple in colour, but already after 24 hours the colour begins to get yellow as well [7]

In cases of alleged accident the following questions have to be answered concerning their plausibility:

– Could the injuries be caused by this accident?
– Does the type of injury correspond to the reported accidental mechanism?
– Is the accidental cause of the injury possible given the child's stage of development?
– Do the injuries originate from different points of time and can not be caused by a single accident?

Child abuse – some aspects for neurosurgeons

Table 5. *Examinations are decisive from a forensic point of view in order to disprove defensive statements. According to Ref. [49]*

Injuries	Defensive statement	Examination
multiple haematomas	constitutional haemorrhagic diathesis	coagulation status
(multiple) fractures	constitutional bone fragility	X-ray examination, possibly additional biochemical examinations
skull fractures	fall (from changing table, at attempts at walking, from playground equipments), fall down the stairs	CCT (possible intracranial injuries)

In cases of alleged falls the plausibility of the history can be checked regarding the following points [34, 98]:

– Are the injuries localized at areas that are exposed to falling?
– Does the reported height of the fall correspond to the degree of the injuries (not only bone injuries but also cerebral injuries)?

Explanations offen used by carers and examinations needed are summarized in Table 5.

In many cases clear medical opinion and distinct judgement can be difficult; it is often easier to exclude the given version of carers (bruises that do not match with the reported history) than to find a reliable answer to the question how injuries arose. Thus, the criminal prosecution of a case might be complicated, too, especially if the given explanations are adapted to the medical findings.

Bone injuries

Fractures due to abuse are mostly seen in younger children (<3 years). A massive act of violence is necessary to break an infantile bone since these are still flexible. In children which present with fractures, the most commonly involved bones are the skull, ribs, the humerus, the femur and the tibia (Fig. 11a–f and Table 6).

Fractures and bony injury [34, 39, 78, 86, 89, 90]:

– Fractures are sudden, painful and lead to immediate loss of function. The children are crying.
– If children are said by the carers not to cry or express pain, ask why. Abused children are sometimes too frightened to complain and the frozen and watchful child can be recognized in the Accident and Emergency department [73]. But this behaviour is seen in cases of chronic child abuse.

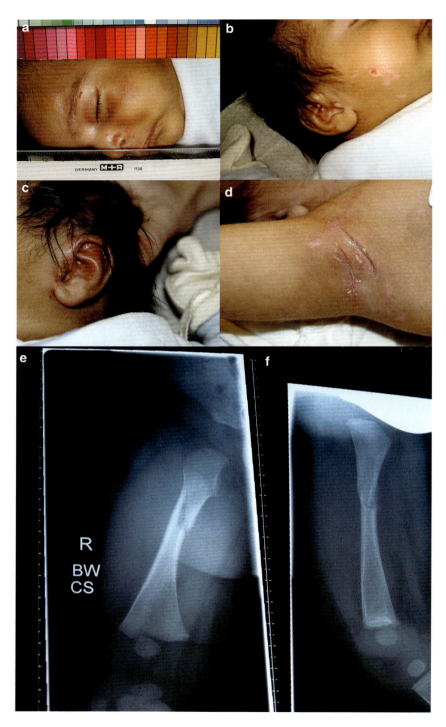

Table 6. *Radiological findings and possible cause of injuries. According to Ref. [49]*

Radiological findings	Cause of injuries
Soft tissue oedema	Contusion, forceful gripping, tractive forces, twisting
Periosteal calcification of the long bones	Calcification of subperiosteal haematomas (see above)
Ruptures of metaphysis (corner signs), detachment of epiphysis	Overstreching and overexpanding of joints (ruptures derive from traction of joint capsule at the osseous base)
(Paravertebral) rib fractures	E.g. in cases of shaking of babies caused by crude compression of the thorax; in older infants caused by foot kicks
Horizontal fractures of long bones	Direct impact of force, bending
Diagonal fractures of long bones	Bending or compression
Spiral fractures	Axial turn
Horizontal fractures of long bones	Bending or axial turn with axial impact

- Children do not continue to walk or play in a normal way with a fracture, but parents who have abused may ignore the injury.
- Pain is at a maximum at the beginning and swelling, bleeding and bruising take a while to fully develop. As these develop, pain may lessen.
- Many fractures show no bruising.
- Though many of the fractures in abused children involve areas of bone dislodged from the main shaft or incomplete (greenstick) breaks, all the classic signs of fracture are not always present. Loss of function is the most important sign of a recent fracture.
- Accidental bone injury is uncommon under the age of 12 months and requires further investigation.

Patterns of fractures and bony injury in abuse (Table 7):

- Single fracture, e.g. humerus with excessive unexplained bruising.
- Multiple fractures in various bones, different stages of healing (classic battered baby syndrome).

Fig. 11. Two months old child, hospitalization due to suspected child abuse with haematomas of the left cheek, right cheek, left ear, scratches of the left upper eyelid and right axillar (a–d). The child was released from hospital and the court ordered a daily supervision of the family by a child-protection agency. Two weeks later the child was brought to different hospital again with a fracture of the right thigh (e–f)

Table 7. *Fractures associated with non-accidental injury. From Ref. [98]*

Bone	Fracture	Accident	Abuse
Rib	Posterior more than anterior/lateral	Rare – road traffic accident, not cardiopulmonary resuscitation	+++
Humerus	Spiral/oblique	+	++
	Metaphysis	Rare	+++
Forearm	Shaft	Common	Direct blow
Femur	Spiral/oblique	Uncommon	++
	Metaphysis	Rare	+++
Tibia	Spiral	Uncommon	++

The scale +, ++, +++ indicates the strength of the association with abusive fractures. Skull: long, wide, branched fractures that cross suture lines (+ depression are associated with abuse.
"Toddler fracture" is a non-displaced spiral fracture of the tibia seen in children who have just started to walk/run and fall twisting their legs beneath them. The child has the usual symptoms of pain, disuse and swelling (sometimes bruising).
Metaphysical fractures are important as damage results from indirect trauma through this relatively fragile growing tissue. They have a strong association with abuse, i.e. pulling, twisting, shaking, and are often multiple [39].

— Metaphyseal-epiphyseal fractures at the end of long bones (these are often multiple after violent shaking and associated with head injury including subdural haematoma).
— Rib fractures, single or multiple (Fig. 12).
— Periosteal new bone formation.
— Skull fracture with intracranial injury.

Rib fractures due to resuscitation do not occur in children [86]. Bone fractures can be poor in symptoms or even without symptoms, especially in babies. There may be swelling but no bruising. Characteristic radiological findings and mechanisms of development of these injuries are summarized in Table 6. The periosteum is quite easy to be detached in children, thus subperiosteal haematomas do occur.

X-ray findings indicating a potential child abuse are [39, 89, 90]: single fracture with multiple bruises, multiple fractures of different age, rib fractures.

Higher specifity for abuse have the following fractures [34]:

— Metaphyseal lesions carry a high specificity for abuse.
— Cartilaginous epiphyseal plate injury.
— Transverse, oblique and spiral shaft fractures.
— Subperiosteal new bone formation.

Child abuse – some aspects for neurosurgeons

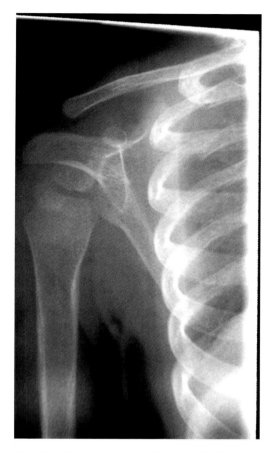

Fig. 12. Rib fracture in a 3-year-old child

These fractures are of lower specificity:

- Narrow, linear, parietal skull
- Shafts of long bones
- Clavicle
- Single fracture.

Dating of injuries and healing of fractures is imprecise. Some advices are given in Table 8.

Head injuries, fractures of the skull

It is assumed that 95% of the severe head injuries in the first year of life are caused by abuse. Abuse with craniocerebral trauma is age dependent a major cause of death in children (Fig. 13). It has to be differentiated between blunt trauma (see Table 3) and the so-called shaken-baby-syndrome (SBS) or non

Table 8. *Healing of fractures. From Ref. [98]*

Feature	Time scale
Soft tissue swelling above the fracture	Immediate-weeks
Periosteal new bone evident	4–21 days
Loss of clarity around fracture site	10–14 days
Soft callus	10–21 days
Hard callus	14–42 days
Remodelling	3–12 months

accidental head injury (NAHI) [3, 5, 17, 18, 22–26, 57–61, 71, 75, 85, 87]. If external head injuries are visible and/or in cases of reduced consciousness further examinations have to take place (CT, MRT) since children have a high risk to develop a malign cerebral oedema.

Skull fractures are a sign of massive blunt violence (hit with the hand, fist, an object or against an object or a counter bearing like a wall) (Fig. 14a–c). The most common fractures are located in the occipito parietal region, however, the location itself is not sufficient to differentiate between fall and hitting [51, 78, 98]. Babies and infants usually do not suffer from life-threatening injuries when falling from heights up to 100 or 150 cm. In 80% of accidental falls from height occured no injuries, in 1% of the cases there was a single linear skull fracture without accompanying intracranial injuries. In contrast, in 55% of non accidental skull fractures there were additional intracranial haemorrhages [78].

When skull fractures are diagnosed reports should include the following: site, which bones; whether suture lines are crossed; configuration of fractures: linear, stellate, branching, depressed; if the fracture is more horizontal, vertical, oblique [34, 98]. The characteristics of injuries are summarized in Table 9. In accidents usually single linear fractures are seen but in abuse cases often multiple complex and depressed fractures occur. A maximum fracture with a

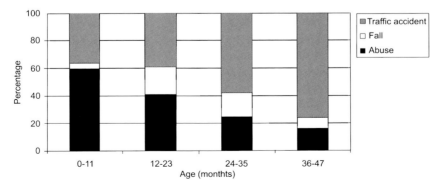

Fig. 13. Age dependent causes of 314 lethal craniocerebral trauma in children below the age of 4 years (according to Ref. [3])

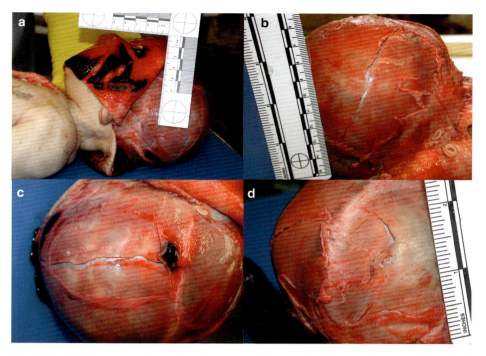

Fig. 14a–d. Severe cranio-cerebral trauma with massive haemorrhages of the skull and multiple fractures (b, c)

Table 9. *Differential diagnosis of skull fractures (according to Hobbs in Meadow 1997). From Ref. [98]*

Characteristics of injury	Accidental fracture	Abuse
Type	singular and linear	multiple, complex, arborescent
Maximal extent of the fracture opening	capillary, narrow, 1–2 mm	broad, increasing, 3 mm and more
Localization	parietal, one cranial bone	occipital, bilateral, parietal, more than one cranial bone
Impression	defined with clear medical history of a fall on a corresponding object	part of a complex fracture, expanded or multiple impressions
Associated intracranial injuries	unusual; do only occur in cases of falls from heights of 2–3 m and above. Epidural haematomas: unusual but serious complications of single fractures	usually subdural haematomas, contusions, intracerebral haemorrhages and brain oedema

width of 3 mm or larger is more often seen in cases of abuse than accidents. One of the main points in skull fractures is the causation: due to abuse or accidental fall. A second point of controversy is the height of a passive fall which can cause a child's skull fracture and cause brain damage [16, 24, 28, 78].

There is meanwhile a huge literature on fatal pediatric head injuries caused by short distance falls [58, 78]. A retrospective analysis of 75,000 reports of falls of children on playing grounds revealed 18 fatal cases. Five children were 1–2 years old, all others were older. No case was reported younger than 1 year of age and only one in the age of 1–2 years with findings comparable to SBS. Two fatal falls from at least 1.5 m while swinging were reported, one case with massive cranial fracture, the other with intensive subdural haematoma without fracture. Other cases were falls from a height of 60 cm without subdural or retinal haemorrhages and another fall from 1.7 m with a depressed fracture and another fall from 70 cm on the floor with subdural haemorrhage and also retinal haemorrhages [58]. Retinal haemorrhages – belonging besides subdural haematoma and encephalopathy to the triad of SBS – are well known in falls from the height, falls downstairs, traffic accidents and other severe craniocerebral traumas. However, it is doubted that they can occur in short distance falls.

In 246 falls of infants under five years from bed or low structures less than 90 cm height [28] no serious injuries or deaths were found. In altogether three cases skull fractures were observed.

In 76 childhood falls in hospital – 75 children were younger than five years – from a height of fall between 30 and 91 cm only one doubtful skull fracture occurred. Williams [99] reported on 398 falls, 106 were observed by independent witnesses. There were 14 severe injuries in falls between 4.5 and 12.20 m, but below 3 m there were no life threatening injuries, but three skull fractures were detected. Weber found three skull fractures in infants who had died after witnessed short distance falls of less than 1 m. Again Hall confirmed that severe or fatal damage can occasionally arise from low falls [28]. In a 4-year-study 18 deaths following falls from less than 0.9 m were observed. Chatwick et al. analyzing 317 childhood falls reported about 7 deaths in 100 falls from less than 1.2 m [16]. However, they doubted the veracity of the histories and their was only one death in those who fell between 3 and 13.7 m. Altogether there is enough evidence both from witnessed falls as well as the experiments from Weber [96, 97] that skull fractures can occur in infant skulls from very low passive falls including heights not exceeding chair or table level [78]. However, skulls fracture often are without any significant internal brain damage (Table 10). According to pediatric statements, falls from a standing position may cause skull fractures, however, without specific symptoms.

Since there is already anecdotal evidence that skull fractures can occur from low passive falls also from heights not exceeding chair or table level, postmortem experiments were carried out.

Child abuse – some aspects for neurosurgeons

Table 10. *Expected injury type with accidental mechanism in very young children. From Ref. [19]**

Mechanism	Injury types
Fall <4 ft <1.2 m	Concussion/soft tissue injury
	Linear fracture
	Epidural haematoma
	Ping-Pong fracture
	? Depressed fracture
Fall >4 ft >1.2 m	Injuries listed above plus the following:
	Depressed fracture
	Basilar fracture
	Multiple fractures
	Subarachnoid haemorrhage
	Contusion
	? Subdural haematoma
	? Stellate fracture
Motor vehicle accident	Injuries listed above plus the following:
	Subdural haematoma
	Diffuse axonal injury

* Injury types preceded by question marks are uncommonly associated with the given mechanism.

Weber [96, 97] experimentally dropped dead infants from a horizontal position of only table height onto a variety of surfaces.

Experimental test series concerned with the stumbling height (82 cm in free fall) and the three various types of floor-stone, carpet, and foam-backed linoleum – were carried out. In each case skull fractures were seen. In three cases the fractures crossed the sutures. Following these experiments (falls from 82 cm heights onto stone (A), carpet (B) and foam-backed linoleum (C)) in another series 35 further falling tests were carried out onto softly cushioned ground. In 10 cases a 2 cm thick foam rubber mat (D) was chosen and in 25 further cases a double-folded (8 cm-thick) camel hair blanket (E). Hence the results of altogether 50 tests could be evaluated.

In test groups A–C on a relatively hard surface, skull fractures of the parietal bone were observed in every case; in test group D this fracture was seen in one case and in test group E in four cases.

Measurements along the fracture fissures showed bone thicknesses of 0.1–0.4 mm. The fracture injuries originated in paper-thin single-layer bone areas without diploe, which can also be considered the preferred regions for skull fractures of older infants following falls from heights. These results indicated that it is no longer possible to assume that the skull of infants is not damaged after falls from table height. However, skulls often fracture without

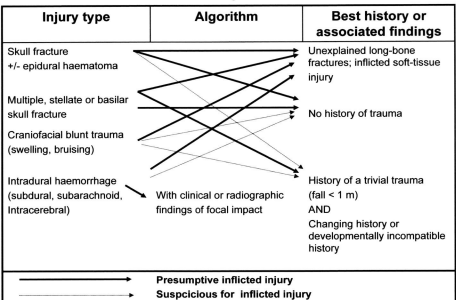

Fig. 15. Algorithm for determination of inflicted skull injury

any significant internal brain damage. Figure 15 shows an algorithm for determination of inflicted skull injury in very young children [61]. If skull fracture and epidural haematoma is combined with long bone fractures the probability of inflicted injury is very high.

Non-accidental head injury/shaken-baby-syndrome

Non-accidental head injury (NAHI) and the shaken-baby-syndrome (SBS) are the most common causes of unnatural death in toddlers and infants. It is estimated that between 15 and 30/100,000 children suffer from NAHI or SBS per year. Traumatic brain injury, in particular the shaken-baby-syndrome leads to significant neurological disability in more than two-thirds of surviving victims and is fatal in 12–27% of cases [3, 5, 23–25, 34, 32, 57, 59–61, 78, 87, 93, 98].

Shaken-baby-syndrome (SBS)

The shaken-baby-syndrome is a typical combination of injuries (subdural haematoma, retinal haemorrhages) resulting from rude shaking of the child (mostly babies, rarely infants) [87, 98].

Child abuse – some aspects for neurosurgeons

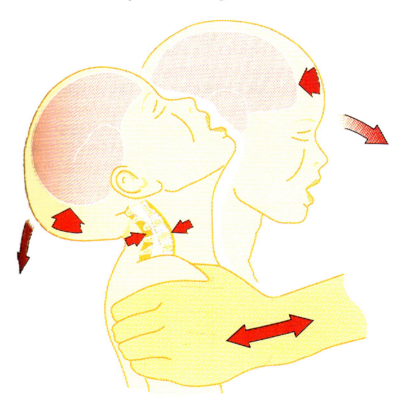

Fig. 16. Mechanism of shaken-baby-syndrome with rupture of bridging veins [49]

The child is gripped at its shoulders, arms or chest and heavily shaken back and forth. The cervical muscles are too weak compared to the head's weight and they are unable to hold the head stable. Thus, the head swings back and forth uncontrollably (see Fig. 16). The moment of inertia of the brain leads to a strain of the pontine veins and/or of vessels of the leptomeninx which often causes – in case of rupture – subdural or subarachnoidal haemorrhages (often bilateral) (Fig. 17). Additionally, retinal haemorrhages occur in 80% of cases; it is not yet known how they develop. If the head does not hit a surface or if it hits a flexible, soft surface, there are no external injuries.

The developing symptomatology (lethargy, vomiting, cerebral spasm, hypothermia, bradycardia, hypertonia, hypotonia, somnolence, prolonged asphyxia, coma) is mainly caused by axon damage accompanied by cerebral oedema and increasing haemorrhage [45, 68, 71].

Ophthalmologic findings: haemorrhages are usually dispersed diffusely and can occur either in front of, behind or within the retina. They are

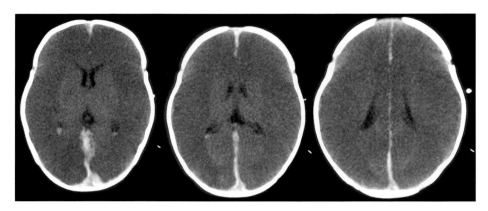

Fig. 17. Subdural haemorrhage interhemispheric in a case of SBS

mostly verifiable on both sides. Additionally retinal detachment or atrophy of the optic nerve might occur. Haemorrhages within the vitreous body which are not fully reabsorbed might cause ablepsia (Table 11).

Table 11. *Ophthalmic injuries in abuse. From Hobbs, Hanks, Wynne 1999*

Structure	Result	Lesion	Effects
Eyelids, periorbital tissue	Blunt trauma, e.g. fist	Bruising – "black eye"	Recovers
Cornea, conjunctiva	Blunt or penetrating trauma, burns, chemicals	Haemorrhage, laceration, abrasion, ulceration, scarring	Variable, depending on severity in visual axis
Lens, anterior structures	Blunt or penetrating trauma	Iris sphincter rupture. Dislocated lens	Vossius ring glaucoma, intraocular scar formation, cataract
Posterior structures, vitreous, retina	Anterior injury transmitted to back of eye. Whiplash, shaking	Vitreous haemorrhage, retinal haemorrhage. Retinal detachment	Retinal scarring, papilloedema, optic atroply
Visual cortex	Head injury. Contrecoup	Cerebral contusion, haemorrhage	Cortical blindness

Longterm outcome of the shaken-baby-syndrome

- Blindness (caused by injuries of the eyes or as central blindness);
- Severe mental and/or physical disablement up to apallic syndrome due to direct cerebral injury (e.g. contusions) or as consequences of the intracranial pressure (hypoxic brain damage);
- Epilepsy;
- Cerebral atrophy with chronic hygroma and
- accompanying injuries of the cerebral spine (dislocation, haemorrhages of the cervical ligaments).

Lethal cases:

Approximately 10% of all lethal cases of child abuse are assumed to be caused by shaken-baby-syndrome. Up to 25% of the shaken-baby-syndrome victims die. Death due to shaken-baby-syndrome might be misinterpreted as SIDS cases since external injuries are totally missing [6].

The NAHI is characterized by a constellation of subdural haematoma and mostly marked retinal haemorrhages with severe diffuse brain injury. Usually other external signs of violence are missing. Haematomae of the skin caused by gripping on the chest or on the outer arms may occur but are not necessarily present. Clinically the infants present with neurological symptoms as lethargy or loss of consciousness shortly after the event, with respiratory failure or fits. SBS resulting in significant brain damage and clinical symptoms requires extensive violent shaking of a child leading to uncontrolled rotation of the head. After hospitalization the correct diagnosis is made rapidly and reliably and is based mostly on the combination of subdural and retinal haemorrhages. However, these haemorrhages are not important for the prognosis. Far more important for the clinical outcome are the combination of diffuse axonal injury and initial traumatic apnoea leading to hypoxia, ischemia and intracranial hypertension [45, 57, 68]. If the infants die immediately after shaking and external signs of violence like grip marks are missing on the chest it may be impossible to make the correct diagnosis at the scene of crime. In fatal cases extensive neuropathological investigations including brain, spinal cord, dura mater as well as the eye balls have to be carried out by experienced forensic neuropathologists.

However, the concept of SBS first described by Guthkelch [27] and Caffey (1972) about 40 years ago is not undisputed. The scientific debate on the specifity of findings like subdural haematoma, retinal haemorrhages and diffuse brain injury [20–23] being caused by shaking has been carried into court rooms and lead to considerable uncertainty amongst lay persons and jurists [85]. Even the concept of SBS was doubted: "...we need to reconsider the diagnostic criteria if not the existence of shaken baby syndrome" [24]. The discussion is due to the fact that Geddes [20–23]

Table 12. *Four predominant types of clinical features, morphological findings and causation in non-accidental head injury according to Ref. [58, 60]*

Types of inflicted brain injury/frequency	Clinical presentation	Morphological findings	Pathomechanism	Outcome
A: hyperacute encephalopathy/ cervicomedullary syndrome (6%)	Acute respiratory failure/death/brain death after partially successful reanimation	Severe brain swelling, hypoxic brain injury, little axonal shearing, only thin subdural haemorrhage	Acute respiratory failure due to broken brain stem after extreme whiplashing	Death
B: acute encephalopathy (53%)	Depressed conscious state, raised intracranial pressure, fits, apnoea, hypotonia, anaemia, shock	Convexity subdural haemorrhages (as well as interhemispheric, subtemporal, suboccipital and in the posterior fossa), cerebral oedema, haemorrhagic contusions, widespread haemorrhagic retinopathy	Repetetive rotational injury with or without impact; classic shaken baby syndrome with coexistent rib or metaphyseal fractures	Up to 60% serious longterm morbidity
C: subacute non-encephalopathic presentation (19%)	Unspecific findings	Less intense brain injury without swelling, various combinations of subdural and retinal haemorrhages, rib fractures, other bone fractures and bruising	Like B but without severe primary traumatic or secondary hypoxic brain damage	Outcome better than in B
D: Chronic extracerebral presentation (22%)	Rapidly expanding head circumference, irritable, vomiting, failure to thrive, hypotonic, fits	Isolated, often chronic (>3 weeks) subdural haemorrhage, retinal haemorrhages originally present have disappeared	Trauma some weeks ago with secondary injury from raised intracranial pressure, hypoperfusion and oedema. Difficulty in attributing a causative mechanism to such late presenting subdural haematoma	Good prognosis with recognition and appropriate treatment

over-interpreted her findings on dural haemorrhages. At the court of appeal where 4 out of 297 cases were reinvestigated she said "I would be very unhappy to think that cases were being thrown out on the basis that my theory was fact." [85]. However, another part of the problem is due to the principle impossibility to carry out evidence based research in this particular field. The present discussion focuses on the following items [85]:

- Can we diagnose a shaken-baby-syndrome?
- Is a non-traumatic etiology of the triad subdural haematoma, encephalopathy and retinal haemorrhages possible or likely?
- How much force is required to produce a shaking injury?
- Do low-level falls cause fatal head injuries?
- Is there a lucid interval in infants who sustain significant inflicted head trauma?
- What is the diagnostic significance of retinal haemorrhages?

In conclusion there is still substantial evidence for the diagnosis of a non-accidental head injury. Based on a data collection for more than five years Minns and Busuttil [60] postulated that a spectrum of clinical features is related to the intensity and type of injury in babies with inflicted brain injury. According to the data base, several patterns of presentation allow delineation of cases into four predominant types (Table 12) (see also [58, 60]):

- hyperacute encephalopathy (cervicomedullary syndrome),
- acute encephalopathy,
- subacute non-encephalopathic presentation,
- chronic extracerebral presentation.

Based on the typing of inflicted brain injury, Minns and Busuttil suggested that the general term "non-accidental head injury" or "inflicted traumatic brain injury" should be used in preference to shaken-baby-syndrome which implies a specific mechanism of injury. Several literature reviews and evaluation of their own case material revealed that if an infant is brought to hospital or dies in a deep coma with several bridging vein ruptures and minor subdural bleeding these findings are not compatible with an alleged minor fall and there is no justification for a fundamental change in the position to interpret such cases as a consequence of severe trauma caused by another person [58].

Thermal injuries

Ten percent of all abused children show injuries caused by the impact of heat. It is assumed that up to 25% of all children with treated thermal injuries are victims of abuse.

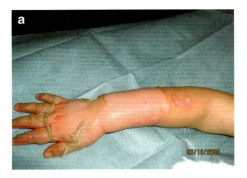
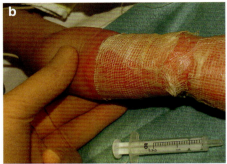

Fig. 18. Typical immersion injury, sharp margin between healthy and injured skin corresponding to the water level

The characteristic pattern of thermal injuries usually allows a "visual diagnosis". It has to be differentiated between the impact of wet heat (scalds) (Fig. 18) and dry heat (contact burns by pressing on hot items, e.g. cigarettes) (Fig. 19); the impact of flames, of current, injuries caused by rubbing, chemical burns and impact of heat by heat emission are rather rare causes of thermal injuries in children. Scalds are more frequently seen than burns.

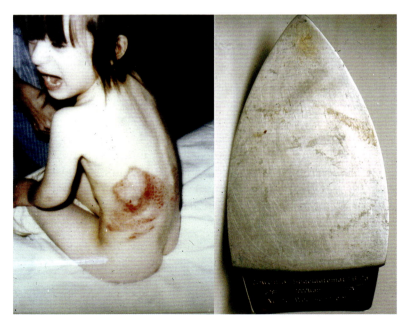

Fig. 19. Contact burn with complete reproduction of the hot surface of a flat iron on the skin (from Ref. [7])

Child abuse – some aspects for neurosurgeons   111

The depth of a lesion (degree of cutaneous burn) depends on the temperature and the duration of the impact of the heat [46, 63, 64] (Fig. 20). It is assumed that infantile skin which is exposed to temperatures above 60°C gets

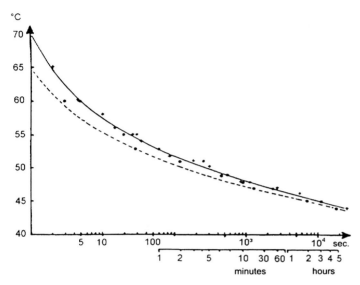

Fig. 20. Time-surface temperature thresholds at which cutaneous burning (scalding) occurs. The broken line indicates the threshold at which irreversible epidermal injury occurs in porcine skin. The solid line indicates the threshold at which epidermal necrosis of porcine skin occurs. The results of critical experimental exposures of human skin are indicated by points. Exposure time in seconds, surface temperature of skin. Original data from Moritz and Henriques (from Ref. [49])

Table 13. *Differential diagnosis of accidental and non accidental scaldings. From Ref. [49]*

Accidental scalds	Immersion
Unsteady pattern of the injury (scalds of different depth)	Steady depth of scald
Diffuse limitation between scalds and healthy skin (at the borders the scalds are rather less pronounced due to cooling of the water)	Sharp margin between healthy and affected skin (water level might be reproduced on skin like a map)
Extremities show rather scalds in form of splashes (e.g. on feet)	In case of immersion of extremities: scalds in form of gloves or socks
In case of scald of the thorax the scald usually is configured like an arrow (water running down the body)	In case of immersion of the face there are no signs of running water

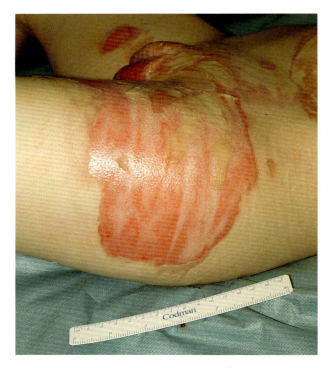

Fig. 21. Irregular shape of scald when hot liquids have fallen on the body

injured four times faster than adults' skin [6, 7]. Large-scale skin damages in children rapidly become life-threatening because of the fluid loss.

Typical accidental scalds occur when children start to straighten up and e.g. lift themselves with the help of a table-cloth and, thus, items lying on the table fall down on the child (cups with hot liquids, etc.). The scalds show characteristic criteria (see Table 13) and affect the face, the shoulders, upper arms and chest [7]. Typical are splash marks when hot liquids fall on the child or the child falls into a bathtub (Fig. 21). Even young children do not stay in their original position when unintentionally exposed to hot water. Rescue efforts might be uncoordinated due to the stage of development which also causes an unsteady pattern of the injury.

The intentional scalds are subdivided into two forms: the intentional sousing of hot liquid or the intentional immersion into hot liquid. Immersion can concern either the extremities (see Fig. 18), the face or even the whole body (e.g. bathing in water being too hot). In these cases typical symmetrical scaldings are seen. Forced immersion scalds show clear lines of demarcation. If cloths are worn this leads to a deeper scald since wet cloths conserve heat. A differentiation between an intentional or accidental sousing based on the described characteristics might be difficult.

Table 14. *Characteristics of accidental and non-accidental contact burns. From Ref. [49]*

Accidental contact burns	Intentional contact burns
Partial reproduction of the item, potentially the item only grazed the skin Lower depth of the wound since the body or the item was not fixed	Complete reproduction with clear outline (cigarette, electric iron, hotplate, ...) Constant depth of the wound due to pressing the child on the item or pressing the item on the child's body

Table 15. *Differential diagnosis of symptoms of child abuse. From Ref. [49]*

Symptoms	Pathological reasons	Examination
Haematomas	Congenital or acquired coagulation defects, e.g. haemophilia, haemorrhagic diathesis, purpura Schoenlein-Henoch, leukemia, vasculitis	Haemogram, coagulation disorders?
Discolouration of skin	Naevi, haemangioma	Dermatolgical examination
Questionable thermic changes	Eczema, erythema nodosum, erythema multiforme, photodermatitis, staphylococcal impetigo, Lyeyell's syndrome, bullous dermatosis, papular urticaria, diaper dermatitis, contact dermatitis	Dermatological examination
Questionable signs of hair pulling	Jonstons's alopecia	Dermatological examination
Patchy distribution of retinal haemorrhages	Acute hypertonia, fulminant meningitis, vasculitis, sepsis, endocarditis, coagulopathies, leukemia, cyanotic congenital cardiac defect, status after vaginal birth (rarely persistent for longer than 2 weeks)	Appropriate additional examinations
Fractures	Osteogenesis imperfecta, copper deficiency, pathological fractures, rachitis, scurvy, congenital syphilis, osteomyelitis, neurological diseases, hyperostosis corticalis	X-ray pictures, bone scan, appropriate additional examinations

Burns are caused by impact of hot items or flames. The characteristics of injuries caused by contact burns are summarized in Table 14.

Accidental impacts by flames can e.g. be caused at barbecues in summer (inadequate use of methylated spirits). Since this is a dramatic incident it is rarely unobserved and results in a direct admission to hospital. Injuries caused by flames (matches, cigarette lighters) are smaller and more irregular.

Injuries by intentional exposition to cold (e.g. showering with cold water, locking in non-heated rooms) are extremely rare.

Cases of hypothermia were described in children who were neglected.

Injuries of the eyes

In rare cases injuries of the eyes are the first symptom of child abuse. Injuries of the eyes caused by sexually transmissible diseases are a special case. All traumatic changes of the eyes might be consequences of abuse (haemorrhages in all anatomical structures, ruptures of the eye balls). Retinal haemorrhages are of special importance.

In cases of suspected child abuse of children under the age of 4 an ophthalmologic examination should be made.

Differential diagnoses

A false positive diagnosis of child abuse has dramatic consequences for the family concerned. In order to avoid misdiagnoses differential diagnoses have to be taken into consideration (see Tables 15–17) [34, 78, 83, 98].

Table 16. *Differential diagnosis of some morphological changes encountered in the abused child. From [68]*

Sign	Confounding diseases
Fractures	Osteogenesis imperfecta
	Menkes' syndrome
	Atypical skull suture line
Scars	Chickenpox lesions resembling cigarette burns
Bruising	Haemophilia
	Hypersensitivity vasculitis
	Bacteremia with DIC
	Folk medicine ("Pseudobattering syndrome")
	Oriental folk medicine phytophotodermatitis
	Mongolian spot
	Erythema multiforme
Retinal haemorrhages	Resuscitation retinopathy (Purtscher's retinopathy)

Table 17. *Differential diagnosis of bruising (a) and recommended haematologic investigations (b) From Wynne 2003*

(a) Differential diagnosis of bruising

Presentation	Differential diagnosis	Features	Investigation
Bruise?	Blue spots, haemangioma, café-au-lait	Static lesion no evolution over time	Follow-up
Bruise?	Bleeding disorder – ITP, haemophilia	Bruise easily	Low platelets, factor VIII ↓
Bruise?	Allergy – periorbital swelling	History of allergy	↑ IgE, eosinophilia
Bruise?	Ink, paint, dirt	Washable	Soap and water

(b) Is it a haematologic disorder?

Disease	Platelet count	Bleeding time	Partial thromboplastin time (PTT)	Prothrombin time (PT)	Factor VIII level	Factor IX level
Idiopathic thrombocytopenic purpura (ITP)	Low	Normal	Normal	Normal	Normal	Normal
Haemophilia	Normal	Normal	Prolonged	Normal	Low	Normal
von Willebrand's disease (defective platelet aggregation)	Normal	Prolonged	Normal/ prolonged	Normal	Low	Normal
Factor IX deficiency	Normal	Normal	Prolonged	Normal	Normal	Low

The application of complimentary or traditional cures, e.g. of Asian or African origin [84], might cause dermal changes that resemble – seen with the eyes of a person with European cultural background -consequences of abuse (e.g. formed haemorrhages, formed burns caused by cupping, etc.). Also rare diseases have to be taken into account, e.g. Gardner-Diamond-syndrome (painful bruising syndrome, Fig. 22) [10, 21].

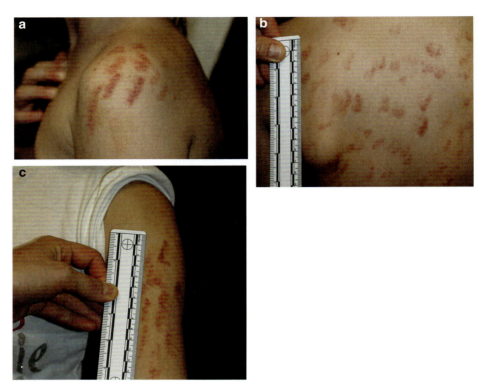

Fig. 22a–c. Painful bruises in 3 brothers and sisters on shoulder, back and arm; probably Gardner-Diamond-syndrome; etiology unclear, probably induced by psychological stress. No report of violence by the children, they complained of similar findings when they had some sort of psychological stress

Münchausen syndrome by proxy

The Münchausen syndrome by proxy is a disorder in which one of the parents (often the mother) affirms that the child has symptoms of an illness or symptoms of an illness are caused ("fabricated") by this person by manipulation (giving non prescribed drugs, especially hypnotics and sedatives, provoking of life-threatening situations (partly suffocation)). The attention gained by the mother seems to be of main relevance. The perpetrators seem to be amenable, caring and rather overprotective. The incidence is not known. Withdrawal of the children can be necessary since other solutions are lacking. The symptoms most commonly seen include: vomiting, diarrhoea, bleeding, fever, convulsions, drowsiness, coma [66, 67].

Infliction of drugs can only be proved by chemical-toxicological examinations (thus, prompt taking of blood and urine samples is necessary). There are some clinical features suggesting abusive poisoning (Table 18) and differential

Child abuse – some aspects for neurosurgeons 117

Table 18. *Clinical features suggestive of abusive poisoning. From Oehmichen et al. (2003)*

Age
  Younger than 1 year or between 5 and 10 years
History
  Non-existent, discrepant, inconsistent or changing
  Does not fit child's development
  Previous poisoning of the child
  Previous poisoning of siblings
  Circumstances or scene do not fit
  Third party (sibling) is blamed
  Delay in seeking medical care
Toxin
  Multiple toxins
  Substances of abuse
  Bizarre substances
Presentation
  Unexplained seizures
  Life-threatening events
  Apparent sudden infant death syndrome
  Death without obvious cause
  Chronic unexplained symptoms that resolve when the child is proctected
  Other evident of abuse or neglect

diagnostic criteria for accidental vs. deliberate poisoning (Table 19) [37, 65, 67, 76].

Characteristics of the Münchausen syndrome by proxy are:

– The symptoms do only occur in presence of the person who is reporting
– The symptoms frequently diminish in hospital after separation from the parent
– Missing verification of pathological findings beside intensive, even invasive diagnostics.

A pathognomonic feature is the perpetrator's motivation to achieve the sick role and intense access to health care via the manipulation of symptoms in the child and its repeated presentation for outpatient and inpatient assessment and treatment. This psychological gain distinguishes MbpS from simulation and malingering as well as from distorted health anxiety in mothers with exaggerated health care behaviour.

There has always been a confusion about who should make the diagnosis of Munchausen syndrome by proxy: a psychiatrist or pediatrician? Is it a diagnosis applied to the parent or the child? Is it a pediatric or a mental health diagnosis? To alleviate confusion, the American Professional Society

Table 19. *Poisoning – is it accident, neglect or deliberate? From Hobbs, Hanks, Wynne (1993)*

	Accident	Neglect	Deliberate
Age	2–3 years rarely older child	2–3 years rarely older child	infancy – 3 years may be any age
History	Usually clear – makes sense	Variable – due to social chaos	a) None – but ill child b) History of accidental ingestion c) Recurrent symptoms
Symptoms	Uncommon <15%	Uncommon <15%	Common a) Seizures, drowsy, vomiting diarrhoea
	>1% need intensive care rarely fatal	>1% need intensive care rarely fatal	b) Dead
Substance	Drugs – analgesics, anxiolytics, cough medicine, oral contraceptive, iron		Drugs – analgesics, antidepressants, anxiolytics, anticonvulsants, insulin, etc.
	Household – bleach, detergent, petroleum product		Other – salt, bicarbonate of soda, corrosives, etc.
Past history	Nil	Repeated ingestions Increased incidence SIDS Known to SSD	Other unexplained child deaths in family including SIDS Other abuses
Diagnosis	History equates with clinical signs Confirmed if necessary by toxicological investigation	As accidental	History usually at variance with clinical signs Ask advice of toxicologist – blood, urine samples think of possibility – parents behaviour may be bizarre – but present as caring and concerned

on the Abuse of Children has recently made a more explicit distinction between the abuse (pediatric *condition falsification*) and the presumed motive behind most such cases (factitious disorder by proxy). Whatever it is called, it is important to remember that harm incurred when a caregiver exaggerates, fabricates, or induces symptoms of a medical *condition* may still simply be termed "child abuse, which happens to occur in a medical setting". This appellation reminds us that the focus of our intervention should always be to identify and minimize harm to the child regardless of the motivation of the perpetrator [88].

Clinical features suggestive of abuse poisoning are summarized in Table 18. In appropriate cases detailed toxicological investigations have to be carried out on blood (serum), urine and hair (hair growth appr. 1 cm/month; verification of deliberate poisoning over a longer time period). Diagnostic criteria which may be helpful in the differential diagnosis of poisoning is shown in Table 19.

Lethal child abuse

Lethal child abuse comprises cases of death caused by external violence or by intoxication. Although death is not intended in most cases it is nevertheless accepted as a possible consequence of the act of abuse. Intentional murder (in cases of extended suicide, murder of newborn babies or homicide in order to conceal another crime) is no form of lethal child abuse [6, 12, 47–49, 53, 55, 69, 79, 80].

There are 10–12 reported cases of lethal child abuse in Germany per year and an estimated number of 10–600 up to 1000 not reported cases [6].

The victims are usually children younger than 4 or 5 years and the perpetrators are in the majority of cases male (father, friend of the mother).

In case of any signs of external violence at the postmortem examination of a child a lethal child abuse has to be taken into consideration.

In about 10% of all cases of lethal child abuse there are no external signs of violence/injuries. In cases of suspicion there is a duty to inform the police of an unnatural or unclear manner of death.

Frequent autopsy findings:

Cranio-cerebral injuries caused by blunt violence or shaking are dominating as causes of death. Beside the actual injuries leading to death there are often signs of preceeding violence. Postmortal X-ray examination should take place.

Physical neglect

Deprivation of necessary care including sufficient nourishment and hydration (passive form of child abuse).

The incidence of physical neglect is not known.

In most cases of physical neglect the perpetrators are female since it is usually the mother who cares for the child. In particular unwanted children or children of ill mothers (addictive disorders, psychiatric disorders) are at risk.

Cases of physical neglect affect almost exclusively babies or infants who are – due to their stage of development – dependent on the care of others (under the age of 3).

The registration of the care condition of a child is a visual diagnosis. In particular there has to be paid attention to untreated dermal alterations. In order to evaluate the physical development of a child it should be compared to normal percentiles with regard to weight and height. The Waterlow-classification provides further information regarding the degree of chronic growth retardation and acute malnutrition.

Starvation

Although one of the leading causes of death worldwide, starvation is comparatively rarely seen in industrialized countries, but this entity may become of major medicolegal importance if death results from deliberate withholding of food, especially in infants. In such cases, the task of the forensic pathologist and the medical examiner, respectively, is not only to clarify the cause of death but also to give an expert opinion on degree and duration of starvation. Several classification systems have been developed to estimate protein-energy malnutrition (PEM) in third world countries (e.g. Waterlow classification, Gomez classification). More simple classifications (e.g. the Gomez classification of PEM) use the weight expected for the respective age group as standard. When applying this standard, small infants will always be light infants. Following the Waterlow classification (Table 20), a stunted physical condition (referring to retardation in cases of chronic malnutrition) is calculated by using the ratio of the measured body height to the one expected for the actual age). Body weight can be used as a sign of acute malnutrition ("wasting"). However, body weight should be related to the respective weight for the actual height. Using such classification

Table 20. *Classification of nutritional status according to the Waterlow classification. From Ref. [47]*

Grade	0	1	2	3
Stunting (chronic)				
actual length in % of normal length for age	>95	95–87.5	87.5–80	<80
Wasting (acute)				
actual weight in % of normal weight for length	>90	90–80	80–70	<70

Using this table a grading as well of the chronic malnutrition (stunting) as of acute malnutrition (wasting) can be achieved.

systems, a grading of stunting and wasting can be achieved which is of great value for the assessment of a child's nutritional status in legal cases. The application of the Waterlow classification to own case material and cases published in literature revealed that in fatal cases the actual weight in percentage of normal weight was always below 60%, the weight in percent of ideal weight for height below 70% [48, 50]. While in very young children (weeks to months old) the actual height in percent of normal height was about or above 90% in older children (months to 2.5 years old) the actual height in percent of normal height for respective age was below 90%, marking chronic starvation with stunting. The Waterlow classification is not only of importance for grading the final stage in cases of fatal starvation but also for the chronological development of the nutritional status, if anthropometrical data have been recorded repeatedly from the affected individual *in vivo*.

Causes of death caused by neglect: in these cases children mostly die of thirst [47] in combination with starvation, intercurrent illnesses (infections, especially pneumonias) or hypothermia. The frequency of cases of death caused by neglect is unknown.

Cases of suspicion of death caused by neglect have to be reported to the police as cases of a possible unnatural manner of death.

Taking the case history

When the history of a case of suspected child abuse is taken the vital sources of information in cases of child abuse are:

– Information of pretreating physicians (general practitioner, accident and emergency doctor or nurse)
– Health visitor, school nurse or midwife
– Paediatric nurse (if child in hospital)
– other individuals – e.g. probation officer, obstetrician, adult psychiatrist and staff, pathologist – can occasionally help
– other sources – other hospitals, towns, armed forces units.

Suspicion of child abuse is raised under the following conditions [68, 74]:

– Unexplained delay in seeking treatment although severe injuries are obvious
– Consultation of different pediatricians (doctor hopping)
– Submitted history (presenting symptoms) is changed after initial presentation
– Discrepancy in the stories given by each parent or caregiver
– A history incompatible with (or very unlikely) the age and development of the child
– Explanation given inconsistent with physical findings

- Ambivalence or hostility in the parent or caregiver
- Injuries blamed on a sibling or on another child

Common stories told by carers to explain injuries suffered by infants or children under their care are [38, 68]:

- Child fell from a low height (<1.25 m or 4 feet) such as couch, crib, bed, chair or down stairs or a compact object fell on child (accident)
- Alleged traumatic event, one day or more before death (accident)
- Unexpectedly found dead (SIDS?)
- Child choked while eating or suddenly turned blue or stopped breathing, and was then shaken (resuscitation)
- Sudden seizure activity
- Aggressive or inexperienced CPR to a child who suddenly stopped breathing
- Injury inflicted by sibling

Structured forensic, investigative interview with the child

Research on appropriate forensic interview protocols showed that perhaps the most important single factor predicting successful interview results pertains to the interviewer's ability to elicit information and the child's willingness and ability to express it, rather than the child's ability to remember it [42]. Experts agree that children should be interviewed as soon as possible after the alleged offences by interviewers who themselves introduce as little information as possible while encouraging children to provide as much information as possible in the form of narratives elicited using open-ended prompts ("Tell me what happened."). Before substantive issues are discussed, interviewers are typically urged to explain their roles, the purpose of the interview, and the "ground rules" (for example, ask children to limit themselves to descriptions of events "that really happened" to them and to correct the interviewer, request explanations or clarification, and acknowledge ignorance, as necessary). Investigators are consistently urged to give priority to open-ended recall prompts and use recognition prompts ("Did he touch you?") as late in the interview as possible and only when needed to elicit undisclosed forensically relevant information.

Interviewers are also routinely advised to avoid the "yes/no" questions which are especially likely to elicit erroneous information from young children.

Researchers at the National Institute of Child Health and Human Development (NICHD) developed a structured interview protocol designed to translate professional recommendations into operational guidelines [42]. The structured NICHD protocol guides interviewers through all phases of the investigative interview, illustrating free-recall prompts and techniques to maximize the amount of information elicited from free recall memory.

After an introductory and rapport-building phase the child is invited to recall a particular allegation ("Tell me everything ...."). As soon as this first narrative is completed, the interviewer prompts the child to indicate whether the incident occurred "one time or more than one time" and then proceeds to secure incident-specific information using follow-up ("What happened then") and cued (e.g., "Earlier you mentioned a [person/object/action] invitations. Tell me everything about that") making reference to details mentioned by the child to elicit uncontaminated free-recall accounts of the alleged incident/s.

Only after exhaustive free-recall prompting do interviewers proceed to directive questions such as "When did it happen?" or "What colour did the car have?". If crucial details are still missing, interviewers then ask limited option-posing questions (mostly yes/no or forced-choice questions). Suggestive utterances, which communicate to the child what response is expected, are strongly discouraged.

Documentation

A clear documentation of all findings is of utmost importance for the further management of the case (Table 21). The following points have to be documented in clinical records:

- condition of care (abused children are often neglected and undernourished)
- height, head circumference, weight (comparison with percentiles)
- stage of development (appropriate to age?)

Injuries have to be documented in a reproducible and easy to understand manner (photos with measuring unit, colour scale, graphs). The documentation should be of descriptive character since premature interpretations are not helpful.

The description has to contain:

- type of injury, dimension and localization
- colour and potentially form (especially for haematomas) (Table 3)

Clinically necessary supplementary examinations like sonography, X-ray, etc. are at the same time a documentation of the severity of the injuries.

The description of an injury is of utmost importance for the interpretation of causation and legal consequences. In case of doubt a detailed description allows conclusions at a later time which could not have been made primarily.

General symptoms in cases of child abuse

Reduced general condition, inadequate care, reduced weight ("failure to thrive"), nanism.

Table 21. *Important points for examination and documentation. According to Hobbs, Hanks, and Wynne*

1. Full paediatric history, including careful note explanations of injury, times, details, etc.
2. Developmental history
3. Parent's expressed difficulties with child – behaviour, health, development
4. Detailed examination of whole child to clued:
    - Growth – height, weight, arm circumference, head circumference (plotted)
    - Nutrition
    - General demeanour and appearance
    - Signs of neglect, sexual abuse, emotional disturbance
    - Development including language, social skills
5. Documentation of injuries. Descriptions should be brief but detailed and include:
    a. Probable nature of the lesion and approximate age (colour for bruises)
    b. Site
    c. Shape
    d. Size (in cm)
    e. Any unusual distinguishing features
    f. An estimate of causation if possible

Possible behavioural characteristics of abused children are:

- Anxiety, jumpiness, tractableness, apathy
- depressive-tense attitude, passive-observant behaviour
- seeking help, clinging, provoking, devious behaviour
- observing attention, frozen watchfulness, regression (relapse in overcome stages of development like wetting one's bed, dirtying oneself, eating disorders)
- these behavioural disorders are not a proof of child abuse but should raise the awareness.

(Long-term) consequences of child abuse depend on different variables. Of significant importance are manner, duration and severity, age of the child at the beginning of the abuse and the presence of a stabilising person to whom the child is closely attached. Physical consequences of severe injuries have to be considered, too.

Proceeding in cases of suspected child abuse

- Extensive documentation of findings.
- In cases of ambulant consultation: admission to hospital? (relief of the situation)
- Documentation of explanation for injuries; no premature confrontation!

Child abuse – some aspects for neurosurgeons

- Work-up of differential diagnoses.
- Potentially additional consulting of a coroner.

  Proceeding in cases of confirmed diagnosis

- Dialogue with the parents or the person presenting the child (cooperative, dismissive, ...); dialogues have to be witnessed! A protocol has to be prepared.
- Getting in contact with the youth welfare office, the child protection ambulance, etc.
- In cases of severe or repeated injuries possibly criminal complaint

Child protection team

To manage a case of suspected child abuse a multidisciplinary team of physicians, psychologists, social workers and nurses is recommended. In addition the help of legal profession is useful. Since many years so called child protection teams (CPT) are working effectively in the US, Canada, parts of Asia and in a few European countries. The first multidisciplinary CPT was founded by Henry Kempe in Denver, Colorado in 1958. In 2008, 89% of all children hospitals in the US support CPT. One of the first CPT in Europe was established in the Children University Hospital in Zurich in 1969. Today all children hospitals in Switzerland and Austria have CPTs, most in cooperation, because of legal regulations. In Germany, one of the first CPTs was

Table 22. *Professions of the CPT in Bonn*

Medical profession	Dermatology
	Forensic medicine
	Gynecology
	Neurosurgery
	Odontology
	Pediatrics
	Radiology
	Surgery
	– Children
	– Traumatology
	Toxicology (Poison Control Center)
	Urology
Care	
Psychology	
Social work	
Theology	

founded at the University Hospital in Bonn in 2006. The Bonn CPT consists of several different medical disciplines and non-medical professions (Table 22). To reconcile so many different specialists in revealing a solid diagnosis of child abuse a schedule is needed. On the other hand the first contact with the child is mainly made by nurses and residents. But how many consultants have seen children who were abused? A guideline should be used by hospital staff to handle cases of suspected child abuse in a reliable way. Thus, it is advantageous to implement in a CPT a guideline, especially in form of a Clinical Pathway.

Clinical pathway

Clinical pathways are multidisciplinary programs of best clinical practice for specified groups of patients with a particular diagnosis that aid the coordination and delivery of high quality care. The clinical pathway originally used in the USA and Australia was aimed at shortening the hospital stay and reducing healthcare costs, which has become an increasingly important issue in medicine. Furthermore, it is an appropriate tool to standardize medical care and increase patient satisfaction. Clinical pathways are able to standardize care for patients with a similar diagnosis, procedure, or symptom. There are four essential components of a clinical pathway: a timeline, the categories of care or activities and their interventions, intermediate- and long-term outcome criteria, and the variance record. In contrast to practice guidelines, protocols, and algorithms, clinical pathways are utilized by a multidisciplinary team and focus on quality and coordination of care.

Definition of Clinical Pathway

A multidisciplinary set of daily prescriptions and outcome targets for managing the overall care of a specific type of patient, e.g., from pre-admission to post-discharge for patients receiving inpatient care. Clinical pathways often are intended to maintain or improve quality of care and decrease costs for patients in particular diagnosis-related groups. [From National Information Center on Health Services Research and Health Care Technology (NICHSR) 2009]

Clinical pathways are used in different disciplines such as visceral surgery, neurosurgery, joint surgery, urology, internal medicine, emergency medicine, neurology and some pediatric subspecialties. A recent Medline search reveals 8771 hits on the search item: clinical pathways, for the years 2007–2009. Only 89 hits handle with Clinical Pathways, thereof 30 studies as clinical trials or meta-analyses. Most studies show a shortening of length of stay (LOS) and cost reduction. But no study has enough power to show a benefit when analysed with the help of the Cochrane Data base or similar evidence based medicine tools. It is an immanent problem that with the implementation of clinical

Child abuse – some aspects for neurosurgeons

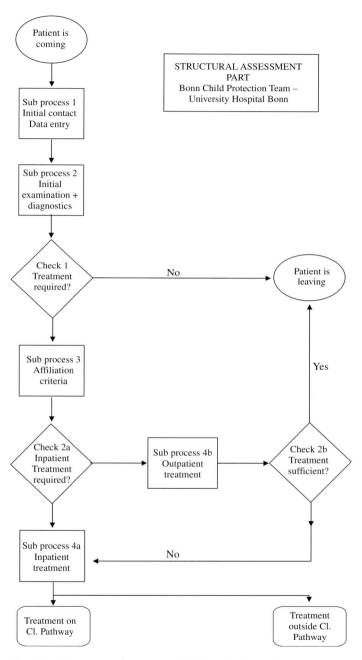

Fig. 23. Structure of a general Clinical Pathway (assessment part)

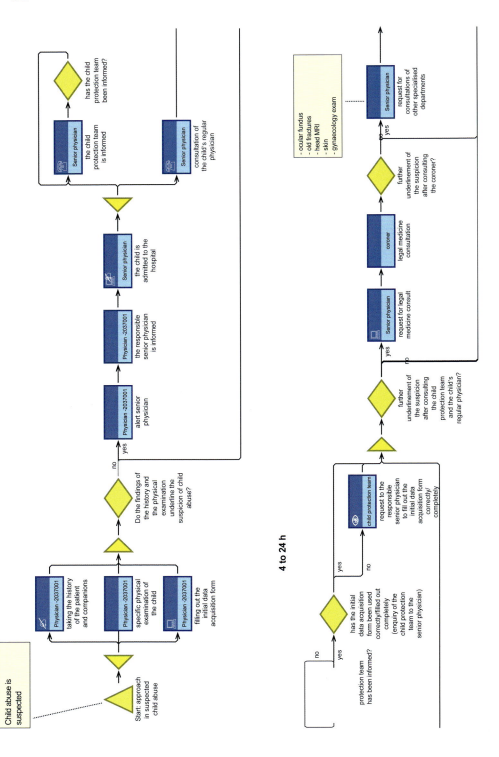

Child abuse – some aspects for neurosurgeons

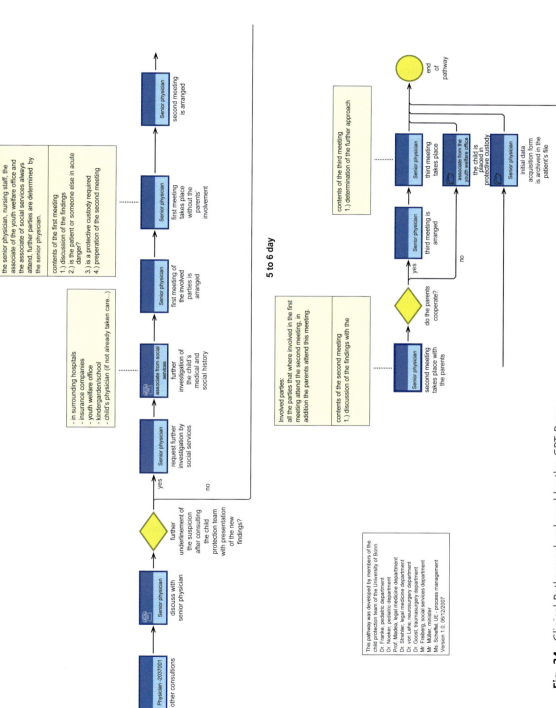

Fig. 24. Clinical Pathway developed by the CPT Bonn

pathways a randomized clinical trial (RCT) is debarred. Most studies compare treatment of patients before and after the adoption of clinical pathways, often in a retrospective view. Nevertheless clinical pathways facilitate the opportunities of a structural, based on best clinical practice, multidisciplinary team working on a timetable. To our knowledge the following clinical pathway is the first of its kind (in 2008 the presentation of this Clinical Path won the first poster price of the 104th annual meeting of the German Society of Paediatrics).

Bonn child protection team clinical pathway for suspected child abuse

Figure 23 shows the structure of a general Clinical Pathway (assessment part). In general the Clinical Pathway is split in 2 parts: 1. Assessment part 2. Treating part.

The Bonn CPT developed a Clinical Pathway to treat suspected abused children (Fig. 24). Since children are often presented in different policlinics, it is of great importance, that the whole staff knows the leading signals of child abuse and the Clinical Pathway. To avoid medical malpractice the first step of the Clinical Pathway for suspected child abuse should be the simple question: do you inform the CPT? The second question should be: have you got the special suspected child abuse sheet? The next steps in process take place automatically. Different consultants and examinations take place in a given order, if necessary. At the end of the Clinical Pathway the child is reported to the youth welfare office. In a conference with the parents or other caretakers of the child, clinicians and members of the CPT and of the youth welfare office decide the further inhabitation of the child in or outside the family. In cases of apparently life threatening abuse police or prosecution should be informed.

References

1. Allen Gamman J (1981) Ophthalmic manifestation of child abuse and neglect. In: Ellerstein NS (ed) Child Abuse and Neglect. A Medical Reference. J. Wiley, New York, pp 121–39
2. American Academy of Pediatrics (2000) Diagnostic imaging of child abuse (Statement from the Section on Radiology). Pediatrics 105: 1345–48
3. Arbogast KB, Margulies SS, Christian CW (2005) Initial neurologic presentation in young children sustaining inflicted and unintentional fatal head injuries. Pediatrics 116: 180–84
4. American Academy of Pediatrcis (2001) Committee on Child Abuse and Neglect. Shaken Baby Syndrome: Rotational cranial unjuries. Technical report. Pediatrics 108: 206–10
5. Bajanowski T, Neuen-Jacob E, Schubries M, Zweihoff R (2008) Nichtakzidentelles Schädel-Hirn-Trauma und Schütteltrauma. Rechtsmedizin 18: 23–28
6. Banaschak S, Schmidt P, Madea B (2003) Smothering of children older than 1 year of age – diagnostic significance of morphological findings. Forensic Sci Int 134: 163–68

Child abuse – some aspects for neurosurgeons 131

7. Banaschak S, Madea B (2007) Kindesmisshandlung. In: Madea B (Hrsg) Praxis Rechtsmedizin, 2. Aufl. Springer, Berlin Heidelberg New York, S 265–76

8. Barnes PM, Norton CM, Dunstan FD, *et al.* (2005) Abdominal injury due to child abuse. Lancet 366: 234–35

9. Bays J, Feldmann KW (2001) Child abuse by poisoning. In: Reece RM, Ludwig S (eds) Child Abuse – Medical Diagnosis and Management, 2nd edn. Lippincott Williams & Wilkins, Philadelphia Baltimore New York London, pp 405–42

10. Berendt C, Goos M, Thiel H, Hengge UR (2001) Painful-Bruising-Syndrom. Hautarzt, 52: 634–37

11. Brinkmann B, Banaschak S (1998) Verbrühungen bei einem Kleinkind. Unfall oder Kindesmisshandlung? Monatsschr Kinderheilkd 146: 1186–91

12. Byard RW, Cohle SD (1999) Sudden death in infancy, childhood and adolescence. Cambridge University Press, Cambridge

13. Caffey J (1946) Multiple fractures in the long bones of infants suffering from chronic subdural hematomas. Am J Roentgenol 56: 163–72

14. Cameron JM, Johnson HR, Cams FE (1966) The battered child syndrome. Med Sci Law 6: 2–21

15. Chapman S (1992) The radiological dating of fractures. Arch Dis Child 67: 1067–65

16. Chatwick DL, Chin S, Salerno C, *et al.* (1991) Deaths from falls in children: how far is fatal? J Trauma 31: 1353–55

17. Debertin AS, Sperhake JP (2008) Untersuchung und Dokumentation des nichtakzidentellen Schädel-Hirn-Traumas im Säuglings- und Kleinkindalter. Rechtsmedizin 18: 17–22

18. Duhaime AC, Christian CW, Rorke LB, Zimmermann RA (1998) Nonaccidental head injury infants – the "shaken baby syndrome". N Engl J Med 338: 1822–29

19. Duhaime AC, Alario AJ, Lewander WJ, Schut L, Sutton LN, Seidl TS, *et al.* (1992) Head injury in very young children: mechanisms, injury types, and ophthalmologic findings in 100 hospitalized patients younger than 2 years of age. Pediatrics 90: 179–85

20. Gaines BA, Schultz BS, Morrison K, Ford HR (2004) Duodenal injuries in children: Beware of achild abuse. J Pediatr Sur 39: 600–02

21. Gardner FH, Diamond LK (1955) A form of purpura producing painful bruising following autosensitisation in red blood cells in certain women. Blood 10(7): 675–90

22. Geddes JF, Hackshaw AK, Vowles GH, Nichols CD, Whitwell HL (2001) Neuropathology of inflicted heas injury in children. I. Patterns of brain damage. Brain 124: 1290–98

23. Geddes JF, Vowles GH, Hackshaw AK, *et al.* (2001) Neuropathology of inflicted head injury in children II. Microscopic brain injury in infants. Brain 124: 1299–306

24. Geddes JF, Plunkett J (2004) The evidence base for shaken baby syndrome. BMJ 328: 719–20

25. Gilliland MGE (1998) Interval duration between injury and severe symptoms in nonaccidental head trauma in infants and young children. J Forensic Sci 43: 723–25

26. Glaser D (2000) Child abuse and the brain – a review. J Child Psychol Psychiat 41: 97–116

27. Guthkelch AN (1971) Infantile subdural haematoma and its relationship to whiplash injuries. BMJ 2: 430–31

28. Hall JR, Reyes HM, Horvat M, Meller JL, Stein R (1989) The mortality of childhood falls. J Trauma 29: 1273–75

29. Helfer RE, Kempe CA (1968) The Battered Child. The University of Chicago Press
30. Helfer ME, Kempe RS, Krugmann RD (Hrsg) (2002) Das Misshandelte Kind. 5. Aufl. Suhrkamp, Frankfurt/M. (Übersetzung von: Helfer ME, Kempe RS, Krugmann RD (eds) (1999) The Battered Child, 5th edn. University of Chigaco Press)
31. Herrmann B (2002) Körperliche Misshandlung von Kindern. Somatische Befunde und klinische Diagnostik. Monatsschr Kinderheilkd 150: 1324–38
32. Herrmann B (2008) Nichtakzidentelle Kopfverletzungen und Schütteltrauma. Klinische und pathophysilogische Aspekte. Rechtsmedizin 18: 9–16
33. Hobbs CJ, Hanks HGI, Wynne JM (1999) Child Abuse and Neglect. A Clinician's Handbook, 2nd edn. Churchill Livingstone, Edinburgh
34. Hobbs CJ, Hanks HGI, Wynne JM (1999) Chapter 4, Physical abuse. In: Hobbs CJ, Hanks HGI, Wynne JM (eds) Child Abuse and Neglect. A Clinician's Handbook, 2nd edn. Churchill Livingstone, London, pp 47–75
35. Jacobi G (Hrsg) Kindesmisshandlung und Vernachlässigung. Epidemiologie, Diagnostik und Vorgehen. Verlag Hans Huber, Bern
36. Kempe CH, Silverman FN, Steele BF, Droegemueller W, Silver HK (1962) The battered child syndrome. JAMA 181: 17–24
37. Kirschbaum K, Musshoff F, Madea B (2009) Unclear loss of consciousness after clobutinol intake. Forensic Sci Int 189: 37–40
38. Kirschner RH, Wilson H (2001) Fatal child abuse: the pathologists perspective. In: Reece RM, Ludwig S (eds) Child Abuse: Medical Diagnosis and Management, 2nd edn. Lippincott Williams and Wilkins, Baltimore, pp 467–90
39. Kleinman PK (ed) (1998) Diagnostic imaging of child abuse, 2nd edn. Mosby, St. Louis Balitmore
40. Knight B (1986) The history of child abuse. Forensic Sci Int 30: 135–41
41. Krug EG, Dahlberg LL, Mercy JA, Zwi AB, Lozano R (2002) World report on violence and death. Genf World Health Organization
42. Lamb ME, Orbach Y, Hershkowitz I, Esplin PW, Horowitz D (2007) A structured forensic interview protocol improves the quality and informativeness of investigative interviews with children: a review of research using the NICHD Investigative Interview Protocol. Child Abuse Negl 31: 1201–31
43. Lazoritz S, Palusci VJ (eds) (2001) The Shaken Baby Syndrome. A Multidisciplinary Approach. The Haworth Maltreatment and Trauma Press, Binghamton; co-published as Journal of Aggression, Maltreatment and Trauma. Vol. 5, No. 1(#9) 2001
44. Lee LY, Ilan J, Mulvey T (2002) Human biting of children and oral manifestations of abuse. A case report and literature review. J Dent Child 69: 92–95
45. Leestma JE (2009) Forensic Neuropathology. CRC-Press, Boca Raton
46. Ludwig S (2001) Visceral injury manifestations of child abuse. In: Reece RM, Ludwig S (eds) Child Abuse – Medical Diagnosis and Management, 2nd edn. Lippincott Williams & Wilkins, Philadelphia Baltimore New York London, pp 157–76
47. Madea B (2005) Postmortem diagnosis of hypertonic dehydration. Forensic Sci Int 155: 1–6
48. Madea B (2005) Death as a Result of Starvation – Diagnostic Criteria. In: Tsokos M (ed) Forensic Pathology Reviews, Vol. 2. Humana Press, Totowa NJ, pp 1–23
49. Madea B (Hrsg) (2007) Praxis Rechtsmedizin, 2. Aufl. Springer, Berlin Heidelberg New York

50. Madea B, Banaschak S (2007) Verhungern. In: B. Madea (Hrsg) Praxis Rechtsmedizin. Befunderhebung – Rekonstruktion – Begutachtung. 2. Aufl. Springer, Berlin Heidelberg, S 196–200

51. Madea B, Preuß J (2005) Sturzverletzungen und ihre rechtsmedizinische Beurteilung. In: Bockholdt B, Ehrlich E (eds) Der Sturz: Morphologie. Forensische Begutachtung. Fallbeispiele. Festschrift für Volkmar Schneider. Berliner Wissenschafts-Verlag, Berlin, S 9–32

52. Madea B, Schmidt P (2007) Hitze: Lokale Hitzeschäden, Verbrennungen und Verbrühungen. In: Madea B (Hrsg) Praxis Rechtsmedizin. Befunderhebung – Rekonstruktion – Begutachtung. 2. Aufl. Springer, Berlin Heidelberg, S 175–85

53. Madea B, Henssge C, Berghaus G (1991) Fahrlässige Tötung eines Säuglings durch Fehlernährung. Arch Kriminol 189: 33–38

54. Madea B, Michalk DV, Lignitz E (1994) Verhungern infolge Kindesvernachlässigung. Kasuistik und gutachterliche Aspekte. Arch Kriminol 194: 29–38

55. Madea B, Preuß J, Lignitz E (2003) Unterkühlung: Umstände, morphologische Befunde und ihre Pathogenese. Rechtsmedizin 14: 41–49

56. Maguire S, Mann MK, Sibert J, Kemp A (2005) Can you age bruises accurately in children? A systematic review. Arch Dis Child 90: 187–89

57. Matschke J, Glatzel M (2008) Neuropathologische Begutachtung des nichtakzidentellen Schädel-Hirn-Traumas bei Säuglingen und Kleinkindern. Rechtsmedizin 18: 29–35

58. Maxeiner H (2008) Das Schütteltrauma von Säuglingen: Eine schwerwiegende Diagnose auf unsicherem Fundament? Archiv für Kriminologie 221: 65–86

59. Minns RA (2005) Shaken baby syndrome: Theoretical and evidential controversies. J Royal Coll Phys Edinburgh 35: 5–15

60. Minns RA, Busuttil A (2004) Patterns of presentation of the shaken-baby-syndrome: four types of inflicted brain injury predominate. BMJ 328: 766

61. Minns RA, Brown JK (eds) (2005) Shaking and Other Non Accidental Head Injuries in Children. Clinics in Developmental Medicine No. 162, Cambridge University Press/Mc Keith Press, Cambridge

62. Montelecone JA, Brodeur AE (1998) Child Maltreatment, Vol. 1: A Clinical Guide and Reference, Vol. 2: A Comprehensive Photographic Reference Identifying Potential Child Abuse, 2nd edn. C.W. Medical, St. Louis

63. Moritz AR, Henriques FC (1947) Studies of thermal injury II. The relative importance of time and surface temperature in the causation of cutaneous burns. Am J Pathol 23: 695–720

64. Moritz AR (1947) Studies of thermal injury III. The pathology and pathogenesis of cutaneous burns. An experimental study. Am J Pathol 23: 915–41

65. Musshoff F, Kirschbaum KM, Madea B (2008) Zwei Fälle von vermutetem Münchhausen-Syndrom-by-proxy. Arch Kriminol 222 (5/6): 162–69

66. Noeker M, Keller KM (2002) Münchhausen-by-Proxy-Syndrom als Kindesmisshandlung. Monatschr Kinderheilkd 150: 1357–69

67. Noeker M, Franke F, Musshoff F, Madea B (2010) Münchhausen-by-proxy-Syndrom. Rechtsmedizin 20: 223–37

68. Oehmichen M, Auer RN, König HG (2005) Forensic Neuropathology Associated Neurology. Springer, Berlin

69. Oehmichen M, Gerling I, Meissner C (2000) Petechiae of the baby's skin as differentiation symptoms of infanticide versus SIDS. J Forensic Sci 45: 602–07

70. Oehmichen M, Meissner C, Saternus KS (2005) Sturz oder Schütteln: Kindliches Schädel-Hirn-Trauma als Folge von Unfall oder Misshandlung. In: Bockholdt B, Ehrlich E (eds) Der Sturz. Morphologie, forensische Begutachtung, Fallbereichte. Berliner Wissenschaftsverlag, Berlin, pp 165–73
71. Oehmichen M, Schleiss D, Pedal I, et al. (2008) Shaken baby syndrome: re-examination of diffuse axonal injury as cause of death. Acta Neuropathol 116: 317–29
72. Olbing K, Bachmann KD, Gross R (1989) Kindesmisshandlung. Eine Orientierung für Ärzte, Juristen, Sozial- und Erziehungsberufe. Deutscher Ärzte-Verlag
73. Ounstead C (1975) Gaze aversion and child abuse. World Med 12: 27
74. Pearn J (1989) Physical abuse of children. In: Mason JK (ed) Pediatric Forensic Medicine and Pathology. Chapman and Hall Medical, London, pp 204–20
75. Püschel K, Richter E (2008) Schütteltrauma. Rechtsmedizin 18: 53–55
76. Reece RM, Christian CW (eds) (2008) Child Abuse: Medical Diagnosis and Management, 3rd edn. American Academy of Pediatrics, Elk Grove Village
77. Roaten JB, Prtrick DA, Bensard DD, et al. (2005) Visceral injuries in nonaccidental trauma: Spectrum of injury and outcomes. Am J Surg 190: 827–29
78. Saukko P, Knight B (2004) Fatal child abuse. In: Saukko P, Knight B (eds) Knight's Forensic Pathology, 3rd edn. Edward Arnold, London, pp 461–79
79. Schmidt P, Madea B (1995) Death in the Bathtub involving children. Forensic Sci Int 72: 147–55
80. Schmidt P, Grass H, Madea B (1996) Child homicide in cologne. Forensic Sci Int 79: 131–44
81. Schmitt BD (1987) The child with non accidental trauma. In: Helfer RE, Kempe RS (eds) The Battered Child. University of Chicago Press, pp 178–96
82. Schwartz AJ, Ricci LR (1996) How accurately can bruises be aged in abused children? Literature review and synthesis. Pediatrics 97: 254–57
83. Smarty S (2009) Battered child syndrome. In: Jamieson A, Moenssens A (eds) Wiley Encyclopaedia of Forensic Science, Vol. 1, pp 263–69
84. Sperhake J, Gehl A (2001) Cao Gio – Kindesmisshandlung oder Heilbehandlung? Rechtsmedizin 11: 101–03
85. Sperhake J, Herrmann B (2008) Schütteltrauma (nicht akzidentelle Kopfverletzung). Aktuelle Kontroversen. Rechtsmedizin 18: 48–52
86. Spevak MR, Kleinmann PK, Belanger PL, Primack C, Richmond JM (1994) Cardiopulmonary resuscitation and rib fractures in infants. A postmortem radiologic-pathologic study. JAMA 272: 617–18
87. Squier (2009) Shaken baby syndrome. In: Jamieson A, Moenssens A (eds) Wiley Encyclopaedia of Forensic Science, Vol. 5, pp 2339–50
88. Stierling and the American Academy of Pediatrics Committee on Child Abuse and Neglect (2007) Beyond Munchausen syndrome by proxy: identification and treatment of child abuse in a medical setting. Pediatrics 110: 985–88
89. Stöver B (2007) Bildgebende Diagnostik der Kindesmisshandlung. Radiologe 47: 1037–49
90. Stöver B (2008) Bildgebende Diagnostik der Kindesmisshandlung. Monatsschr Kinderheilkd 156: 385–98
91. Tardieu A (1860) Etude medico legal sur les services et mauvais traitments sur les enfants. Ann Hyg Pub Med Leg 13: 361–98

Child abuse – some aspects for neurosurgeons

92. Thyen U (1993) Kindesmisshandlung und Missbrauch als Ausdruck von Gewalt in der Familie. In: Kruse K, Oehmichen M (Hrsg) Kindesmisshandlung und sexueller Missbrauch. Rechtsmedizinische Forschungsergebnisse, Bd. 5 Schmidt-Römhild, Lübeck, S 11–24

93. Thyen U, Tegtmeyer FK (1991) Das Schütteltrauma des Säuglings – eine besondere Form der Kindesmisshandlung. Monatsschrift Kinderheilkunde 139: 292–96

94. Trube-Becker E (1982) Gewalt gegen das Kind. Kriminalistik Verlag, Heidelberg

95. UNICEF Innocenti Report Card Issue No. 5 September 2003

96. Weber W (1984) Experimentelle Untersuchungen zu Schädelbruchverletzungen des Säuglings. Z Rechtsmed 92: 87–94

97. Weber W (1985) Zur biomechanischen Fragilität des Säuglingsschädels. Z Rechtsmed 94: 93–101

98. Wynne J (2003) Child physical and emotional abuse. In: Payne-James J, Busuttil A, Smock W (eds) Forensic Medicine: Clinical and Pathological Aspects. Greenwhich Medical, London, pp 469–85

99. Williams RA (1991) Injuries in infants and small children resulting from witnessed and corroborated free falls. J Trauma 31: 350–52

Technical standards

Prophylactic antibiotics and anticonvulsants in neurosurgery

B. Ratilal[1] and C. Sampaio[2]

[1] Department of Neurosurgery, Hospital de São José, Centro Hospitalar de Lisboa Central, Lisboa, Portugal
[2] Laboratório de Farmacologia Clínica e Terapêutica, Faculdade de Medicina da Universidade de Lisboa, Lisboa, Portugal

With 8 Figures and and 3 Tables

Contents

Abstract 140
Introduction 140
Antibiotic prophylaxis 142
  Antibiotics for craniotomies 142
  Antibiotics for spinal surgeries 142
  Antibiotics for basilar skull fractures 143
    Background 143
    Clinical material and methods 143
    Results 146
  Non-RCTs that have been systematically reviewed 149
    Discussion 150
    Conclusions 151
  Antibiotics for cerebrospinal fluid shunts 151
    Background 151
    Clinical material and methods 152
    Results 153
    Discussion 166
    Conclusions 167
Anticonvulsant prophylaxis 168
  Anticonvulsants for subarachnoid hemorrhages 168
  Anticonvulsants for acute traumatic brain injuries 168
  Anticonvulsants for chronic subdural hematomas 169
    Background 169
    Clinical material and methods 169

Results 170
Discussion... 170
Conclusions 171
Anticonvulsants for brain tumors 172
Background 172
Clinical material and methods 172
Results 173
Discussion... 177
Conclusions 178
Commentaries 178
References... 178

Abstract

The prophylactic administration of antibiotics to prevent infection and the prophylactic administration of anticonvulsants to prevent first seizure episodes are common practice in neurosurgery. If prophylactic medication therapy is not indicated, the patient not only incurs the discomfort and the inconvenience resulting from drug treatment but is also unnecessarily exposed to adverse drug reactions, and incurs extra costs. The main situations in which prophylactic anticonvulsants and antibiotics are used are described and those situations we found controversial in the literature and lack further investigation are identified: anticonvulsants for preventing seizures in patients with chronic subdural hematomas, antiepileptic drugs for preventing seizures in those suffering from brain tumors, antibiotic prophylaxis for preventing meningitis in patients with basilar skull fractures, and antibiotic prophylaxis for the surgical introduction of intracranial ventricular shunts.

In the following we present systematic reviews of the literature in accordance with the standard protocol of *The Cochrane Collaboration* to evaluate the effectiveness of the use of these prophylactic medications in the situations mentioned. Our goal was to efficiently integrate valid information and provide a basis for rational decision-making.

Keywords: Antibiotics; anticonvulsants; brain tumor; chronic subdural hematoma; epilepsy; infection; prophylaxis; skull base fracture; systematic review; ventricular shunt.

Introduction

There are several conditions in neurosurgical practice in which prophylactic anticonvulsants for the prevention of first seizure episodes and prophylactic antibiotics for the prevention of infection are administered empirically, without satisfactory scientific support.

The use of prophylactic antibiotics in neurosurgery has long been controversial. Pennybacker *et al.* reported the first trial of a modern antibiotic in brain and spinal surgery in 1947, in which 501 craniotomies and 169 spinal operations performed during World War II were included [87]. The infection rate in penicillin-treated patients (0.9%) seemed to be inferior to historical controls (4.4%). After an initial period of enthusiasm, prophylactic antibiotics were abandoned by many neurosurgeons based on nonrandomized studies that suggested no benefit in their use. However, several trials published in the 1980s and early 1990s showed a consistent benefit for prophylactic antibiotics in neurosurgery [5, 7, 94, 95], although the use of prophylactic antibiotics also encourages the emergence of antibiotic-resistant bacterial strains [91]. Prophylactic antibiotics are used regularly in craniotomies, in spinal surgeries, in patients with basilar skull fractures, and in patients with cerebrospinal fluid (CSF) shunts.

Seizures are a burden, as they have a negative impact on quality of life, including effects on daily activities, independence, work, and driving. On the other hand, anticonvulsants can impair cognitive function in healthy volunteers and in patients with brain impairments [74, 119]. The negative effects of these drugs in children may persist even after drug withdrawal [69], and babies born to mothers exposed to antiepileptic drugs are at increased risk for major congenital malformations, cognitive impairment and fetal death [8]. Furthermore, cognitive dysfunction worsens with increases in anticonvulsant dosage, higher serum levels and polytherapy [111]. The incidence of acute side-effects can occur in up to 10% of the patients and include: cognitive impairment, myelosuppression, liver dysfunction, and dermatologic reactions – ranging from minor rashes to the life-threatening Stevens-Johnson syndrome. Anticonvulsants are frequently used to prevent first seizure episodes in patients with subarachnoid hemorrhages, in patients with acute traumatic brain injuries, in patients with chronic subdural hematomas, and in patients with brain tumors.

Traditional reviews are subject to bias introduced through incomplete literature searches, weighing evidence without a formal evaluation of its quality, and other forms of overt and covert bias that may influence the reader. The need for a systematic review – an overview of primary studies which includes explicit statements as to its objectives, materials and methods, and which has been conducted according to explicit and reproducible methodology – has been widely recognized. *The Cochrane Collaboration* focuses systematic review efforts on randomized controlled trials (RCTs) of therapeutic intervention. The strict methodology of a Cochrane systematic review includes a comprehensive literature search, an evaluation of the quality of studies therein, extraction and presentation of the relevant data, meta-analysis routines if possible, and an analysis of the reasons for variability in results. Meta-analysis is not simply the combining or averaging of the results of many studies but transforms results into standardized scores that can be compared and possibly combined across trials.

The goal of this article was to conduct high-quality, systematic reviews according to *The Cochrane Collaboration* standards to provide a basis for rational decision-making for those identified controversial issues that required further investigation [93–96, 115]. A description of each topic follows, highlighting the actual evidence of its effectiveness.

Antibiotic prophylaxis

Antibiotics for craniotomies

The effectiveness of prophylactic antibiotics in craniotomies was evaluated in a meta-analysis of published randomized studies comparing prophylactic antibiotics to a placebo [5]. This revision included eight RCTs of good methodological quality, each indicating that the treatment prevents wound infection. This meta-analysis allowed the confident conclusion that antibiotic prophylaxis reduces the wound infection rate in craniotomies by roughly fourfold. In fact, trials carried out later compare proposed new antibiotic regimens with one of those already demonstrated to be effective and not with placebo [89, 123]. Also, another systematic review that included 6 RCTs suggested a beneficial effect of antibiotics on postoperative meningitis, although not as strong as their effect on all deep infections combined [5].

Thus, a consensus appears to be developing that the question facing neurosurgeons is no longer whether to administer prophylactic antibiotics or not, but which antibiotics to use. Also, research on techniques for obtaining dural sealants and watertight skin closures is likely to make a larger contribution to eliminating post-craniotomy meningitis.

Antibiotics for spinal surgeries

Infection rates for spinal procedures are low, even without antibiotic prophylaxis. The benefit of prophylactic antibiotic therapy in spinal surgery was evaluated by a meta-analysis in which 12 clinical studies were included [5]. From these, six were RCTs and all reported a lower wound infection rate for antibiotic-treated patients, although the results were not statistically significant for any individual trial. Results strongly supported the practice of administering at least a single preoperative dose of an antibiotic active against Gram-positive organisms for spinal operations. In fact, recent trials are consistent with these findings [88]. The meta-analysis also concluded that the low risk associated with prophylactic antibiotic use and the substantial patient morbidity and financial costs of postoperative spinal infections justify treatment even when many patients must be treated to prevent a single infection and recommended that future trials of antibiotic prophylaxis in spinal surgery use an active control arm, rather than placebo treatment.

Antibiotics for basilar skull fractures

Background

The estimated incidence of basilar skull fracture (BSF) from non-penetrating head trauma varies between 7 and 15.8% of all skull fractures, with associated CSF leakage occurring in 2–20.8% of patients [16]. Clinical signs that may lead a physician to suspect a BSF include: CSF otorrhea or rhinorrhea; bilateral periorbital ecchymosis; Battle's sign; peripheral facial nerve palsy; hemotympanum or tympanic membrane perforation with blood in the external auditory canal; hearing loss; evidence of vestibular dysfunction; and anosmia. High-resolution bone computed tomographic (CT) scans have dramatically improved the radiological diagnosis of this type of fracture. BSFs are of special significance because the dura mater may be torn adjacent to the fracture site, placing the central nervous system (CNS) in contact with bacteria from the paranasal sinuses, nasopharynx or middle ear. If the dura mater is torn, CSF leakage can occur. BSF will predispose the patient to meningitis. A greater associated risk has been reported when CSF leakage exists, in particular, if it persists for more than seven days [65].

The role of prophylactic antibiotics in preventing bacterial meningitis in patients with BSF is disputed. Growing concern about the emergence of resistant organisms argues against their use. In addition, there are reports of higher incidences of meningitis in patients with BSF who have received prophylactic antibiotics [21].

Two meta-analyses yielded conflicting results. Brodie showed a statistically significant reduction in the incidence of meningitis with prophylactic antibiotic therapy for patients with posttraumatic CSF leakage [15]. Villalobos *et al.* concluded that antibiotic prophylaxis after a BSF does not appear to decrease the risk of meningitis, independent of whether or not CSF leakage has occurred [118]. These studies did not include an extensive review of the literature, both searched papers only until 1995 and 1996 respectively, and their conclusions were based mainly on retrospective and observational studies.

Clinical material and methods

We identified relevant trials following the optimal search strategy devised for The Cochrane Collaboration [30] through electronic searches of the Cochrane Central Register of Controlled Trials (CENTRAL) (The Cochrane Library, Issue 3, 2005), MEDLINE, EMBASE, and LILACS, from inception to September 2005. We also electronically searched meeting proceedings from the American Association of Neurological Surgeons (AANS) (1997 to June 2005) and hand-searched the abstracts from the

Table 1. *Characteristics of included studies ('Antibiotics for basilar skull fractures')*

Author and year	Type of stydy	No. of patients	Treatment group (No.)	Control group (No.)	Inclusion/exclusion criteria	Intervention	Primary outcomes	Allocation conceal-ment
Demetriades 1992 [28]	single center, controlled	37	14 + 11	12	Inclusion: open skull fracture or BSF (diagnosed radiologically or clinically). Exclusion: GCS < 6, neurosurgical intervention or major extracranial injuries. 196 patients enrolled, 39 withdrews (31 lost to follow up, 5 violations of the protocol, 3 deaths within 5 days). 37 patients with BSF included. Groups well matched for age, sex, cause of injury, type of fracture, GCS, bladder catheterization, endotracheal intubation.	group A: no AB; group B: ceftriaxone 1 g IV daily for 3 days; group C: combined ampicillin (1 g IV 6-hourly dose)/sulphadiazine (0.5 g IV 6-hourly dose for 3 days)	intracranial or extracranial infection: meningitis, brain abscess, wound sepsis, pneumonia, urinary tract infection.	unclear
Eftekhar 2004 [32]	single center, controlled, not blinded	109	53	56	Inclusion: acute traumatic pneumocephalus verified by CT scan. Exclusion: AB therapy for other reasons, penetrating traumatic brain injury/open skull fracture, surgery for any reason, discharge from hospital without doctor's approval, life-threatening lesions including severe brain, abdominal or vascular injuries, death from other causes. 2 groups well balanced with respect to their characteristics.	PAT + group: ceftriaxone 1 g twice a day for 5 days; PAT − group: no AB	meningitis (based on clinical and CSF findings)	unclear
Hoff 1976 [55]	single center, controlled,	160	NS	NS	Inclusion: BSF based on clinical or radiographic evidence. Exclusion: allergy to penicillin;	group 1: no AB; group 2: penicillin 1.2 million units IV	CNS infection	unclear

	blinded				CSF leakage immediately after injury.	daily for 3 days; group 3: penicillin 20 million units IV daily for 3 days.		
Ignelzi 1975 [57]	single center, controlled, blinded	10	5	5	Inclusion: BSF. Exclusion: NS.	treatment group: ampicillin or cephalothin 1 g 6-hourly dose for 10 days; control group: no AB.	CNS infection and change in posterior nasopharyngeal flora	unclear
Klastersky 1976 [60]	single center, placebo-controlled, double-blinded	52	26	26	Inclusion: recent cranial trauma and rhinorrhoea or otorrhoea. Exclusion: NS. 2 groups well matched for age, sex, presence of diseases other than cranial trauma, prognosis at time of admission.	treatment group: 5 mega units of penicillin G IV 6-hourly with a mean duration of 7.7 days (range 4–13 days); placebo group.	meningitis (positive CSF culture), possible CNS infection, other serious infection (pulmonary, urinary tract), death from brain damage, bacterial colonizations of bronchial secretions/urine	unclear

No. Number; AB antibiotic; PAT+ prophylactic antibiotic treatment given; PAT− prophylactic antibiotic treatment not given; NS not specified.

meeting proceedings of the European Association of Neurosurgical Societies (EANS) (1995–2003). In addition, we contacted researchers active in the field for information regarding unpublished trials and contacted authors of published trials for further information and unpublished data. We did not apply any language restrictions.

We considered for analysis RCTs comparing the use of prophylactic antibiotics versus placebo or no intervention in patients with basilar skull fractures. We also identified the non-RCTs to perform a separate meta-analysis to compare results. We included patients of any age with a recent BSF, independent of the presence and severity of CSF leakage. The type of intervention considered was either of the following: any antibiotic adminis-tered at the time of primary treatment of the BSF compared with placebo or no antibiotic. Trials comparing different antibiotics, different antibiotic dosages, routes of administration, or differences in the timing or duration of administration were excluded. The following outcome measures were evaluated: (1) frequency of meningitis: suspected clinically (fever, neck stiff-ness, deterioration of neurological status, headache) and confirmed by lum-bar puncture (CSF analysis including biochemistry, Gram stains and/or bacteriological cultures); (2) all-cause mortality/meningitis-related mortality; (3) need for surgical correction in patients with CSF leakage; and (4) non-CNS infection. Subgroup analyses for meningitis were performed if suffi-cient relevant information was available to determine differences in patients with versus without CSF leakage.

We analyzed clinical heterogeneity qualitatively, taking into account factors such as the population studied, type and dose of antibiotic used, methodologi-cal quality, number of patients excluded or lost to follow-up, and the outcome measures stated in the protocol. Sources of bias were investigated.

We performed statistical analyses using the statistical software provided by the Cochrane Collaboration [97].

Results

We found five RCTs comparing prophylactic antibiotics in BSF with placebo or no antibiotics (Table 1) [28, 32, 55, 57, 60]. All trials included patients with a clinical or radiological diagnosis of BSF. All studies stated that patients were randomized between the treatment and control groups although the precise methods of randomization and details as to the concealment of allocation were considered to be unclear in all trials. Entry criteria did not differ considerably. Exceptions were one trial [55] in which CSF leakage was an exclusion criterion, and another [60] in which patients had to have evidence of CSF leakage in order to be included. Two other trials [28, 32] included patients with and without CSF leakage. There was only one study in which the presence of CSF leakage was not specified [57]. The primary outcome for all trials included the occurrence of meningitis. Criteria for these diagnoses were based on clinical grounds, and further investigations and prophylactic medication were commenced as soon as the diagnosis of BSF was made in all trials. None of the studies reported data on outcomes as to the safety and tolerability of prophylactic antibiotics.

Overall, 368 patients were enrolled in these five studies. Two of them [32, 55] enrolled 73% of these patients. Since we could not access the number of patients included in each group of the Hoff trial [55], we could not include it in the meta-analysis. A total of 208 patients were analyzed from four RCTs: 109 patients in the treatment group and 99 in the control group. Only one study [60] was double-blind throughout, using identical appearance interventions (antibiotics or placebo). The other studies were not placebo-controlled and did not measure outcomes blindly. In addition, only two studies [28, 60] reported the number of and reasons for patients leaving the trials. In three trials [28, 32, 60] patients were well matched between the treatment and control arms for demographics, clinical status at admission and presence of rhinorrhea or otorrhea. The other trials [55, 57] did not describe the characteristics of the population included in each group. Data was analyzed on a per-protocol basis in all trials. The global quality of included trials was assessed by Jadad score [58]: one study scored 4 [60], two studies scored 2 [28, 55] and two studies scored 1 [32, 57].

We tested statistical heterogeneity between trial results using the I^2 test and found no evidence of heterogeneity in all the outcomes measured ($I^2 = 0\%$). Therefore we used fixed-effect models to synthesize data.

1. *Frequency of meningitis with subgroup analysis* (Figs. 1 and 2)
No significant differences were found for this outcome (Peto OR: 0.68; 95% CI: 0.28–1.65) (Fig. 1). In addition, no differences were found in the subgroups of patients with (Peto OR: 0.37; 95% CI: 0.06–2.24) or without (Peto OR: 0.77; 95% CI: 0.25–2.38) CSF leakage (Fig. 2).

2. *All-cause mortality/meningitis-related mortality* (Fig. 3)
We accessed relevant data from the four trials. No significant differences were found for all-cause mortality (Peto OR: 1.76; 95% CI: 0.41–7.60) or for meningitis-related mortality (Peto OR: 1.03; 95% CI: 0.06–16.44).

3. *Need for surgical correction in patients with CSF leakage*
Only one study [32] provided data for this secondary outcome and no patients in either the treatment or control group underwent surgical correction for CSF leakage in this trial.

4. *Non-CNS infection*
Only one study [60] provided data for this outcome. No significant differences were found (Peto OR: 0.62; 95% CI: 0.16–2.41).

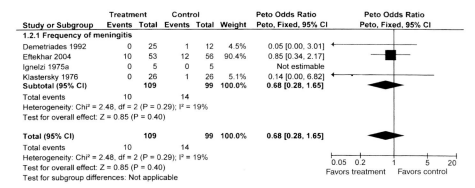

Fig. 1. Forest plot showing the effect of antibiotic prophylaxis *versus* placebo or no antibiotic for frequency of meningitis. *Squares* denote the point estimate of treatment effect (the area of the *squares* is proportional to the weight given to the information from the trial). *Horizontal lines* indicate 95% CI for individual trials. When the horizontal line crosses the vertical line marking no treatment effect, the individual study has not shown statistically significant evidence for the treatment effect. *Arrows* denote that the 95% CI extends beyond the values in the plot. The *diamond* represents the subtotal and total results of the meta-analysis, including the point estimate of treatment effect and the 95% CI

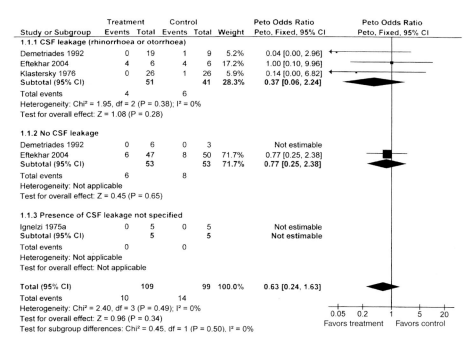

Fig. 2. Forest plot showing subgroup analysis for frequency of meningitis comparing patients with and without evidence of CSF leakage

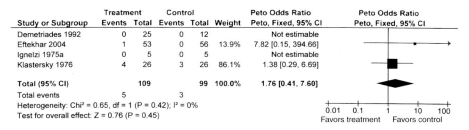

Fig. 3. Forest plot showing the effect of antibiotic prophylaxis for all-cause mortality

Non-RCTs that have been systematically reviewed

In order to study the consistency of these results we performed a meta-analysis of the 17 controlled non-randomized studies identified. Of these, 15 were retrospective controlled studies [3, 21, 24, 26, 34, 35, 41, 42, 52, 71, 72, 92, 112, 114, 130] and two were prospective observational studies with a historical control group [46, 57]. Overall, 2168 patients were included in these 17 studies, in which 1141 patients were treated with antibiotics and 1027 patients were not. Tests for heterogeneity were not statistically significant (Chi-squared $P=0.16$; $I^2 = 26\%$). Globally, the frequency of meningitis in the treatment group was 6.92% and in the control group 6.52% ($P=0.65$) (random-effects model OR: 1.13; 95% CI: 0.67–1.88). Individually, only one study [35] showed a significant difference favoring the treatment group (OR: 0.47; 95% CI: 0.25–0.88). This study contributed most to the results (weight 19.4%), but it did not significantly impact the direction of the results.

Additionally, we performed a subgroup analysis for patients with CSF leakage (529 patients in the treatment group and 260 in the control group) and without CSF leakage (334 patients in the treatment group and 292 in the control group). In five studies [3, 46, 52, 57, 114] the presence of CSF leakage was not specified (278 patients in treatment groups and 475 in control groups). The OR (random-effects model) for patients with CSF leakage was 0.61 (95% CI: 0.37–0.99) and for patients without CSF leakage it was 0.86 (95% CI: 0.27–2.78). In the subgroup of patients for which no data was available regarding the presence of CSF leakage, the OR was 2.01 (95% CI: 0.91–4.44). No statistically significant differences were found for all causes of mortality in the eight studies in which relevant data were available [3, 57, 34, 41, 42, 71, 72, 130]. These included 460 patients in the treatment group and 265 in the control group (random-effects model OR: 0.78; 95% CI: 0.26–2.28). No significant differences were found for meningitis-related mortality (random-effects model OR: 0.43; 95% CI: 0.08–2.29).

Discussion

The quality of the controlled evidence available to evaluate the use of prophylactic antibiotics in BSF was indicated by the identification of only five RCTs that we considered suitable for this review. Even these had important methodological shortcomings. In general, the quality of the trials included was poor, as reflected in the Jadad score [58]. In one trial [32] we had access to unpublished data that allowed us to perform some comparisons. We were able to study a total of 208 patients.

Curiously, the frequency of meningitis in one trial [32] was significantly higher than in the other trials. The diagnosis of meningitis was based on CSF analysis in patients with compatible clinical findings and was comparable with the other trials. However, this trial [32] included only the subset of patients with BSF and pneumocephalus, which is associated with a dural tear with an open communication of air in the paranasal sinuses, mastoid air cells or petrous temporal regions and the central nervous system (CNS). These patients with pneumocephalus may have had an additional risk factor for developing meningitis that was independent of CSF leakage. Further investigations are necessary to clarify this issue.

Given the current data, it is not possible to recommend the use of prophylactic antibiotics in patients with BSF. Our results did not show that the administration of antibiotics had an effect on the frequency of meningitis. No significant difference was found in the subgroup of patients with CSF leakage, although there was a tendency in favor of the treatment group. Again, no significant difference was found for all-cause or meningitis-related mortality. Although no significant differences were found, the CIs of all outcomes were wide. This is partially explained by the relatively small number of patients enrolled and the small number of events recorded.

The global results of the analysis of data extracted from the excluded studies are in agreement with the randomized data. Subgroup analysis within the excluded trials suggests a benefit from antibiotic prophylaxis in patients with CSF leakage. However, treatment interventions caused significantly more meningitis in the subgroup of patients without specification regarding CSF leakage status. These analyses should be read with caution, as they are based mostly on retrospective studies and the data is not randomized. Additionally, the type of participants, interventions, diagnoses and outcome measures were significantly different between these studies. This makes the data difficult to interpret. Nevertheless, we thought it would be interesting to compare data from RCTs with non-RCTs since non-randomized studies tend to overestimate treatment effect size, which may be the case here.

According to the frequencies of events in the treatment and control groups, and the relative risk of meningitis in the subgroup of patients with CSF leakage (0.64), a sample size of 798 patients was needed in order to show a statistically significant result between the two interventions, with a power of 90% and the probability of a type I error of 5%. This figure is similar when considering the data from the non-randomized case-controlled studies for the subgroup of patients with CSF leakage, for which the sample size necessary to show a significant result was 737 patients.

Conclusions

This systematic review did not show that prophylactic antibiotics had an effect on the prevention of meningitis in patients with BSF, regardless of CSF leakage. Currently available evidence from RCTs does not support the use of prophylactic antibiotics in patients with BSF. Future trials should evaluate all clinically relevant outcomes (all-cause mortality, need for surgical correction in patients with CSF leakage, disability), not merely CNS infection endpoints, and should pay attention to subgroups of patients, such as those with CSF leakage and/or pneumocephalus.

Antibiotics for cerebrospinal fluid shunts

Background

Approximately 40 of every 100,000 individuals in the United States have shunts in place, the majority of them children [75]. The most significant complication resulting from intracranial ventricular shunts is infection, and it affects from 1.5 to 38% of patients [23]. Age seems to be an important risk factor, with infection rates among young children of up to 20% [13, 108]. It is believed that younger people have higher morbidity rates because of infection, which is a cause for concern. The symptoms of shunt infection are variable; they may be related to the type of infective organism and may also be dependent on age. Shunt infection may be associated with increased risk of death, increased risk of seizure disorders, and decreased mental performance. Treatment usually requires prolonged hospitalization for antibiotic administration and repeated surgery.

It is not clear what mechanism predisposes a shunt to infection, given that the device is recognized by the body as a foreign object [14]. It is likely that the initial step in this process is a bacterial colonization of the device during the surgical procedure. A reduction of normal defense mechanisms and local immunity caused by the foreign object follows, as does a complex and effective adhesion process between the bacteria and device. These have a role in postoperative device-related infections. However, the benefit of systemic antibiotic prophylaxis is not generally accepted, and its use is frequently a matter of discussion. In fact, some authors found no relationship between infection and the use of systemic prophylactic antibiotics [105, 113]. A meta-analysis performed by Langley *et al.* showed a 50% reduction in the risk of infection for internal shunts if perioperative prophylaxis was used, that is, if prophylaxis was maintained for 24–72 hours after surgery [63]. Another meta-analysis focused on data that was strongly correlated with a high baseline infection rate [51]. The benefit associated with antibiotics was no longer apparent when the baseline infection was less than or equal to 5%. These studies did not constitute an extensive and comprehensive review of the literature, and the papers included were searched until 1990 in the former study and 1993 in the latter.

Nevertheless, continuous prophylactic antibiotics are widely administered to patients with external ventricular drains (EVDs), despite a paucity of data supporting their use. There is no evidence of a difference in the rate of CSF infection in patients with EVDs who received continuous prophylactic antibiotics for the duration of drain placement compared with those who received only periprocedural dosing (started immediately before placement of the drain and continued for no more than 3 doses or less than 24 hours) [1]. The advent and growing use of the newly developed antibiotic-impregnated shunts (AIS) also demanded an evidence-based investigation of their effectiveness and safety compared with standard shunt systems.

Clinical material and methods

We identified relevant trials following the optimal search strategy devised for The Cochrane Collaboration [30] through electronic searches of CENTRAL (The Cochrane Library, Issue 3, 2005), MEDLINE, EMBASE, and LILACS, from inception to June 2005. We also electronically searched meeting proceedings from the AANS (1997 to June 2005) and hand-searched the abstracts from the meeting proceedings of the EANS (1995–2003). In addition, we contacted researchers active in the field for information regarding unpublished trials and contacted authors of published trials for further information and unpublished data. We did not apply any language restrictions.

We considered for analysis randomized and quasi-randomized studies comparing the use of prophylactic antibiotics in intracranial ventricular shunt procedures with placebo or the standard treatment. We included patients of any age who had undergone any type of intracranial ventricular CSF shunt surgical procedure. We excluded patients with either suspected or confirmed preexisting infection. Infection was defined according to the study investigator's criteria. The types of intervention considered were the following two: systemic administration of any antibiotic(s), at any dosage, beginning prior to or at the time of the surgical procedure and prolonged for any duration of time compared with placebo or no antibiotics; or use of AIS systems compared with standard shunt systems. Trials comparing different antibiotics, different dosages, different routes of administration, or differences in the timing or duration of administration were excluded. The following outcome measures

Prophylactic antibiotics and anticonvulsants

were evaluated: (1) evidence of infection in at least 1 of the following: shunt equipment, overlying wound, CSF, or site related to the distal drainage route; organism identification by tissue cultures from material in or around the shunt; or cultures from fluid or CSF drawn from the shunt system itself; (2) death resulting from central nervous system infection or other cause of death including progression of the primary disease process and multisystem failure; (3) shunt revision (part or all of a shunt system); and (4) adverse events caused by antibiotics according to the original authors' categorization. Subgroup analyses for shunt infection were performed if sufficient relevant information was available to determine differences in the following: (1) the risk of infection developing in ventriculo-peritoneal (VP) shunts versus ventriculo-atrial (VA) shunts; (2) the risk of infection developing in children versus all ages; and (3) the risk of infection when using periprocedural antibiotics versus continuous antibiotics.

We analyzed clinical heterogeneity qualitatively, taking into account factors such as the population studied, surgical procedure, and technique. We performed statistical analyses using the statistical software provided by the Cochrane Collaboration [97]. We investigated for statistical heterogeneity between trial results using the I^2 statistic [53]. We calculated the number needed to treat based on meta-analysis estimates, and did not treat the data as if it arose from a single trial, given that the latter approach is more prone to bias [2]. We assessed the difference between subgroups by calculating a two-tailed z-score. Because there is evidence that the quality of allocation concealment particularly affects the results of studies, we scored this quality on the scale used by Schulz *et al.* [106].

Results

We identified 21 potentially eligible trials, of which 17 were included in the review (Table 2) (3 excluded [36, 107, 110] and one duplicate citation [77]). We conducted different analyses to reflect the clinical heterogeneity resulting from interventions that are fundamentally different, separating systemic antibiotics from AIS systems and internal shunts from external drains. Overall, 1684 patients were enrolled in the 15 studies that were included in a meta-analysis in which the effectiveness of systemic antibiotic prophylaxis for internal shunts was evaluated [9, 11, 12, 17, 31, 50, 82, 99, 100, 105, 120, 121, 124, 126, 128]. Two other trials identified evaluated the use of antibiotic-impregnated catheters for the surgical introduction of ventricular drains, one of which studied the benefit of AIS for internal shunts (110 shunts) [47] and the other evaluated its benefit for external drains (288 drains) [127]. Entry criteria did not differ considerably between the trials included. Shunt infection was a primary outcome in all trials and was always based on clinical and laboratory grounds. Sufficient information on the withdrawals and dropouts to determine the number of patients in each treatment group entering and completing the trial

Table 2. *Characteristics of included studies ('Antibiotics for cerebrospinal fluid shunts')*

Author and year	Type of study	No. of patients	Treatment group (No.)	Control group (No.)	Inclusion/exclusion criteria	Intervention	Primary outcomes	Allocation concealment
Bayston 1975 [9]	single center, controlled, not blinded	132	54	78	Inclusion: children undergoing shunt operation. Exclusion: NS. Characteristics of each group not described. Baseline for variables between groups not performed.	1st phase: control group and AB group (cloxacillin IM 1 hour preop and 6 hours after); 2nd phase: control group and AB group (gentamicin IM 1 hour preop and 6 hours after)	wound infection and colonized shunts	unclear
Blomstedt 1985 [11]	single center, placebo-controlled, double-blinded	174	62 + 25	60 + 27	Inclusion: all patients > 12 yrs undergoing a ventriculoatriostomy or external ventriculostomy. Exclusion: patients < 12 yrs, allergy to sulfa/trimethoprim, patients receiving antibiotics during preceding week, patients already with shunt in place. 174 patients enrolled in the trial (62 in group 1, 60 in group 2, 25 in group 3 and 27 in group 4); 26 excluded (19 regimen not completed, 6 received other AB, 1 suspected allergic reaction). Age, sex, incidence of malignant tumors similar in 2 treatment groups.	for shunting procedures: Group 1 (trimethoprim 90 mg sulphametoxazole 400 mg×3 12-hourly); Group 2 (placebo). For external ventriculostomies: Group 3 (trimethoprim 90 mg-sulphametoxazole 400 mg 12-hourly until drainage tube removal); Group 4: (placebo)	shunt infection	unclear

Prophylactic antibiotics and anticonvulsants   155

Study	Design				Inclusion / Exclusion	Intervention	Outcome	Quality
Blum 1989 [12]	single center, placebo-controlled, single-blinded	100	50	50	Inclusion: all children >14 yrs operated for hydrocephalus. Exclusion: hypersensitivity to drug selected, AB therapy in previous 7 days or another AB in posterior 10 days, concurrent infections, immunosuppressive therapy/immunodeficiency, agammaglobulinemia, agranulocytosis, leukemia, severe anemia, lymphoma, thymus aplasia, liver cirrhosis, burns, uremia, diabetes mellitus and factors impairing wound healing. 100 of 169 patients met inclusion criteria. Age and sex similar in 2 treatment groups.	treatment group: single-dose cefazedone 50 mg/kg body-weight; placebo group	shunt infection	inadequate
Bullock 1988 [17]	single center, placebo-controlled, double-blinded	104	48	56	Inclusion: patients (regardless of age) undergoing elective neurosurgical procedure. Exclusion: piperacillin hypersensitivity/allergy, neurosurgical op in previous month, any AB therapy previous 7 days. 417 patients enrolled in which 104 were VP shunts. 2 groups well matched for age, sex, hospital stay,	treatment group: piperacillin 2 g IV commenced between 30 and 60 min prior to op incision and 2 further 6-hourly doses; placebo group	sepsis	inadequate

(continued)

Table 2 *(continued)*

Author and year	Type of study	No. of patients	Treatment group (No.)	Control group (No.)	Inclusion/exclusion criteria	Intervention	Primary outcomes	Allocation conceal-ment
Djindjian 1986 [31]	single center, controlled, not blinded	60	30	30	op time and duration of vacuum drainage. Inclusion: patients (regardless of age) receiving 1st shunt. Exclusion: no AB in previous 14 days, previous ventricular drainage, replacement of previously implanted shunt. Baseline for variables between groups not performed.	treatment group: oxacillin 200 mg/kg/day IV 4-hourly for 24 hours (6×2 g for adult); control group	CSF infection	unclear
Govender 2003 [47]	multicenter, controlled, single-blinded	153	50	60	Inclusion: patients (regardless of age) with hydrocephalus identified primarily as uninfected. Exclusion: CSF infection before or at time of shunt insertion, pregnancy/lactancy, sensitivity to rifampicin/clindamycin, or open and uncorrected myelomeningocele/encephalocele. 153 patients enrolled, 43 excluded (19 died before appropriate follow-up period, 7 protocol violations, 2 CSF infection	AIS group: patients receiving AIS with clindamycin and rifampicin; control group: patients receiving standard unishunt system that lacked any AB agent.	shunt infection	unclear

					at the time of shunt insertion, 15 missed follow-up). No difference in median follow-up period between groups.		
Haines 1982 [50]	single center, placebo-controlled, double-blinded	76	35	39	Inclusion: children < 17 yrs for insertion/revision of CSF shunts. Exclusion: allergy to penicillin, patients on AB therapy. 76 patients enrolled. 2 excluded due to CSF infection at time of op. 2 groups well matched for age, sex, previous shunt infection, presence of spina bifida, 1st shunt placement, CSF glucose, protein or WBC values.	AB group: methicillin 12.5 mg/kg 6-hourly beginning 6 hours preop, during induction of anaesthesia, and continuing for 72 hours; placebo group	shunt unfection and shunt malfunc-tion	inadequate
Odio 1984 [82]	multicenter, placebo-controlled, double-blinded	37	18	17	Inclusion: children undergoing shunt procedures. Exclusion: laboratory evidence of hepatic/renal disease, AB received in previous 72 hours. 37 patients enrolled. 2 excluded because of adverse reactions to AB in 1st dose. Baseline for variables between groups not performed.	treatment group: vancomycin 15 mg/kg IV one hour preop and 6 hours later; placebo group	shunt infection and adverse effects of AB	adequate
Rieder 1987 [99]	single center, placebo-controlled,	63	31	32	Inclusion: children for elective VP shunt insertion. Exclusion: evidence of	treatment group: cephalothin 25 mg/kg or 2 g max IV	shunt infection and shunt	adequate

(continued)

Table 2 *(continued)*

Author and year	Type of study	No. of patients	Treatment group (No.)	Control group (No.)	Inclusion/exclusion criteria	Intervention	Primary outcomes	Allocation conceal-ment
	double-blinded				active infection, previous shunt infection, immunosuppressed, corticosteroid therapy, allergies to penicillin/cephalothin, AB therapy in previous 4 weeks. 2 groups well matched for age, sex, history of CSF infection and duration of surgery.	preincision and 3 further 6-hourly doses; placebo group	malfunc-tion	
Rocca 1992 [100]	single center, controlled	27	13	14	Inclusion: patients (regardless of age) submitted to craniotomy or shunt placement. Exclusion: infection or AB in previous 15 days, allergy to β-lactams, urgent ops and reinterventions. 78 patients enrolled in which 27 shunt procedures. Baseline for variables between groups not performed.	treatment group: cefamandole 1.5 g IV 1 hour preop and 3 8-hourly doses; control group	local and remote infections	unclear
Schmidt 1985 [105]	multicenter, controlled, not blinded	152	79	73	Inclusion: patients (regardless of age) for shunt insertion/revision. Exclusion: AB given or signs of infection in	AB group: methicillin 200 mg/kg in 6 doses during 24 hours starting at induction of anaesthesia;	shunt infection	adequate

						control group		
					preceding 4 weeks. 2 groups well matched for age, sex, aetiology of hydrocephalus, observation time, method of shunt and duration of op.			
Walters 1992 [120]	single center, placebo-controlled, double-blinded	294	130	113	Inclusion: children undergoing CSF shunt procedure. Exclusion: shunt infection, concomitant systemic infection, allergies to rifampicin/trimethoprim. 294 enrolled, 51 withdrew (15 lost to follow-up and 36 infected at time of initial op); Baseline for variables between groups not performed.	treatment group: rifampicin 20 mg/kg and trimethoprim 5 mg/kg per day in divided doses, the 1st 2 hours preop and 8-hourly for further 48 hours; placebo group	shunt infection	unclear
Wang 1984 [121]	single center, placebo-controlled, double-blinded	127	55	65	Inclusion: children undergoing VP shunt op. Exclusion: shunt infection in preceding month, AB within previous week, allergy to trimethoprim/ sulfamethoxazole. 127 patients enrolled, 7 withdrew (unsuspected shunt infection diagnosed at time of op); 2 groups were well matched for age, sex, history of shunt infection and duration of op.	treatment group: trimethoprim 5 mg/kg/ sulfamethoxazole 25 mg/kg IV during 1 hour preop and 2 more 8-hourly doses; placebo group	shunt infection and shunt malfunction	adequate
Yogev	single center,	190	106	84	Inclusion: all children for	treatment group:	shunt	unclear

(continued)

Table 2 *(continued)*

Author and year	Type of study	No. of patients	Treatment group (No.)	Control group (No.)	Inclusion/exclusion criteria	Intervention	Primary outcomes	Allocation conceal-ment
1985 [124]	placebo-controlled				VP shunt replacement/ revision. Exclusion: NS.	nafcillin alone or nafcillin and rifampicin 200 mg/kg/day and 20 mg/kg/day started 13 hours preop and continued for 48 hours; placebo group	infection	
Young 1987 [126]	multicenter, controlled, single blinded	133	64	69	Inclusion: clean neurosurgical procedure (regardless of age). Exclusion: evidence of concurrent infection, AB in previous week, allergies to cephalosporin/aminoglyco-noglycosides. 846 patients enrolled, 16 excluded (8 in each group and none had infection – 4 used AB in prior week, 2 inadvertent administration of AB follow-ing op, 4 unsuspected brain abscess, 1 preop infection and 5 inability to verify that study was performed according to protocol. 2 groups well matched for sex, and duration of op.	treatment group: cefazolin 1 g and gentamicin 80 mg or 1 mg/kg and 25 mg/kg in children, IV, 1 hour preincision and repeated 6-hourly throughout op; control group	postop infection	adequate
Zabramski 2003	multicenter, controlled	288	149	139	Inclusion: all hospitalized patients (>18 yrs) for	treatment group: catheter impregnated	CSF infection	adequate

| [127] | | | | | placement of EVD. Exclusion: pregnancy, allergies tetracycline/ rifampicin, dermatitis/ infection at catheter insertion site, CSF shunt within previous 30 days, known/suspected CSF infection, need for placement of >1 ventricular catheter, and uncorrected coagulopathy. 306 patients enrolled, 18 excluded (14 with EVD less than 24 hours, 4 CSF culture revealed infection). 2 groups well matched for age, sex, indication for catheter placement and length of time catheter remained in place. | with minocycline and rifampicin; control group: standard non-impregnated silicone catheter. | | |
| Zentner 1995 [128] | single center, controlled | 129 | 67 | 62 | Inclusion: all patients (regardless of age) undergoing CSF shunting. Exclusion: NS. 2 groups well matched for age, aetiology of hydrocephalus, shunting procedure, shunt type, risk factors, duration of op, and duration of preop hospitalization. | treatment group: cefotiam 150 mg/kg IV for children and 2 g for adults after induction of anaesthesia and before skin incision; control group | shunt infection | adequate |

NS not specified; AB Antibiotic; AIS antibiotic-impregnated system.

was only available in 4 trials [82, 105, 121, 126]. Data was presented on a per-protocol basis in all trials. Missing data precluded the conducting of some planned analysis in this systematic review, although we contacted the authors of the studies whenever we deemed this necessary.

Assuming that significant statistical heterogeneity is not present if $I^2 = 50\%$, we found no evidence of heterogeneity for any of the groups in the outcomes measured. Therefore we used fixed-effect models to synthesize data.

1. *Shunt infection*
1.1 Systemic antibiotic prophylaxis
1.1.1 Systemic antibiotic prophylaxis for internal shunts (Fig. 4)
Analysis of the 15 trials included (1684 patients) found a statistically significant difference for shunt infection that favored treatment (OR: 0.51, 95% CI: 0.36–0.73; number needed to treat 12, 95% CI: 7–30). Individually, only 1 trial was statistically significant [11]. Two trials favored the control group, although they were not significant [100, 105].

1.1.2 Systemic antibiotic prophylaxis for external shunts
Authors of only 1 trial [11] evaluated the benefit of antibiotic prophylaxis in external shunts and did not find any difference between groups.

1.2 Antibiotic-impregnated catheters
1.2.1 Antibiotic-impregnated catheters for internal shunts
One trial [47] was found that showed a trend that favored the treatment group, although it was not statistically significant (OR: 0.32, 95% CI: 0.08–1.23).

Study or Subgroup	Treatment Events	Total	Control Events	Total	Weight	Odds Ratio M-H, Fixed, 95% CI
2.1.1 Internal shunts						
Bayston 1975	1	54	4	78	3.7%	0.35 [0.04, 3.21]
Blomstedt 1985	4	62	14	60	15.3%	0.23 [0.07, 0.73]
Blum 1989	3	50	7	50	7.6%	0.39 [0.10, 1.61]
Bullock 1988	1	48	3	56	3.1%	0.38 [0.04, 3.74]
Djindjian 1986	1	30	6	30	6.7%	0.14 [0.02, 1.23]
Haines 1982	2	35	5	39	5.1%	0.41 [0.07, 2.27]
Odio 1984	3	18	4	17	4.0%	0.65 [0.12, 3.46]
Rieder 1987	2	31	3	32	3.2%	0.67 [0.10, 4.29]
Rocca 1992	1	13	0	14	0.5%	3.48 [0.13, 93.30]
Schmidt 1985	7	79	4	73	4.4%	1.68 [0.47, 5.98]
Walters 1992	15	130	21	113	22.9%	0.57 [0.28, 1.17]
Wang 1984	4	55	5	65	4.9%	0.94 [0.24, 3.69]
Yogev 1985	2	106	6	84	7.6%	0.25 [0.05, 1.27]
Young 1987	1	64	2	69	2.2%	0.53 [0.05, 6.01]
Zentner 1995	5	67	8	62	8.9%	0.54 [0.17, 1.76]
Subtotal (95% CI)		**842**		**842**	**100.0%**	**0.51 [0.36, 0.73]**
Total events	52		92			

Heterogeneity: Chi² = 10.02, df = 14 (P = 0.76); I² = 0%
Test for overall effect: Z = 3.66 (P = 0.0002)

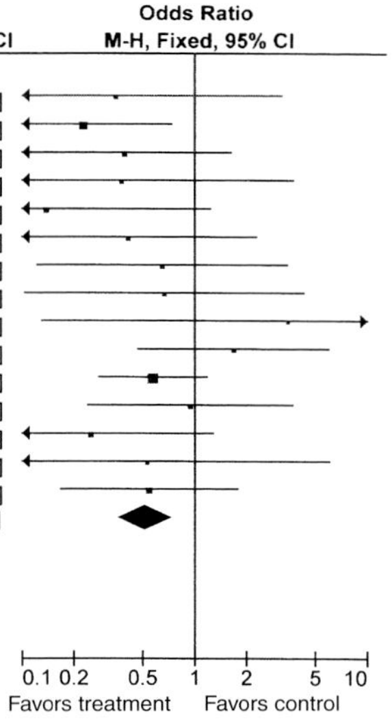

0.1 0.2   0.5   1   2   5   10
Favors treatment   Favors control

Fig. 4. Forest plot showing the effect of systemic antibiotic prophylaxis *versus* placebo or no antibiotic for shunt infection

Prophylactic antibiotics and anticonvulsants 163

1.2.2 Antibiotic-impregnated catheters for external shunts
The only trial [127] identified found a benefit favoring the treatment group (OR: 0.13, 95% CI: 0.03–0.60).

2. *Death from any cause*
2.1 Systemic antibiotic prophylaxis
We could not analyze this outcome because there was only 1 trial [105] in which the authors reported this outcome, and there were no events.
2.2 Antibiotic-impregnated catheters
We were able to access relevant data from the two trials [47, 127] that evaluated antibiotic-impregnated catheters, and neither one showed differences between groups.

3. *Shunt revision*
3.1 Systemic antibiotic prophylaxis
3.1.1 Systemic antibiotic prophylaxis for internal shunts
Three trials [50, 99, 121] involving 248 patients provided relevant data regarding the outcome "need of shunt revision" in both treatment and control groups. We found no significant difference between groups (OR: 0.76, 95% CI: 0.42–1.36).
3.1.2 Systemic antibiotic prophylaxis for external shunts
No data available.
3.2 Antibiotic-impregnated catheters
3.2.1 Antibiotic-impregnated catheters for internal shunts
Govender *et al.* [47] reported the only eligible trial (9 of 50 occurrences *versus* 15 of 60 controls), and we found no significant difference between the groups (OR: 0.66, 95% CI: 0.26–1.67).
3.2.2 Antibiotic-impregnated catheters for external shunts
No data available.

4. *Adverse events of antibiotics*
Only 2 trials [82, 128] enrolling 163 patients reported the incidence of the adverse events of systemic antibiotics in internal shunts (8%, 7 of 87 occurrences). The eventual adverse effects of systemic antibiotics from external shunts or antibiotic-impregnated shunts were not reported in the eligible trials.

Subgroup analyses

1. *Ventriculo-peritoneal shunts versus ventriculo-atrial shunts*
1.1 Systemic antibiotic prophylaxis
We were able to include 13 trials in this subgroup analysis, which enrolled 1416 patients. Subgroup analyses for the effect of prophylactic systemic antibiotics of

different types of internal shunts found a significant difference between treatment and control groups for both VA shunts (OR: 0.46, 95% CI: 0.23–0.94) and VP shunts (OR: 0.54, 95% CI: 0.34–0.85). No difference was found between the two subgroups (systemic antibiotics for VP *versus* VA shunts; $P = 0.2$).

1.2 Antibiotic-impregnated catheters
We did not find any relevant data.

2. *Children (under 18 years of age) versus all ages*

2.1 Systemic antibiotic prophylaxis
Subgroup analyses regarding the effect of prophylactic systemic antibiotics for internal shunts found a significant difference between treatment and control groups for both the subgroup of trials that included only children (OR: 0.52, 95% CI: 0.33–0.83) and the subgroup of trials that included patients of all ages (OR: 0.52, 95% CI: 0.30–0.90). No difference was found between the two subgroups (systemic antibiotics for children *versus* all ages; $P = 0.06$).

2.2 Antibiotic-impregnated catheters
No data available.

Study or Subgroup	Treatment Events	Total	Control Events	Total	Weight	Odds Ratio M.H, Fixed, 95% CI
Bayston 1975	1	54	4	78	3.7%	0.35 [0.04, 3.21]
Blomstedt 1985	4	62	14	60	15.3%	0.23 [0.07, 0.73]
Blum 1989	3	50	7	50	7.6%	0.39 [0.10, 1.61]
Bullock 1988	1	48	3	56	3.1%	0.38 [0.04, 3.74]
Djindjian 1986	1	30	6	30	6.7%	0.14 [0.02, 1.23]
Odio 1984	3	18	4	17	4.0%	0.65 [0.12, 3.46]
Rieder 1987	2	31	3	32	3.2%	0.67 [0.10, 4.29]
Rocca 1992	1	13	0	14	0.5%	3.48 [0.13, 93.30]
Schmidt 1985	7	79	4	73	4.4%	1.68 [0.47, 5.98]
Wang 1984	4	55	5	65	4.9%	0.94 [0.24, 3.69]
Young 1987	1	64	2	69	2.2%	0.53 [0.05, 6.01]
Zentner 1995	5	67	8	62	8.9%	0.54 [0.17, 1.76]
Subtotal (95% CI)		571		606	64.4%	0.53 (0.34, 0.83)

Total events 33 60
Heterogeneity: Chi² = 9.06, df = 11 (P = 0.62); I² = 0%
Test for overall effect: Z = 2.81 (P = 0.005)

5.1.2 Continuous antibiotics

Haines 1982	2	35	5	39	5.1%	0.41 [0.07, 2.27]
Walters 1992	15	130	21	113	22.9%	0.57 [0.28, 1.17]
Yogev 1985	2	106	6	84	7.6%	0.25 [0.05, 1.27]
Subtotal (95% CI)		271		236	35.6%	0.48 (0.26, 0.88)

Total events 19 32
Heterogeneity: Chi² = 0.88, df = 2 (P = 0.65); I² = 0%
Test for overall effect: Z = 2.37 (P = 0.02)

Total (95% CI)		842		842	100.0%	0.51 (0.36, 0.73)

Total events 52 92
Heterogeneity: Chi² = 10.02, df = 14 (P = 0.76); I² = 0%
Test for overall effect: Z = 3.66 (P = 0.0002)

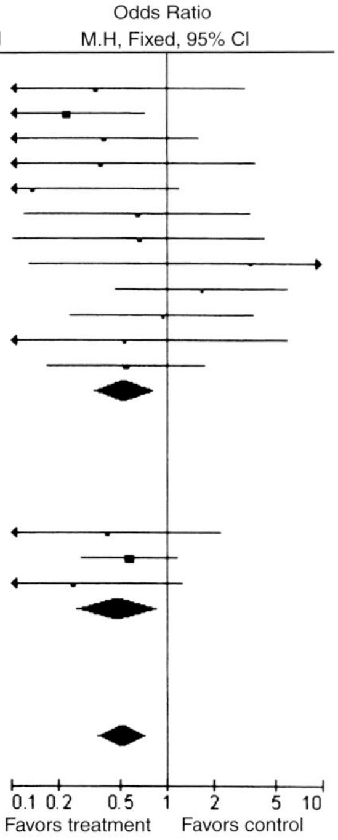

0.1 0.2   0.5   1   2   5 10
Favors treatment   Favors control

Fig. 5. Forest plot showing subgroup analysis for internal shunt infection comparing periprocedural and continuous systemic antibiotics

3. *Periprocedural systemic antibiotics (less than 24 hours postoperatively) versus continuous systemic antibiotics (prolonged for more than 24 hours postoperatively)*

3.1 Systemic antibiotic prophylaxis

We were able to include the 15 trials that used systemic prophylactic antibiotics for the subgroup analysis of prophylactic periprocedural systemic antibiotics versus continuous systemic antibiotics for internal shunts (Fig. 5). Both subgroups showed a significant difference compared with placebo/no antibiotics (OR: 0.53, 95% CI: 0.34–0.83 and OR: 0.48, 95% CI: 0.26–0.88). No additional benefit was found when continuous antibiotics were compared with periprocedural administration ($P = 0.0002$).

No sufficient available data for evaluating periprocedural *versus* continuous antibiotics for external ventricular drains.

3.2 Antibiotic-impregnated catheters
Not applicable.

Sensitivity analysis

We performed a sensitivity analysis for well-allocated as opposed to poorly or unclearly allocated trials regarding the use of systemic antibiotics for internal

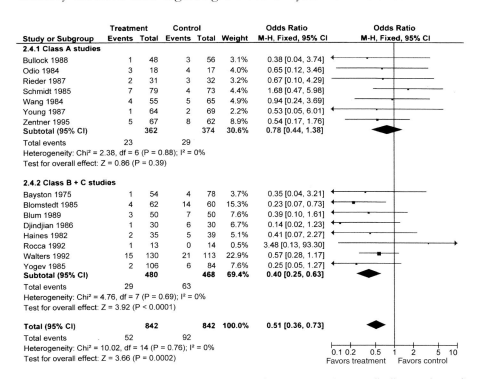

Fig. 6. Forest plot showing sensitivity analysis comparing well-allocated studies (Class A) versus unclear (Class B) or poorly allocated (Class C) studies

shunt infection (Fig. 6). Authors of trials deemed to have taken adequate measures to conceal allocation [17, 82, 99, 105, 121, 126, 128] enrolled 736 patients and showed a non-statistically significant effect for shunt infection regarding the use of systemic antibiotics (OR: 0.78, 95% CI: 0.44–1.38). Trials in which the authors either did not report an allocation concealment approach at all or trials in which concealment was inadequate [11, 12, 31, 50, 100, 120, 124] enrolled 948 patients and found a statistically significant difference for shunt infection and for the other studied end points that favored the treatment group (OR: 0.40, 95% CI: 0.25–0.63).

We also performed a separate analysis for placebo-controlled trials versus standard care-controlled trials for shunt infection, regarding the use of systemic antibiotics in internal shunts, that showed a statistical significance only for placebo-controlled trials (OR: 0.46, 95% CI: 0.30–0.71 and OR: 0.66, 95% CI: 0.34–1.26, respectively).

Funnel plots [33] for shunt infection regarding the use of systemic antibiotics did not suggest selective reporting of trials.

Discussion

We included 17 randomized controlled trials in this systematic review. However, these studies have certain methodological shortcomings. For example, none of the trials included used an intention-to-treat analysis, and ~50% of the trials either did not describe the randomization method or it was inadequately described. Only 7 of the studies were double-blinded using identical-appearance interventions [11, 17, 50, 82, 99, 120, 121]. The attrition rate was ~5%. With the data available, we considered it appropriate to perform a meta-analysis that compared systemic prophylactic antibiotics with placebo or no antibiotics for internal shunts. Although we intended to test other endpoints aside from shunt infection, such as death due to any cause, shunt revision, and the adverse events of antibiotics, we were able to include only a few trials for each one.

Based on subgroup analyses, the benefit of systemic antibiotic prophylaxis (that is, periprocedural [given for 24 hours postoperatively] or continuous intravenous antibiotic therapy) was similar for children compared with a subgroup of patients of all ages and for VP shunts *versus* VA shunts. Accordingly, there is no support for administration of prophylactic antibiotics for more than 24 hours postoperatively. It would be desirable to have a head-to-head comparison of these two strategies. It should be emphasized that the lack of evidence of difference between the groups is consistent with either there being no difference between these groups in terms of effect size or that there are too few people in the studies to allow a clear conclusion to be made because of lack of power. Also, a head-to-head comparison between a single dose of antibiotic given immediately prior to an operation and multiple doses continued postoperatively is critical.

The validity of the review may be weakened by the fact that, when we performed the sensitivity analysis for adequate allocated trials regarding the use of systemic antibiotics for internal shunts that included seven randomized controlled trials, we found a non-significant effect for shunt infection (OR: 0.78, 95% CI: 0.44–1.38), because it occurred with the remaining endpoints studied. However, it is worth noting that the two subgroups maintained the same trend. The group of well-allocated trials was smaller, which may account for the loss of statistical significance. In addition, all studies presented the data on a per-protocol basis, which may also inflate the effect size. This aspect may be particularly important in the studies by Walters *et al.* [120] and Rocca *et al.* [100], in which they report a high dropout rate (31% [24 of 78] and 17% [51 of 294], respectively), although the former had less weight (0.49%), and the latter study was important but below the critical 20% level. Overall, systemic antibiotics in internal shunts do have a beneficial effect, but it is possible that the effect size is smaller than that estimated in our review.

Presently, there are insufficient trials to permit definite conclusions regarding the benefit of the use of prophylactic systemic antibiotics for external shunts or the benefit of AIS systems compared with standard systems. Only individual trials evaluated the effect of systemic antibiotics in patients with EVDs, the benefit of AIS systems in patients with external drains, or the benefit of AIS systems in patients with internal shunts.

Conclusions

Given the current data, it is possible to recommend in current practice the use of periprocedural systemic prophylactic antibiotics in patients undergoing implantation of internal ventricular shunts regardless of their age and the type of internal shunt used. Nonetheless, it was not possible to clearly evaluate the incidence of the antibiotics' adverse effects. The available mortality data is sparse and the type and dose of antibiotics need to be optimized. Currently the available evidence only suggests a benefit for the use of prophylactic antibiotics for the first 24 hours postoperatively. No conclusions can be reached regarding the administration of prophylactic antibiotics for EVDs.

Future randomized controlled trials should study relevant outcomes such as death, adverse events caused by antibiotics, and shunt revision. There is also a need to evaluate the effectiveness of systemic prophylactic antibiotics for EVDs and the effectiveness of different regimens of systemic prophylactic antibiotics rather than placebo for internal ventricular shunts, namely the duration of administration. The evidence suggests that antibiotic-impregnated catheters reduce the incidence of shunt infection, although no strong recommendation can be made given the data available. This evidence is only limited by the small number of studies and participants. Even though our results suggest that the AISs are effective across populations – and heterogeneity of populations across studies can make results more universal – further well-conducted randomized controlled trials are required to clarify this issue.

Anticonvulsant prophylaxis

Anticonvulsants for subarachnoid hemorrhages

The long-term use of anticonvulsant medication to prevent seizures in patients with subarachnoid hemorrhages (SAH) was once an accepted medical practice, based on early investigations that suggested the risk of seizures in these patients was as high as 22% [20]. Not surprisingly, more recent series show a decline in the incidence of postoperative epilepsy with aneurysm surgery (~5%), likely a reflection of the advances in the surgical/endovascular techniques, and in the neurocritical intensive care units [4]. Because of the strong association of adverse effects in patients with aneurismal SAH, particularly the possible aggravation of cerebral vasospasm or the increased risk of fever, itself strongly associated with poor functional and cognitive outcome [125], the continued and generalized use of these drugs in SAH could no longer be justified. The idea of limiting anticonvulsant prophylaxis to a necessary minimum emerges, especially because most seizures occur with the ictus or within few hours of the hemorrhage [68, 98]. After this initial period the incidence of seizures is low [18]. Chumnavej *et al.* demonstrated that a 3-day regimen of phenytoin prophylaxis is safer and equally effective in comparison with arbitrary longer-term phenytoin coverage, as the incidence of significant side effects is greatly reduced without a concomitant increase in the risk of seizures, even if 80% of patients received aneurysm repair by craniotomy [22]. This data is consistent with that of traumatic head injury patients in whom early anticonvulsant use did not change the incidence of late seizures. Whether or not anticonvulsant prophylaxis is necessary is still debatable [101], although until an aneurysm is treated even a rare seizure may be catastrophic, predisposing the patient to rebleeding, and there is insufficient controlled data to recommend withholding antiepileptics altogether in the acute stage.

Anticonvulsants for acute traumatic brain injuries

The occurrence of seizures may result in accidental injury and cause cognitive and social constraints on work performance, school performance, and driving. In the acute period following a head injury (within seven days post-injury), seizures may precipitate additional secondary neuronal injury due to elevations in intracranial pressure, blood pressure changes, changes in oxygen delivery, or excess neurotransmitter release. In addition, there are several studies demonstrating the neuro-protective effects of anticonvulsants in both hypoxia-ischemia 'in vitro' and 'in vivo' models [86]. On the other hand, the incidence of unwanted side effects of antiepileptic drugs should not be disregarded. A well-conducted, systematic review that evaluated 10 RCTs on acute traumatic brain injury concluded that prophylactic anticonvulsants are effective in reducing early post-traumatic seizures, but there is neither any evidence that this treatment reduces the occurrence of late seizures, nor that it has any effect on mortality or neurological disability [104]. Insufficient evidence is available to establish the net benefit of prophylactic treatment at any time after injury.

Anticonvulsants for chronic subdural hematomas

Background

Chronic subdural hematomas (CSHs) are usually caused by minor head injuries and most often result from the tearing of a bridging vein. The frequency of pre- and post-operative seizures in these patients is not established. The overall incidence of seizures in patients with CSH has been reported to vary from 2.3 to 17% [70, 83] with an incidence of post-operative seizures reported from 1.0 to 23.4% [48, 54]. The wide variation in these numbers is probably related to the severity of the head injury and the type of surgical procedure performed in each study.

CSH typically occurs in people with prior brain atrophy, such as elderly people or chronic alcoholics, who are also more vulnerable to the potential side-effects of anticonvulsant drugs [90]. The efficacy of prophylactic anticonvulsive medication in this pathology has been debated and there is no consensus on its use. There is a wide variation in practice. For some experts, the low incidence of seizures does not justify an anticonvulsant prophylaxis in patients with CSH caused by minor head injury [83]. Others suggest that this prophylactic medication should be considered only in alcoholic patients because of their higher risk of seizure [102]. Another study verified a significant increase in morbidity and mortality associated with respiratory complications and status epilepticus in patients with new-onset seizures. It recommended the administration of anticonvulsants for a period of six months following diagnosis in all patients with CSH [103].

Clinical material and methods

We searched for relevant trials following the optimal search strategy devised for The Cochrane Collaboration [30] through electronic searches of CENTRAL (The Cochrane Library, Issue 1, 2009), MEDLINE, EMBASE, and LILACS, from inception to March 2009. We also electronically searched meeting proceedings from the AANS and hand-searched the abstracts from the meeting proceedings of the EANS. In addition, we contacted researchers active in the field for information regarding unpublished trials and contacted authors of published trials for further information and unpublished data. We did not apply any language restrictions.

All studies were required to be RCTs comparing any anticonvulsant versus placebo or no intervention in patients with chronic subdural hematomas. We intended to include patients of any age with cranial computerized tomography (CT) or magnetic resonance imaging (MRI) compatible with an old subdural hematoma with radiological or clinical evidence of mass effect. We intended to exclude patients with a history of pre-existing seizures. The type of intervention considered was either of the following: administration of any anticonvulsant drug, at any dosage, beginning at the time of the diagnosis and prolonged for any length of time, compared with placebo or no anticonvulsant. Trial quality and extracted data were to be independently assessed. The following outcome measures were intended to be evaluated: (1) frequency of pre-operative and post-operative seizures; (2) frequency of specific anticonvulsant adverse side-effects (safety of administration); (3) all-cause mortality; (4) other complications: permanent neurological impairment, long term epilepsy, and CSH recurrence.

We intended to analyze clinical heterogeneity qualitatively, taking into account factors such as the type of participants, the type and dose of anticonvulsant used, methodological quality, the number of patients excluded or lost to follow-up, and the outcome measures stated in the protocol. We intended to assess the internal validity of individual trials, using the Cochrane Collaboration's risk of bias tool as described by Higgins and Green [53].

Results

No trials were found that were eligible for inclusion in the review. No data could be analyzed.

Discussion

Given the conflicting results regarding the use of prophylactic anticonvulsants in patients with CSH, it is disappointing that there are no RCTs that evaluate their effectiveness in these patients. Only three retrospective studies with a control group were identified.

Rubin and Rappaport [102] conducted a retrospective analysis of 143 adult patients treated for CSH from January 1979 to July 1991. Surgeries were performed on 138 patients. Before surgery 5.6% of the patients had seizures, whereas after surgery this frequency was 3%. Until July 1986, all patients received prophylactic anticonvulsants from the time of surgery (83 patients). After this date, drug therapy was given only if seizure was present (55 patients). Seizure was noted in 4.8% of patients compared with 3.6% of patients who did not receive anticonvulsants. Of those who received anticonvulsants, eight

(9.6%) had non-serious drug-related adverse effects (mild allergic reaction and phenytoin intoxication). According to the authors, antiepileptic drugs should not be administered prophylactically in patients with CSH because the risk of epilepsy is not high enough to balance the morbidity caused by the anticonvulsants.

In the retrospective analysis of Ohno *et al.* [83], 129 patients treated for CSH between August 1980 and March 1992 were studied. Patients were usually given phenobarbital pre-operatively. Until December 1987, 56 of 59 patients were given anticonvulsant post-operatively. Prophylactic use of these drugs was subsequently discontinued, except in those patients with severe head injury (17 of 70 received prophylaxis). None of the 73 patients in total who were given prophylactic antiepileptic drug treatment developed seizures. Only two of 56 patients not given prophylaxis developed early post-operative seizures. A total of four patients had seizures, none of whom had received anticonvulsant drugs. The incidence of seizures was considered low and similar to that previously reported for minor head injury. Those who conducted the trial suggest that routine use of antiepileptic prophylaxis is not justified in patients with CSH related to minor injuries.

Sabo *et al.* [103] reported a retrospective analysis with historical controls of 98 patients treated surgically for CSH and examined the prevalence of seizure activity, morbidity, mortality and the side-effects of anticonvulsant medication. Of the 92 patients without pre-existing seizure, 42 (46%) received adequate prophylactic phenytoin. Adequate prophylaxis included an initial dose of phenytoin (15 mg/kg) and daily medication to adjust serum drug levels within therapeutic range. The administration of this drug was associated with three non-serious dermatological reactions. One (2.4%) patient among the 42 who received prophylactic anticonvulsants experienced seizure activity in comparison to 16 (32%) of 50 patients who did not receive adequate prophylaxis ($P<0.001$). The onset of new seizures was found in 17 (18.5%) of the 92 patients and was associated with increases in morbidity ($P=0.036$) and mortality ($P<0.005$). Therefore, they recommend the use of phenytoin prophylaxis in patients treated surgically for CSH for six months following diagnosis.

Other retrospective studies considered the incidence of seizures in patients with CSH but did not include any control group for anticonvulsant therapy [54, 70, 61, 73]. Given the lack of high-quality controlled trials and the clinical heterogeneity of the data from the available studies, pointing to the possibility of bias, no meta-analysis was performed.

Conclusions

No conclusions can be reached about the use of prophylactic anticonvulsants in patients with CSH from the information currently available. Non-controlled studies yielded conflicting results. Clinicians must balance the potential benefit against the possible risk of complications in each case.

Randomized clinical trials of prophylactic anticonvulsants in patients with CSH are essential in order to gain a clear idea of the effectiveness of this form of treatment.

Anticonvulsants for brain tumors

Background

Up to 60% of people with brain tumors may display seizures or may have a seizure for the first time after diagnosis of the tumor. Approximately 2% of people with gliomas, and 3–16% of people with meningiomas also seize after surgery [59]. This range of seizure probability and the additional surgical trauma has made seizure prophylaxis a widely accepted practice despite its potential adverse effects and drug interactions.

In people with brain tumors it has been established that: anticonvulsants-induced side effects appear to occur more frequently than in other patient groups [25, 66]; the risk of seizures varies according to the type of brain tumor, its grade and its location [117, 122]; phenytoin, carbamazepine, and phenobarbital reduce the efficacy of corticosteroids, which are administered to almost all brain tumor patients; the ability of anticonvulsants to stimulate the cytochrome P450 enzyme system induces a markedly accelerated metabolism of a wide spectrum of chemotherapeutic agents, causing difficulties in chemotherapeutic dosing [44]; corticosteroids and many chemotherapeutic agents modify the metabolism of anticonvulsants, making anticonvulsant under- and overdosing more common [49, 62, 78]; the potential immuno-suppressive side effect of some anticonvulsants represents an additional risk to these already immuno-compromised patients [79].

For years there has been controversy about the indications and the effectiveness of seizure prophylaxis. Some authors have recommended prophylactic antiepileptics for cerebral metastatic melanoma and also for postoperative patients with specific conditions [19, 29], whereas others have questioned the value of this practice [43]. The Quality Standards Subcommittee of the American Academy of Neurology (AAN) did not recommend the routine use of prophylactic antiepileptics in people with newly diagnosed brain tumors [44], regardless of some pitfalls that weaken the strength of this review's conclusions [116]. However, the reality is that many physicians and particularly neurosurgeons in North America and Europe still prescribe antiepileptic drugs for people with brain tumors who have not had seizures [109].

Clinical material and methods

We identified relevant trials following the optimal search strategy devised for the Cochrane Collaboration through electronic searches of CENTRAL (The

Cochrane Library, Issue 1, 2008), PubMed, EMBASE, CancerLit, and LILACS (1966–2007) that included free-text and MeSH terms. We also hand-searched conference proceedings, textbooks, original and review articles, and contacted clinical researchers who conducted or were conducting identified trials, whenever necessary. We did not apply any language restrictions.

We considered for analysis controlled clinical trials with random allocation, blinded or unblinded, comparing prophylactic antiepileptics with no prophylaxis or prophylaxis with a placebo in patients with diagnosis of glioma, using the World Health Organization (WHO) classification of brain tumors, meningiomas, skull base tumors, and brain metastases from any primary tumor. The drugs of interest in this review were phenytoin, carbamazepine, valproic acid, phenobarbital and newer drugs such as gabapentin, pregabalin, zonisamide, lamotrigine, oxcarbazepine, levetiracetam, topiramate, vigabatrin, and tiagabine. Studies comparing different anticonvulsants were excluded. Participants may have had surgery for the diagnosis or treatment of the underlying tumor. We independently extracted data and assessed trial quality. The following outcome measures were evaluated: (1) proportion of individuals in the treatment and control groups who were free from seizures at the time defined by those who conducted the trial as the time of outcome measurement; (2) adverse effect rate, which included any untoward reaction attributed to the drug of interest regardless of dose and magnitude, causing or not causing withdrawal from the study.

We performed statistical analyses using the statistical software provided by the Cochrane Collaboration [97]. We estimated the relative risk of seizures with 95% confidence intervals (CIs) between participants receiving antiepileptic prophylaxis and individuals treated with the control intervention. We explored heterogeneity using tests for statistical heterogeneity (the Chi-squared and I^2 statistics) and funnel plots. For the analysis of adverse effects we used binary data to estimate the relative risk and the number needed to harm (NNH). There was no opportunity to run sensitivity analyses in this systematic review.

Results

We identified 16 potentially eligible trials, of which 11 studies were excluded: five trials compared two different anticonvulsants [27, 10, 67, 76, 129]; two trials were duplicate studies with fewer patients [39, 81]; two trials evaluated seizure prevention using diazepam after the injection of contrast media in participants with brain tumors [84, 85]; two trials did not provide data on participants with brain tumors [38, 56]. Five trials met our inclusion criteria for analysis (Table 3) [37, 40, 45, 64, 80]. The eligibility criteria were uniform for all studies, overall. The main goal of two of the trials was to investigate whether antiepileptic drugs could prevent seizures in the early or late postoperative periods [40, 64], and a third followed participants for up to 12 months after craniotomy [80]. The remaining two studies assessed the value

Table 3. *Characteristics of included studies ('Anticonvulsants for brain tumors')*

Author and year	Type of study	No. of patients	Treatment group (No.)	Control group (No.)	Inclusion/exclusion criteria	Intervention	Primary outcomes	Allocation conceal-ment
Forsyth 2003 [37]	random allocation, unblinded design	100	46	54	Inclusion: documented brain tumor/metastasis. Exclusion: life expectancy <4 weeks, prior seizures, allergy to anticonvulsants, lactation, drugs/ethanol abuse.	treatment group: phenytoin 15 mg/kg po loading in 3 doses, followed by 5 mg/kg po qd (n=45). If intolerance, phenobarbital used instead (n=1); control group: no treatment.	seizure after start of therapy	adequate
Franceschetti 1990 [40]	random allocation, placebo-controlled, unblinded	63	25+16	22	Inclusion: adult operated on supratentorial tumors. Exclusion:NS	Group A: 65 patients with preop seizures (not considered in the review); Group B: 63 patients without preop seizures, randomized in three subgroups: no treatment (22); phenobarbital 4 mg/kg/day× 5 days, then 2 mg/kg/day po (25); and phenytoin 10 mg/kg/d for 5 days, then 5 mg/kg po once daily (16)	early (1st week) and late (>1 week) postop seizures	not used
Glantz 1996 [45]	random allocation, double-blinded, placebo-controlled	74	37	37	Inclusion: newly diagnosed brain tumor by biopsy or CT/MRI in case of known primary lesion. Exclusion: prior seizures, age< 18 yrs, KPS< 50%, abnormal liver enzymes, previous anticonvulsant use, previous brain surgery, other concurrent intracranial disease.	treatment group: valproic acid po (dose adjusted to levels 50–100 ug/mL); placebo group	first seizure and mortality	adequate

| Lee 1989 [64] | random allocation, double-blinded, placebo-controlled | 86 | 44 | 42 | Inclusion: adults with supratentorial craniotomy with diagnosis of tumor (86 patients included in the review), aneurysm, AVM hypertensive hematoma. Exclusion: prior seizure, heart disease, unclear medical history. | treatment group: phenytoin 15 mg/kg IV before wound closure, then 5–6 mg/kg/day IV 3 times daily during 1st 3 postop days; placebo group | immediate (<24 hours) and early (<3 days) postop seizures | unclear |
| North 1983 [80] | random allocation, double-blinded, placebo-controlled | 81 | 42 | 39 | Inclusion: supratentorial surgery. Exclusion: previous seizure/treatment with anticonvulsant, cerebral abscess. 81 patients with brain tumors included in the review. | treatment group: phenytoin 250 mg twice daily IV, then 100 mg po 3 times daily for 12 months. Doses adjusted accordingly serum levels; placebo group | seizure after start of therapy | not used |

No. Number; *NS* not specified; *KPS* Karnofsky Performance Status Scale.

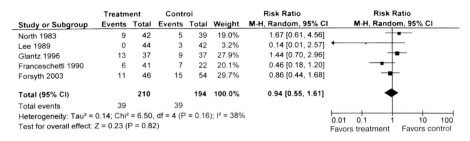

Fig. 7. Forest plot showing the effect of anticonvulsants prophylaxis *versus* placebo or no drug for the occurrence of seizures

of seizure prevention without surgery as a potential confounding variable [37, 45]. We did not identify any prospective, controlled studies (randomized or nonrandomized) of seizure prophylaxis in adults or children with brain tumors using newer antiepileptic drugs.

We rated and summarized study validity [53]. Three of the trials included were highly vulnerable to bias [40, 64, 80]. One trial had a moderate risk of bias because it did not include a placebo intervention [37]. Glantz *et al.* described sequence generation and allocation concealment, did not report results selectively, included information on adverse events and withdrawals from the study, and was the trial with the lowest risk of bias [45].

1. Effectiveness in preventing seizures (Fig. 7)
Four hundred and four participants were considered in the analysis of this outcome. Prophylaxis with the antiepileptic drugs phenytoin, phenobarbital, or divalproex sodium was no better than placebo or observation (RR: 0.94, 95% CI: 0.55–1.61; $P = 0.8$). One trial was the least precise and contributed little to the meta-analysis because the participants were followed for 72 hours after surgery and there were no seizures in the treatment group [64]. Therefore, a sensitivity analysis without this trial was unnecessary. The model was reasonably homogeneous ($I^2 = 38.5\%$) and the funnel plot did not suggest publication bias.

2. Adverse events of anticonvulsants (Fig. 8)
One study did not report adverse events [64] and another reported on this factor but only with overall results [80]. Franchescetti *et al.* reported that three patients in the group allocated to phenytoin and one participant in the group allocated to phenobarbital had adverse neurological effects in the first postoperative week without going into further detail [40]. Two trials detailed the adverse events. Forsyth *et al.* reported that 13 of 46 participants taking antiepileptic drugs had adverse events: nausea (4), rash (3), sore gums (1), myelosuppression (1), increased levels of lactate dehydrogenase (1), vertigo and blurred vision (1), tremor (1), and gait ataxia (1) [37]. Glantz *et al.* reported three patients who developed skin rashes (two receiving divalproex sodium, one

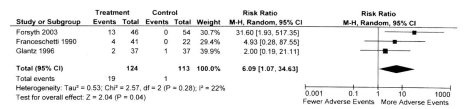

Fig. 8. Forest plot showing the effect of anticonvulsant prophylaxis *versus* placebo or no drug for the adverse event rate

allocated to placebo) [45]. Overall, there were 237 participants with data for this outcome: 124 allocated to the treatment group, and 113 to the control group. The participants who received anticonvulsants were more likely to have adverse effects: 19 events in the treatment group (15%), and one in the control group (0.9%) (RR: 6.09, 95% CI: 1.07–34.63; $P = 0.04$). The number of participants taking anticonvulsants in order for one to experience an adverse effect (NNH) was three. The model was homogeneous and the funnel plot did not suggest publication bias.

Discussion

In these five clinical trials with random allocation, phenobarbital, phenytoin, and divalproex sodium did not prevent seizures in people with brain tumors who had been seizure-free before participation in the study.

The best data we have is from a collection of different brain tumors with different seizure risks, each subgroup with few participants, and is largely based on two trials, of which only one had sufficient statistical power [45]. Evidence of this nature is inconclusive and hence we prefer to say that the best evidence available at present is neither in favor of nor against seizure prophylaxis in brain tumors. However, it is unlikely from these results that there is a clinically important effect of phenytoin, phenobarbital, or divalproex sodium in preventing seizures in the absence of careful drug-level monitoring. Therefore, it is important to test the efficacy of newer antiepileptic drugs in this context, beginning with well-designed phase II studies.

As for the seizure outcome, an analysis of adverse effects is difficult and incomplete because some clinical trials did not routinely report adverse effects. In our review we sought to compare the adverse event rate between treatment with antiepileptic drugs and control interventions. The risk of adverse effects was significantly higher in people taking antiepileptic drugs, although we recognize that older antiepileptic drugs may have a higher rate of adverse events. Therefore, the risk-to-benefit analysis of seizure prophylaxis can improve by using newer antiepileptic drugs. We do not wish to underestimate the toxicity of the older generations of antiepileptic drugs, and decisions about seizure prophylaxis need to weigh up the side-effect profile of these drugs.

Conclusions

The evidence that seizure prophylaxis using phenobarbital, phenytoin, and divalproex sodium in people with brain tumors is inconclusive at best. The clinical heterogeneity between and within trials limits any claim to effectiveness or ineffectiveness. Therefore, there is no data supporting the use of prophylactic antiepileptics, and the risk of adverse events limits their overall potential benefit. Use of these antiepileptic drugs is associated with a higher risk of adverse effects than in a control group, which is a major factor to consider when deciding to start seizure prophylaxis. Neither tumor pathology nor surgical therapy affected the results.

There is a need for trials using adaptive randomization methods that will allow us to test different newer antiepileptics. The active participation of neurosurgeons as investigators may enhance the impact of these trials in changing clinical management paradigms and longstanding dogmas.

Commentaries

The balance of the potential benefit against the possible risk of complications of treatment must always be considered in each individual case. The purpose of this article was to present to clinicians the best available information on controversial subjects so a decision can be made with the best data available, rather than to establish strict rules. With this idea in mind from the outset, we have shown that prophylactic systemic antibiotics are indicated for the surgical introduction of ventricular shunts, while their use is not routinely advised in patients with basilar skull fractures, even in the presence of CSF leakage. Nor can the use of prophylactic anticonvulsants be recommended for people with brain tumors who have not had seizures, even if they are undergoing a craniotomy. Unfortunately, no relevant trial was found and no conclusions could be reached about the use of prophylactic anticonvulsants in patients with CSH – a very good example of an everyday pathology in neurosurgery that requires further research. In addition to the call for further investigation into relevant subjects, the intent of this article was to address major research points for each subject to avoid duplication of work.

References

1. Alleyne CH, Hassan M, Zabramski JM (2000) The efficacy and cost of prophylactic and periprocedural antibiotics in patients with external ventricular drains. Neurosurgery 47: 1124–29
2. Altman DG, Deeks JJ (2002) Metaanalysis, Simpson's paradox, and the number needed to treat. BMC Med Res Methodol 2: 3
3. Ash GJ, Peter J, Bass DH (1992) Antimicrobial prophylaxis for fractured base of skull in children. Brain Inj 6: 521–27

4. Baker CJ, Prestigiacomo CJ, Solomon RA (1995) Short-term perioperative anticonvulsant prophylaxis for the surgical treatment of low-risk patients with intracranial aneurysms. Neurosurgery 37: 863–71
5. Barker FG (1994) Efficacy of prophylactic antibiotics for craniotomy: a metaanalysis. Neurosurgery 35: 484–92
6. Barker FG (2002) Efficacy of prophylactic antibiotic therapy in spinal surgery: a meta-analysis. Neurosurgery 51: 391–401
7. Barker FG (2007) Efficacy of prophylactic antibiotics against meningitis after craniotomy: a meta-analysis. Neurosurgery 60: 887–94
8. Battino D, Tomson T (2007) Management of epilepsy during pregnancy. Drugs 67: 2727–46
9. Bayston R (1975) Antibiotic prophylaxis in shunt surgery. Dev Med Child Neurol (Suppl) 35: 99–103
10. Beenen LFM, Lindeboom J, Kasteleijn-Nolst DGA, Heimans JJ, Snoek FJ, Touw DJ, Ader HJ, van Alphen HAM (1999) Comparative double blind clinical trial of phenytoin and sodium valproate as anticonvulsant prophylaxis after craniotomy: efficacy, tolerability, and cognitive effects. J Neurol Neurosurg Psychiatry 67: 474–80
11. Blomstedt GC (1985) Results of trimethoprim-sulfamethoxazole prophylaxis in ventriculostomy and shunting procedures. A double-blind randomized trial. J Neurosurg 62: 694–97
12. Blum J, Schwarz M, Voth D (1989) Antibiotic single-dose prophylaxis of shunt infections. Neurosurg Rev 12: 239–44
13. Bondurant CP, Jimenez DF (1995) Epidemiology of cerebrospinal fluid shunting. Pediatr Neurosurg 23: 254–59
14. Borges LF (1982) Cerebrospinal fluid shunts interfere with hosts defenses. Neurosurgery 10: 55–60
15. Brodie HA (1997) Prophylactic antibiotics for posttraumatic cerebrospinal fluid fistulae. A metaanalysis. Arch Otolaryngol Head Neck Surg 123: 749–52
16. Buchanan RJ, Brant A, Marshall LR (2004) Traumatic cerebrospinal fluid fistulas. In: Winn HR (ed) Youmans Neurological Surgery. Saunders, Philadelphia, pp 5265–72
17. Bullock R, van Dellen JR, Ketelbey W, Reinach SG (1988) A double-blind placebo-controlled trial of perioperative prophylactic antibiotics for elective neurosurgery. J Neurosurg 69: 687–91
18. Byrne JV, Boardman P, Ioannidis I, Adcock J, Traill Z (2003) Seizures after aneurysmal subarachnoid hemorrhage treated with coil embolization. Neurosurgery 52: 545–52
19. Byrne TN, Cascino TL, Posner JB (1983) Brain metastasis from melanoma. J Neurooncol 1: 313–17
20. Cabral RJ, King TT, Scott DF (1976) Epilepsy after two different neurosurgical approaches to the treatment of ruptured intracranial aneurysm. J Neurol Neurosurg Psychiatry 39: 1052–56
21. Choi D, Spann R (1996) Traumatic cerebrospinal fluid leakage: risk factors and the use of prophylactic antibiotics. Br J Neurosurg 10: 571–75
22. Chumnanvej S, Dunn IF, Kim DH (2007) Three-day phenytoin prophylaxis is adequate after subarachnoid hemorrhage. Neurosurgery 60: 99–102
23. Claus BC (2004) Shunt infection. In: Winn HR (ed) Youmans Neurological Surgery. Saunders, Philadelphia, pp 3419–25

24. Clemenza JW, Kaltman SI, Diamond DL (1995) Craniofacial trauma and cerebrospinal fluid leakage: a retrospective clinical study. J Oral Maxillofac Surg 53: 1004–07
25. Cockey GH, Amann ST, Reents SB, Lynch JB Jr (1996) Stevens-Johnson syndrome resulting from whole-brain radiation and phenytoin (Abstract). Am J Clin Oncol 19: 32–34
26. Dagi TF, Meyer FB, Poletti CA (1983) The incidence and prevention of meningitis after basilar skull fracture. Am J Emerg Med 1: 295–98
27. De Santis A, Villani R, Sinisi M, Stocchetti N, Perucca E (2002) Add-on phenytoin fails to prevent early seizures after surgery for supratentorial brain tumours: a randomized controlled study. Epilepsia 43: 175–82
28. Demetriades D, Charalambides D, Lakhoo M, Pantanowitz D (1992) Role of prophylactic antibiotics in open and basilar fractures of the skull: a randomized study. Injury 23: 377–80
29. Deutschman CS, Haines SJ (1985) Anticonvulsant prophylaxis in neurological surgery. Neurosurgery 17: 510–17
30. Dickersin K, Scherer R, Lefebvre C (1994) Identifying relevant studies for systematic reviews. BMJ 309: 1286–91
31. Djindjian M, Fevrier MJ, Otterbein G, Soussy JC (1986) Oxacillin prophylaxis in cerebrospinal fluid shunt procedures: results of a randomized open study in 60 hydrocephalic patients. Surg Neurol 25: 178–80
32. Eftekhar B, Ghodsi M, Nejat F, Ketabchi E, Esmaeeli B (2004) Prophylactic administration of ceftriaxone for the prevention of meningitis after traumatic pneumocephalus: results of a clinical trial. J Neurosurg 101: 757–61
33. Egger M, Davey Smith G, Schneider M, Minder C (1997) Bias in metaanalysis detected by a simple, graphical test. BMJ 315: 629–34
34. Einhorn A, Mizrahi EM (1978) Basilar skull fractures in children. The incidence of CNS infection and the use of antibiotics. Am J Dis Child 132: 1121–24
35. Eljamel MS (1993) Antibiotic prophylaxis in unrepaired CSF fistulae. Br J Neurosurg 7: 501–05
36. Epstein MH, Kumor K, Hughes W, Lietman P (1982) Use of prophylactic antibiotics in pediatric shunting operations – a double-blind prospective study. In: Presented at the American Association of Neurological Surgeons 1982 Annual Meeting
37. Forsyth PA, Weaver S, Fulton D, Brasher PM, Sutherland G, Stewart D, Hagen NA, Barnes P, Cairncross JG, DeAngelis LM (2003) Prophylactic anticonvulsants in patients with brain tumour. Can J Neurol Sci 30: 106–12
38. Foy PM, Chadwick DW, Raigopalan N, Johnson AL, Shaw, MDM (1992) Do prophylactic anticonvulsant drugs alter the pattern of seizures after craniotomy? J Neurol Neurosurg Psychiatry 55: 753–57
39. Franceschetti S, Binelli S, Casazza M, Croci D, Lodrini S, Panzica F, Solero CL, Avanzini G (1988) Crisi postoperatorie in pazienti operati per neoplasie sopratentoriali: studio prospettico. [Postoperative seizures in patients operated on supra-tentorial neoplasms: a prospective study.] Bolletino della Lega Italiana contro l'Epilepsia 62–63: 413–15
40. Franceschetti S, Binelli S, Casazza M, Lodrini S, Panzica F, Pluchino F, Solero CL, Avanzini G (1990) Influence of surgery and antiepileptic drugs on seizures symptomatic of cerebral tumours. Acta Neurochir (Wien) 103: 47–51
41. Frazee RC, Mucha P Jr, Farnell MB, Ebersold MJ (1988) Meningitis after basilar skull fracture. Does antibiotic prophylaxis help? Postgrad Med 83: 267–74

42. Friedman JA, Ebersold MJ, Quast LM (2001) Post-traumatic cerebrospinal fluid leakage. World J Surg 25: 1062–66
43. Glantz M, Recht LD (1997) Epilepsy in the cancer patient. In: Vinken PJ, Bruyn GW (eds) Handbook of Neurology: Neuro-Oncology, Vol. 25. Elsevier, Amsterdam, pp 9–18
44. Glantz MJ, Cole BF, Forsyth PA, Recht LD, Wen PY, Chamberlain MC (2000) Practice parameter: anticonvulsant prophylaxis in patients with newly diagnosed brain tumours. Report of the Quality Standards Subcommittee of the American Academy of Neurology. Neurology 54: 1886–93
45. Glantz MJ, Cole BF, Friedberg MH, Lathi E, Choy H, Furie K, Akerley W, Wahlberg L, Lekos A, Louis S (1996) A randomized, blinded, placebo-controlled trial of divalproex sodium prophylaxis in adults with newly diagnosed brain tumours. Neurology 46: 985–91
46. Gonzalez JL (1998) Profilaxis con antibioticos en fracturas de base de craneo. Tiene justification esa conducta? [Antibiotic prophylaxis in basilar skull fractures. Is it worth it?] Revista Cubana de Cirugía 37: 5–9
47. Govender ST, Nathoo N, van Dellen JR (2003) Evaluation of an antibiotic-impregnated shunt system for the treatment of hydrocephalus. J Neurosurg 99: 831–39
48. Grisoli F, Graziani N, Peragut JC, Vincentelli F, Fabrizi AP, Caruso G, Bellard S (1988) Perioperative lumbar injection of Ringer's lactate solution in chronic subdural hematomas: a series of 100 cases. Neurosurgery 23: 616–21
49. Grossman SA, Sheidler VR, Gilbert MR (1989) Decreased phenytoin levels in patients receiving chemotherapy. Am J Med 87: 505–10
50. Haines SJ, Taylor F (1982) Prophylactic methicillin for shunt operations: effects on incidence of shunt malfunction and infection. Childs Brain 9: 10–22
51. Haines SJ, Walters BC (1994) Antibiotic prophylaxis for cerebrospinal fluid shunts: a metaanalysis. Neurosurgery 34: 87–92
52. Helling TS, Evans LL, Fowler DL, Hays LV, Kennedy FR (1988) Infectious complications in patients with severe head injury. J Trauma 28: 1575–77
53. Higgins JPT, Green S (2008) Cochrane Handbook for Systematic Reviews of Interventions. The Cochrane Collaboration. Available from www.cochrane-handbook.org
54. Hirakawa K, Hashizume K, Fuchinoue T, Takahashi H, Nomura K (1972) Statistical analysis of chronic subdural hematoma in 309 adult cases. Neurol Med Chir (Tokyo) 12: 71–83
55. Hoff JT, Brewin A, Hoi Sang U (1976) Letter: antibiotics for basilar skull fracture. J Neurosurg 44: 649
56. Holland JB, Stapleton SR, Moore AJ, Marsh HT, Uttley D, Bell BA (1995) A randomised double blind study of sodium valproate for the prevention of seizures in neurosurgical patients. J Neurol Neurosurg Psychiatry 58: 116
57. Ignelzi R, VanderArk G (1975) Analysis of the treatment of basilar skull fractures with and without antibiotics. J Neurosurg 43: 721–26
58. Jadad AR, Moore RA, Carroll D, Jenkinson C, Reynolds DJ, Gavaghan DJ, McQuay HJ (1996) Assessing the quality of reports of randomized clinical trials: is blinding necessary? Control Clin Trials 17: 1–12
59. Ketz E (1976) Brain tumours and epilepsy. In: Vinken PJ, Bruyn GW (eds) Handbook of Clinical Neurology, Vol. 16. North-Holland Publishing Company, Amsterdam, pp 254–69
60. Klastersky J, Sadeghi M, Brihaye J (1976) Antimicrobial prophylaxis in patients with rhinorrhea or otorrhea: a double blind study. Surg Neurol 6: 111–14

61. Kotwica Z, Brzezinski J (1991) Epilepsy in chronic subdural haematoma. Acta Neurochir (Wien) 113: 18–20
62. Lackner TE (1991) Interaction of dexamethasone with phenytoin. Pharmacotherapy 11: 344–47
63. Langley JM, LeBlanc JC, Drake J, Milner R (1993) Efficacy of antimicrobial prophylaxis in placement of cerebrospinal fluid shunts: metaanalysis. Clin Infect Dis 17: 98–103
64. Lee ST, Lui TN, Chang CN, Cheng WC, Wang DJ, Heimburger RF, Lin CG (1989) Prophylactic anticonvulsants for prevention of immediate and early postcraniotomy seizures. Surg Neurol 31: 361–64
65. Leech PJ, Paterson A (1973) Conservative and operative management of cerebrospinal fluid leakage after closed head injury. Lancet 1: 1013–15
66. Lehmann DF, Hurteau TE, Newman N, Coyle TE (1997) Anticonvulsant usage is associated with an increased risk of procarbazine hypersensitivity reactions in patients with brain tumours. Clin Pharmacol Ther 62: 225–29
67. Levati A, Savoia G, Zoppi F, Boselli L, Tommassino C (1996) Peri-operative prophylaxis with phenytoin: dosage and therapeutic levels. Acta Neurochir (Wien) 138: 274–78
68. Lin CL, Dumont AS, Lieu AS, Yen CP, Hwang SL, Kwan AL, Kassell NF, Howng SL (2003) Characterization of perioperative seizures and epilepsy following aneurysmal subarachnoid hemorrhage. J Neurosurg 99: 978–85
69. Loring DW, Meador KJ (2004) Cognitive side effects of antiepileptic drugs in children. Neurology 62: 872–77
70. Luxon LM, Harrison MJG Luxon LM, Harrison MJG (1979) Chronic subdural haematoma. Q J Med 48: 43–53
71. MacGee EE, Cauthen JC, Brackett CE (1970) Meningitis following acute traumatic cerebrospinal fluid fistula. J Neurosurg 33: 312–16
72. McGuirt WF Jr, Stool SE (1995) Cerebrospinal fluid fistula: the identification and management in pediatric temporal bone fractures. Laryngoscope 105: 359–64
73. McKissock W, Richardson A, Bloom WH (1960) Subdural haematoma. A review of 389 cases. Lancet 1: 1365–69
74. Mecarelli O, Vicenzini E, Pulitano P, Vanacore N, Romolo FS, Di Piero V, Lenzi GL, Accornero N (2004) Clinical, cognitive, and neurophysiologic correlates of short-term treatment with carbamazepine, oxcarbazepine, and levetiracetam in healthy volunteers. Ann Pharmacother 38: 1816–22
75. Moss AJ, Hamburger S, Moore RM Jr, Jeng LL, Howie LJ (1991) Use of selected medical device implants in the United States, 1988. Adv Data 191: 1–24
76. Nakamura N, Ishijima B, Mayanagi Y, Manaka S (1999) A randomized controlled trial of zonisamide in postoperative epilepsy: a report of the Cooperative Group Study. Jpn J Neurosurg 8: 647–56
77. Nathoo N, Govender ST, Barnett GH, van Dellen JR (2004) Evaluation of an antimicrobial impregnated shunt system for the treatment of hydrocephalus. In: Presented at the American Association of Neurological Surgeons 2004 Annual Meeting
78. Neef C, Voogd-van der Straaten I (1988) An interaction between cytostatic and anticonvulsant drugs. Clin Pharmacol Ther 43: 372–75
79. Neuwelt EA, Kikuchi K, Hill S, Lipsky P, Frenkel EP (1983) Immune responses in patients with brain tumours. Factors such as anti-convulsants that may contribute to impaired cell-mediated immunity. Cancer 51: 248–55

Prophylactic antibiotics and anticonvulsants

80. North JB, Penhall RK, Hanieh A, Frewin DB, Taylor WB (1983) Phenytoin and postoperative epilepsy. A double-blind study. J Neurosurg 58: 672–77
81. North JB, Penhall RK, Hanieh A, Hann CS, Challen RG, Frewin DB (1980) Postoperative epilepsy: a double-blind trial of phenytoin after craniotomy. Lancet 1: 384–86
82. Odio C, Mohs E, Sklar FH, Nelson JD, McCracken GH (1984) Adverse reactions to vancomycin used as prophylaxis for CSF shunts procedures. AJDC 138: 17–19
83. Ohno K, Maehara T, Ichimura K, Suzuki R, Hirakawa K, Monma S (1993) Low incidence of seizures in patients with chronic subdural haematoma. J Neurol Neurosurg Psychiatry 56: 1231–33
84. Pagani JJ, Hayman LA, Bigelow RH, Libshitz HI, Lepke RA, Wallace S (1983) Diazepam prophylaxis of contrast media-induced seizures during computed tomography of patients with brain metastases. Am J Roentgenol 140: 787–92
85. Pagani JJ, Hayman LA, Bigelow RH, Libshitz HI, Lepke RA (1984) Prophylactic diazepam in prevention of contrast media-associated seizures in glioma patients undergoing cerebral computed tomography. Cancer 54: 2200–04
86. Papazisis G, Kallaras K, Kaiki-Astara A, Pourzitaki C, Tzachanis D, Dagklis T, Kouvelas D (2008) Neuroprotection by lamotrigine in a rat model of neonatal hypoxic-ischaemic encephalopathy. Int J Neuropsychopharmacol 11: 321–29
87. Pennybacker JB, Taylor M, Cairns H (1947) Penicillin in the prevention of infection during operations on the brain and spinal cord. Lancet 2: 159–62
88. Petignat C, Francioli P, Harbarth S, Regli L, Porchet F, Reverdin A, Rilliet B, de Tribolet N, Pannatier A, Pittet D, Zanetti G (2008) Cefuroxime prophylaxis is effective in noninstrumented spine surgery: a double-blind, placebo-controlled study. Spine 33: 1919–24
89. Pons VG, Denlinger SL, Guglielmo BJ, Octavio J, Flaherty J, Derish PA, Wilson CB (1993) Ceftizoxime versus vancomycin and gentamicin in neurosurgical prophylaxis: a randomized, prospective, blinded clinical study. Neurosurgery 33: 416–22
90. Prabhu S, Zauner A, Bullock M (2004) Surgical management of traumatic brain injury. In: Winn HR (ed) Youmans Neurological Surgery. Saunders, Philadelphia, pp 5145–80
91. Price DJ, Sleigh JD (1970) Control of infection due to Klebsiella aerogenes in a neurosurgical unit by withdrawal of all antibiotics. Lancet 2: 1213–15
92. Raskind R. Cerebrospinal fluid rhinorrhea and otorrhea (1965) Diagnosis and treatment in 35 cases. J Int Coll Surg 43: 141–54
93. Ratilal B, Costa J, Sampaio C (2005) Anticonvulsants for preventing seizures in patients with chronic subdural haematoma. Cochrane Database Syst Rev 3: CD004893
94. Ratilal B, Costa J, Sampaio C (2006) Antibiotic prophylaxis for preventing meningitis in patients with basilar skull fractures. Cochrane Database Syst Rev 1: CD004884
95. Ratilal B, Costa J, Sampaio C (2006) Antibiotic prophylaxis for surgical introduction of intracranial ventricular shunts. Cochrane Database Syst Rev 3: CD005365
96. Ratilal B, Costa J, Sampaio C (2008) Antibiotic prophylaxis for surgical introduction of intracranial ventricular shunts: a systematic review. J Neurosurg Pediatr 1: 48–56
97. Review Manager (RevMan) [Computer Program] (2004) Version 4.2 for Windows. The Cochrane Collaboration, Oxford, England
98. Rhoney DH, Tipps LB, Murry KR, Basham MC, Michael DB, Coplin WM (2000) Anticonvulsant prophylaxis and timing of seizures after aneurysmal subarachnoid hemorrhage. Neurology 55: 258–65

99. Rieder MJ, Frewen TC, Del Maestro RF, Coyle A, Lovell S (1987) The effect of cephalothin prophylaxis on postoperative ventriculoperitoneal shunt infections. CMAJ 36: 935–38

100. Rocca B, Mallet MN, Scemama F, Malca S, Chevalier A, Gouin F (1992) Infections à distance du foyer opératoire en neurochirurgie. Rôle de l'antibioprophylaxie. [Perioperative remote infections in neurosurgery. Role of antibiotic prophylaxis.] Presse Med 21: 2037–40

101. Rosengart AJ, Huo JD, Tolentino J, Novakovic RL, Frank JI, Goldenberg FD, Macdonald RL (2007) Outcome in patients with subarachnoid hemorrhage treated with antiepileptic drugs. J Neurosurg 107: 253–60

102. Rubin G, Rappaport ZH (1993) Epilepsy in chronic subdural haematoma. Acta Neurochir (Wien) 123: 39–42

103. Sabo RA, Hanigan WC, Aldag JC (1995) Chronic subdural hematomas and seizures: the role of prophylactic anticonvulsive medication. Surg Neurol 43: 579–82

104. Schierhout G, Roberts I (2001) Antiepileptic drugs for preventing seizures following acute traumatic brain injury. Cochrane Database Syst Rev 4: CD000173

105. Schmidt K, Gjerris F, Osgaard O, Hvidberg EF, Kristiansen JE, Dahlerup B, Kruse-Larsen C (1985) Antibiotic prophylaxis in cerebrospinal fluid shunting: a prospective randomized trial in 152 hydrocephalic patients. Neurosurgery 17: 1–5

106. Schulz KF, Chalmers I, Hayes RJ, Altman DG (1995) Empirical evidence of bias. Dimensions of methodological quality associated with estimates of treatment effects in controlled trials. JAMA 273: 408–12

107. Shapiro M, Wald U, Simchen E, Pomeranz S, Zagzag D, Michowiz SD, Samuel-Cahn E, Wax Y, Shuval R, Kahane Y, Sacks T, Shalit M (1986) Randomized clinical trial of intraoperative antimicrobial prophylaxis of infection after neurosurgical procedures. J Hosp Infect 8: 283–95

108. Simon TD, Riva-Cambrin J, Srivastava R, Bratton SL, Dean JM, Kestle JR; Hydrocephalus Clinical Research Network (2008) Hospital care for children with hydrocephalus in the United States: utilization, charges, comorbidities, and deaths. J Neurosurg Pediatr 1: 131–37

109. Siomin V, Angelov L, Li L, Vogelbaum MA (2005) Results of a survey of neurosurgical practice patterns regarding the prophylactic use of anti-epilepsy drugs in patients with brain tumors. J Neurooncol 74: 211–15

110. Siqueira MG, Koury LS, Silva AD, Jabur A, Rezende Filho CP (1987) Profilaxia antibiótica transoperatória em neurocirurgia: estudo prospectivo controlado. [Intraoperative antibiotic prophylaxis in neurosurgery: a randomized controlled clinical trial.] Arq Bras Neurocirurg 6: 5–12

111. Smith DB (1991) Cognitive effects of antiepileptic drugs. Adv Neurol 55: 197–212

112. Steidtmann K, Welge-Lussen A, Probst R (1997) Antibiotikaprophylaxe bei laterobasalen Frakturen. [Antibiotic prophylaxis in laterobasal fractures.] HNO 45: 448–52

113. Stenager E, Gerner-Smidt P, Kock-Jensen C (1986) Ventriculostomy-related infections: an epidemiological study. Acta Neurochir (Wien) 83: 20–23

114. Tos M (1973) Course of and sequelae to 248 petrosal fractures. Acta Otolaryngol 75: 353–54

115. Tremont-Lukats IW, Ratilal BO, Armstrong T, Gilbert MR (2008) Antiepileptic drugs for preventing seizures in people with brain tumors. Cochrane Database Syst Rev 2: CD004424

116. Tremont-Lukats IW, Teixeira GM (2002) Anticonvulsant prophylaxis in patients with brain tumours: an overview. Neuro-oncol 4: S97

Prophylactic antibiotics and anticonvulsants

117. Vecht CJ, van Breemen M (2006) Optimizing therapy of seizures in patients with brain tumors. Neurology 4: 10–13
118. Villalobos T, Arango C, Kubilis P, Rathore M (1998) Antibiotic prophylaxis after basilar skull fractures: a metaanalysis. Clin Infect Dis 27: 364–69
119. Vining EP, Mellitis ED, Dorsen MM, Cataldo MF, Quaskey SA, Spielberg SP, Freeman JM (1987) Psychologic and behavioral effects of antiepileptic drugs in children: a double-blind comparison between phenobarbital and valproic acid. Pediatrics 80: 165–74
120. Walters BC, Goumnerova L, Hoffman HJ, Hendrick EB, Humphreys RP, Levinton C (1992) A randomized controlled trial of perioperative rifampin/trimethoprim in cerebrospinal fluid shunt surgery. Childs Nerv Syst 8: 253–57
121. Wang EE, Prober CG, Hendrick BE, Hoffman HJ, Humphreys RP (1984) Prophylactic sulfamethoxazole and trimethoprim in ventriculoperitoneal shunt surgery. A double-blind, randomized, placebo-controlled trial. JAMA 251: 1174–77
122. Wen PY, Marks PW (2002) Medical management of patients with brain tumours. Curr Opin Oncol 14: 299–307
123. Whitby M, Johnson BC, Atkinson RL, Stuart G (2000) The comparative efficacy of intravenous cefotaxime and trimethoprim/sulfamethoxazole in preventing infection after neurosurgery: a prospective, randomized study. Brisbane Neurosurgical Infection Group. Br J Neurosurg 14: 13–18
124. Yogev R (1985) Cerebrospinal fluid shunt infections: a personal view. Pediatr Infect Dis 4: 113–18
125. Young B, Rapp RP, Norton JA, Haack D, Tibbs PA, Bean JR (1983) Failure of prophylactically administered phenytoin to prevent early posttraumatic seizures. J Neurosurg 58: 231–35
126. Young RF, Lawner PM (1987) Perioperative antibiotic prophylaxis for prevention of postoperative neurosurgical infections. A randomized clinical trial. J Neurosurg 66: 701–05
127. Zabramski JM, Whiting D, Darouiche RO, Horner TG, Olson J, Robertson C, Hamilton AJ (2003) Efficacy of antimicrobial-impregnated external ventricular drain catheters: a prospective, randomized, controlled trial. J Neurosurg 98: 725–30
128. Zentner J, Gilsbach J, Felder T (1995) Antibiotic prophylaxis in cerebrospinal fluid shunting: a prospective randomized trial in 129 patients. Neurosurg Rev 18: 169–72
129. Zhang Y, Zhou LF, Du GH, Gao L, Xu B, Xu J, Gu YX (2000) Phenytoin or sodium valproate for prophylaxis of postoperative epilepsy: a randomized comparison. Chin J Nerv Ment Dis 26: 231–33
130. Zrebeet HA, Huang PS (1986) Prophylactic antibiotics in the treatment of fractures at the base of the skull. Del Med J 58: 741–48

The dural sheath of the optic nerve: descriptive anatomy and surgical applications

P. FRANCOIS[1,2], E. LESCANNE[3], and S. VELUT[1,2]

[1] Université François Rabelais de Tours, Laboratoire d'anatomie, Tours, France
[2] CHRU de Tours, Service de Neurochirurgie, Tours, France
[3] CHRU de Tours, Service d'Oto-Rhino-Laryngologie, Tours, France

With 3 Figures

Contents

Abstract 187
Introduction 188
  Embryology 188
  The interperiosteodural concept 190
  Intracranial segment 191
  Intracanalicular segment 191
    Relations with bony structures 191
    Meningeal relations 194
  Intraorbital segment 195
Conclusion 197
References 198

Abstract

The aim of this work was to clarify the descriptive anatomy of the optic dural sheath using microanatomical dissections on cadavers. The orbit is the rostral part of the extradural neural axis compartment; the optic dural sheath forms the central portion of the orbit.

In order to describe this specific anatomy, we carefully dissected 5 cadaveric heads (10 orbits) up to the meningeal structure of the orbit and its contents. 1 cadaveric head was reserved for electron microscopy to add to our knowledge of the collagen structure of the optic dural sheath.

In this chapter, we describe the anatomy of the interperiostal-dural concept and the anatomy of the orbit. The optic dural sheath contains three portions: the intracranial, the intracanalicular and the intraorbital segment. Each one has specific anatomic relations which result in particular surgical considerations.

Keywords: Optic nerve; dural sheath; anatomy; skull base surgery.

Introduction

The dural sheath of the optic nerve is a structure which has received little attention in the literature. Nevertheless, it illustrates a broader idea of the dura mater: the interperiostodural concept. This sheath has the particularity of being the longest of the transbasal sheaths. It courses along with the optic nerve from its foramen to the orbit. At this point, it reinforces the sclera and provides the optic globe with its characteristic biomechanical properties. In this chapter we will successively discuss the embryology of optic nerves, the principles of the interperiostodural concept followed by a descriptive anatomy of this dural sheath and try to clarify its relations to nearby structures and the surgical implications at the level of each of its three segments: intracranial, intracanalicular and intraorbital.

Embryology

The optic vesicle begins to form as an evagination on the diencephalic neural fold on day 22. The stem of the optic vesicle narrows to form the optic stalk. The nerve fibers that emerge from the retinal ganglion cells in the sixth week travel through the optic stalk to reach the brain. The optic stalk is transformed into the optic nerve. As the optic vesicle forms, it is surrounded by a sheath of mesenchyme which differentiates to form the two coverings of the optic globe: an inner, pigmented, vascular layer called the choroid (homologous in origin with the pia mater and arachnoid membranes) and an outer, fibrous layer called the sclera (homologous with the dura mater). This latter tissue gives rise to the optic dural sheath whereas the choroid gives rise to the subarachnoid space between the optic nerve and its dural sheath. The subarachnoid space extends through the bony optic canal and along the optic nerve to the globe (Fig. 1A, B). However, the extent of communication in the optic canal showed wide variation from one specimen to another. This subarachnoid space is larger distally (near the globe) than proximally (region of the optic canal). Elevation of intracranial cerebrospinal fluid pressure is transmitted to the subarachnoid space surrounding the optic nerve sheath and thence into the optic nerve parenchyma leading to stasis of normal axoplasmic flow resulting in optic disk swelling. This mechanical theory explains pathogenesis of disk swelling in patients with elevated intracranial pressure.

The dural sheath of the optic nerve 189

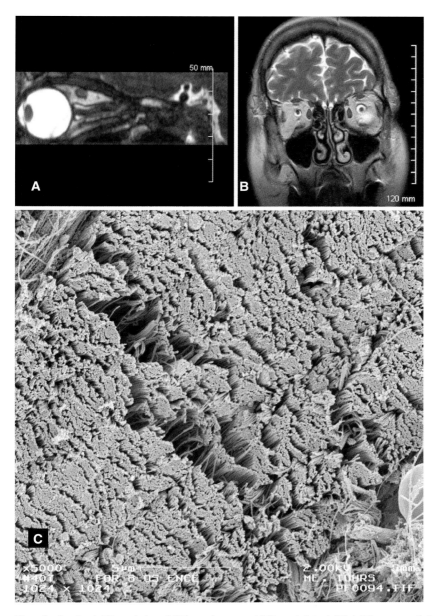

Fig. 1. Sagittal T2-weighted (A) and coronal T2-weighted (B) MRI scans of the orbit. The cerebrospinal fluid is contained in the subarachnoid space surrounding the optic nerve. This subarachnoid space extends through the bony optic canal and along the optic nerve to the globe. (C) An electron micrographic coronal section of the dural sheath of the optic nerve (X5000). The dura mater is composed of fibroblasts and extensive quantities of extracellular collagen

The interperiosteodural concept

The dura mater of the brain is comprised by two layers: an osteoperiostal layer which adheres to the bone and a thicker, encephalic layer which remains in contact to the arachnoid. These two layers adhere to one another at the level of the cranial vault but are separated at the dural sinuses and the interperiosteodural spaces represented by the orbits, the cavernous spaces and the "epidural" spinal space. These interperiosteodural spaces are filled with adipose tissue and veins. The adipose tissue serves to improve movement between the two sheets. The fatty tissue is less developed at the level of the cavernous space [7, 19]. Apart from the area of the sinuses, the venous lacunae are placed between these sheets and are more developed near the clivus where they form the petroclival venous confluence [3]. The internal carotid artery and the abducens nerve pass through this interperiosteodural space [3, 8].

The interperiosteodural concept has been especially studied at the level of the cavernous spaces. Ridley, in 1695, was the first to describe the parasellar region as a venous space surrounding the internal carotid artery [14]. In 1732, Winslow coined the term "cavernous sinus" for this region by analogy with the cavernous body of the penis since it contains fibrous trabeculae within its confines [20]. In 1949, first Taptas followed by Bonnet in 1955 described this sinus as a space located between the two layers of the dura mater [1, 16]. This space has been the object of numerous controversies. Finally, the notion of the cavernous space as being a space located between an osteoperiostal layer and an encephalic layer has since been extended to include the orbit and the spine inasmuch as the interperiosteodural concept has become an accepted anatomical concept extending from the coccyx to the sclera [9–11].

In the cavernous space, the lateral wall is thus constituted by a layer of encephalic dura mater which is continuous with the encephalic layer covering the middle cerebral fossa. This last-mentioned is doubled by a second plane formed by the juxtaposition of the dural sheaths of the cranial nerves coursing along the lateral wall of the cavernous space [4, 12, 18]. Consequently, these dural sheathes accompanying the cranial nerves up to the superior orbital fissure, which they cross in order to join the orbit, participate in forming the thickness of the lateral wall of the space. The medial wall of the cavernous space is formed by the hypophyseal dural sac constituted by the encephalic dura mater [2] dorsally and the periostium which covers the sphenoid ventrally. Between these two layers lie the coronary sinuses which represent intercavernous anastomoses just like the venous space of the clivus space anastomoses with the petroclival venous confluence. At the junction of the cavernous space and the orbit, the osteoperiostal layer continues through the periorbit while the encephalic layer continues through the dural sheath of the optic nerve. Thus, anatomic elements of the orbit annexed to the optic tracts are located between these two structures. The dural sheath of the optic nerve forms a fibrous sleeve which is in fact an invagination of the encephalic layer of the anterior base of the skull at the optic porus.

The orbit is therefore an interperiosteodural space corresponding to the rostral prolongation of the cavernous space. This space contains the vascular and nervous elements of the orbital cone surrounded by intra and extra-conic fatty islets. The dural sheath of the optic nerve is positioned at its center.

Described in this manner, the dural sheath of the optic nerve originates at the level of the optic canal and accompanies the optic nerve to the sclera. It is constituted by a close-knit meshwork of collagen fibers (Fig. 1C). Its collagen architecture provides indisputable mechanical properties since a 1 mm diameter collagen fiber is estimated to have a resistance of 10 kg. The dural sheath of the optic nerve includes three different segments which need to be described: the very short intracranial segment, the intracanalicular segment in the optic canal and an intraorbital segment which extends to the sclera.

Intracranial segment

This segment is very short and is essentially constituted by the invagination of the encephalic layer of the sphenoid planum at the level of the optic canal. This meningeal invagination does not adhere perfectly to the bone and gives rise to the falciform ligament. It can be a few millimeters in length. This ligament normally protects the dorsal surface of the optic nerve although, when an infraoptic tumor is present, it may shear it. Indeed, meningiomas of the tubercule of the sella turcica or of the sellar diaphragm can lift up the visual pathways and as a result, the ligament can leave its imprint on their dorsal surface. This fact may explain some preoperative visual field defects. Accordingly, the surgical approach to these tumors requires opening this falciform ligament before mobilization of the visual pathways.

Intracanalicular segment

At this level, the relations of the dural sheath are mainly with bony structures and the meninges.

Relations with bony structures

The dural sheath of the optic nerve exits the base of the skull through the optic canal which courses obliquely in a lateral and ventral direction. It is located at the junction of the lesser wing and the body of the sphenoid (Fig. 2). It comes into close contact with the anterior clinoid process which forms its lateral border. The anterior clinoid process is attached to the body of the sphenoid by two bony bridges which form the floor and the roof of the optic canal [15]. The roof of the canal is anterior to the floor; this explains why the plane of the

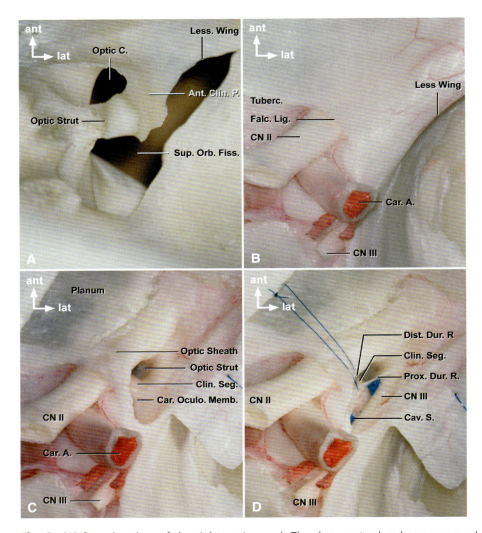

Fig. 2. (A) Superior view of the right optic canal. The dura mater has been removed. The optic canal, which provides passage for the optic nerve and the ophthalmic artery, opens into the orbital apex. It is separated from the superior orbital fissure by the optic strut which forms the floor of the optic canal. The optic strut and the roof of the optic canal constitute the anterior and posterior roots of the lesser wing of the sphenoid bone. (B) Superior view of the roof of the cavernous sinus without dissection. (C) The anterior clinoid process and the optic strut have been drilled to expose the anterior clinoid space. The dura that lines the lower margin of the anterior clinoid process and extends medially above the oculomotor nerve to surround the internal carotid artery and form the proximal dural ring is referred to as the carotidoculomotor membrane. The clinoid segment of the carotid artery is located between the proximal and distal dural rings. Above the distal dural ring, the carotid artery lies in the subarachnoid space and below it the cavernous sinus can be seen. (D) The proximal dural ring around the carotid artery has been opened to expose the oculomotor nerve in the lateral wall of the cavernous sinus (blue latex)

The dural sheath of the optic nerve

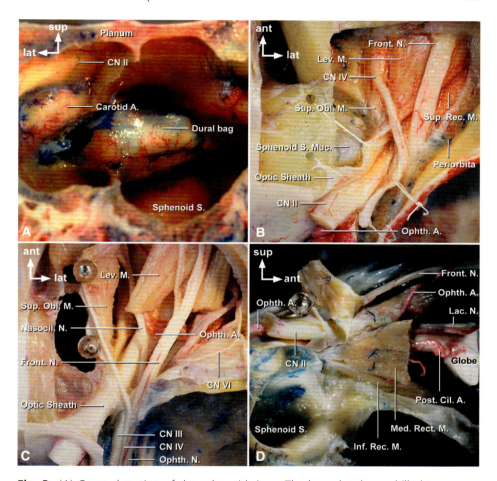

Fig. 3. (A) Coronal section of the sphenoid sinus. The bone has been drilled to expose the hypophyseal dural sac containing the hypophysis. The optic nerve lies above the anterior loop of the carotid artery in the cavernous sinus. (B) Superior view of the right optic canal. The bone has been drilled and the dural sheath of the optic nerve has been opened to expose the optic nerve. The trochlear and frontal nerves cross the optic nerve and lie outside muscles just below the periorbit. The ophthalmic artery arises from the intracranial internal carotid artery and extends along the inferolateral aspect of the optic sheath. (C) Superior view of the right orbit. The frontal nerve and the levator and superior rectus muscles have been divided and reflected to expose the ophthalmic artery and the nasociliary nerve as they pass above the optic nerve. The abducens nerve courses on the medial side of the ophthalmic nerve in the cavernous sinus, but it passes below the ophthalmic nerve in the superior orbital fissure to enter the medial surface of the lateral rectus muscle. (D) Medial view of the left orbit. The levator and medial rectus muscles have been sectioned to expose the distal dural sheath of the optic nerve near the globe. After passing above the optic nerve (85% of the cases), the ophthalmic artery courses between the superior oblique and the medial rectus muscles where it gives rise to the anterior and posterior ethmoidal arteries, the posterior ciliary artery and the meningeal branch for the dural sheath of the optic nerve

optic porus is not coronal. The optic canal has a truncal form and is wider in the back (elliptical shape) than in the front (circular shape). The optic porus is separated from the superior orbital fissure by a bony bridge called the "optic strut". This structure is an important surgical landmark when accessing the extra-dural portion of the anterior clinoid process. The "optic strut" joins the lesser wing of the sphenoid to the lateral wall of the sphenoid sinus. During the surgical treatment of spheno-orbital meningiomas, loss of vision in the patient requires that drilling be extended to the dural sheath of the optic nerve. The optic strut should constitute the medial limit of the drilling process; if drilling is continued further medially the sphenoid sinus will be opened, exposing the patient to postoperative rhinorrhea and possible infectious complications. The floor of the optic canal forms a relief in the sphenoid sinus which is an important landmark during endoscopic surgery of the pituitary gland. At this level, it is located above the anterior bend of the intracavernous carotid, lateral to the floor of the sella turcica. The bone can be very thin or even absent and when that is the case, the dural sheath of the optic nerve is in direct contact with the mucosa of the sphenoid sinus (Fig. 3A).

Meningeal relations

The meningeal relations of the dural sheath of the optic nerve are complex in the region of the sella turcica. In order to clearly understand them, the anterior clinoid process has to be drilled in order to expose the anterior clinoid space. The dura mater covering the ventral surface of the clinoid process forms a "carotidoculomotor membrane" strung between the internal carotid artery medially and the dural sheath of the oculomotor nerve. This membrane forms the meningeal roof of the cavernous space (Fig. 2C). The carotidoculomotor membrane is constituted by encephalic dura mater; medially it forms the proximal and distal carotid rings (Fig. 2D). The clinoid segment of the internal carotid is comprised between these two rings. The internal carotid forms its cavernous segments ventrally to the proximal carotid ring. Dorsally to the distal ring, it penetrates into the subarachnoid spaces. At this point, the dural sheath of the optic nerve is in contact with the distal carotid ring (Fig. 2D). The ophthalmic artery constitutes the first branch of the internal carotid artery, arising medial to the anterior clinoid process. It then joins the orbit after traversing the optic canal.

During the surgical treatment of carotid and ophthalmic aneurysms, the anterior clinoid process should be drilled in order to clearly expose the origin of the ophthalmic artery and allow the aneurysm to be isolated with a clip. Hashimoto [5] insisted on the fact that a preoperative 3D angioscan can help the surgeon determine the exact location of the aneurysm's collar in relation to the optic strut (a radiological landmark) and thereby improve subsequent therapeutic strategy. When the aneurismal collar is dorsal to the optic strut, the aneurysm should most often be treated surgically. However, when the collar is ventral to the optic strut, the aneurysm is intracavernous and should be treated with an endovascular technique.

Yang *et al.* [21] reviewed the principles involved in extradural anterior clinoidectomy when techniques for the post-traumatic decompression of the optic nerve are employed. He underlined the fact that the clinoid segment of the internal carotid is only separated from the medial border of the anterior clinoid process by a thin meningeal sheet: the carotid collar. This meningeal structure is stretched between the carotid rings. The proximal ring is often incomplete while the distal ring is tightly packed. This fact explains why venous blood coming from the cavernous spaces can surround the clinoid segment of the internal carotid. A clinoidectomy using the extradural approach which is indispensable for gaining access to the dural sheath of the optic nerve, can prove to be difficult especially when the sheath is prominent caudally. It should be carefully drilled so as to avoid injury to the internal carotid. After this preparatory bony procedure, the dural sheath of the optic nerve is exposed then incised along the optic nerve from the falciform ligament to the anular tendon (anulus of Zinn) between the insertion of the lateral and superior rectus muscles.

Intraorbital segment

In its orbital segment, the relations of the dural sheath of the optic nerve are essentially with the vascular and nervous elements going to the orbit. At the exit of the optic canal, the meninges of the sheath of the optic nerve become particularly dense (Fig. 3B). At this level, it helps form the anular tendon ring where the muscles providing mobility to the ocular globe and its annexes (eyelid) insert. The anular tendon forms the apex of the orbital cone through which course the dural sheath of the optic nerve dorsally in addition to the abducens nerve, the nasociliary nerve, the superior and inferior branches of the oculomotor nerve and the ophthalmic artery. The dural sheath of the optic nerve is an essential surgical landmark beyond the anular tendon since it represents the central element in the orbital cone formed by the rectus, levator and oblique muscles. It is surrounded by adipose tissue which facilitates eye movements in the three spatial planes.

The ophthalmic artery arises at the medial border of the internal carotid, in general beyond the distal carotid ring, but sometimes at the level of the clinoid segment between the two carotid rings or at the cavernous sinus (8% of the cases) [13, 15], below the proximal carotid ring. When this is the case, it joins the orbit through the superior orbital fissure. The ophthalmic artery accompanies the optic nerve in its sheath, traveling along its inferomedial border (Fig. 3D). Beyond the optic canal, it travels obliquely through the sheath of the optic nerve and joins the orbital apex lateral to the optic nerve. Occasionally, it gives off a recurrent branch in the optic canal which takes part in the vascularization of the intracanalicular segment of the optic nerve [17]. In 85% of the cases, the ophthalmic artery crosses the dural sheath of the optic nerve dorsally where it lies between the medial rectus and superior oblique muscles before giving rise to the anterior and posterior ethmoid arteries. The ophthalmic artery also gives rise to the lacrymal, the ciliary, the supraorbital, the medial palpebral, the infratrochlear and the dorsal nasal arteries. The central retinal artery is the smallest of its branches considering its diameter but the most important according to its function since it is a terminal branch which provides vascularization to the macula. The central retinal artery enters the lower surface of the optic nerve at the junction between the anterior $1/3$ and median $1/3$ about twenty millimeters from the optic canal following a short, serpiginous trajectory. There it passes to the center of the optic nerve up to the globe and vascularizes the retina. The central retinal artery can present anatomical variations: origin by a common trunk along with the posterior ciliary or muscular arteries, a proximal origin with a long intraorbital trajectory before penetrating the dural sheath of the optic nerve, or finally, with a distal origin and a very short intraorbital trajectory. The intraorbital portion of the optic nerve derives its blood supply from a rich anastomotic vascular network located in the pia mater which is supplied by the ciliary arteries. Optic nerve meningiomas are derived from arachnoidal cap cells and may grow in a subdural, extradural or combined location. It may focally enlarge or may extend axially along the nerve to the intracranial compartment. Optic sheath meningioma in the posterior orbit are virtually impossible to resect completely without resulting in blindness. Optic neuropathy after surgical treatment may be due to inadvertent retraction, vascular compromise or heat transmission from bipolar coagulation energy or drilling.

In summary, five different elements cross the orbital segment of the dural sheath of the optic nerve dorsally:

- The trochlear nerve in the back of the orbit which exits the cavernous space through the superior orbital fissure. It has an extra-conic trajectory under the periorbit and joins to the superior oblique muscle which it innervates (Fig. 3B).
- The frontal nerve, the dorsal dividing branch of the ophthalmic nerve, which arises at the superior orbital fissure outside the common tendon ring and lies under the periorbit in front of the trochlear nerve. It courses above the levator muscle and gives off the supratrochlear and supraorbital nerves (Fig. 3C).
- The nasociliary nerve is the second dividing branch of the ophthalmic nerve. It also arises at the superior orbital fissure ventrally to the frontal nerve. It travels in the orbital cone and joins the anteromedial compart-

ment of the orbit. It gives off the long ciliary nerves and distributes sympathetic fibers to the dilator muscle of the pupil. These fibers course around the intracavernous carotid and join the ophthalmic nerve at the cavernous space.

- The ophthalmic artery crosses over the optic nerve's dural sheath. It sometimes crosses the dural sheath of the optic nerve ventrally before reaching the anteromedial compartment of the orbit.
- The superior ophthalmic vein receives anastomoses from the facial and supraorbital veins. It travels under the superior rectus muscle and crosses over the dural sheath of the optic nerve before taking up a position along the sheath's lateral border. It empties into the cavernous space by exiting the orbit through the superior orbital fissure, outside the anular tendon.

Orbital lesions can be approached by the transcranial, transmandibular, transnasal, transethmoid, or finally, the lateral or transconjunctival orbital route [13]. The choice of surgical approach depends on the lesion's localization, size, and characteristics as well as the operator's experience and preference. Most of the time, two approaches are available to neurosurgeons: the transcranial and the lateral approach. The transcranial provides access to the orbital apex through its dorsal wall and to the compartment located medial to the dural sheath of the optic nerve when the space between the levator muscles of the eyelid and the superior oblique are open. In order to treat lesions which have appeared in front of the superior orbital fissure or along the lateral border of the dural sheath of the optic nerve, the surgeon must open the space located between the superior and the lateral rectus muscles [6]. These upper approaches require a craniotomy and drilling of the roof of the orbit. The trochlear and frontal nerves are particularly exposed to injury due to their extraconic location, under the periorbit. In contrast, the central retinal artery is protected by the dural sheath of the optic nerve. In lateral approaches to the orbit, drilling removes the lateral wall of the orbit and provides access to the inferolateral quadrant of the orbit by passing under the lateral rectus muscle. This approach minimizes the risks of injury to the trochlear and frontal nerves but opens the door to injuring the central retinal artery or the short ciliary nerves.

Conclusion

The optic dural sheath is the longest dural sheath. It describes an intracranial, intracanalicular and intraorbital segments with specific surgical implications. The optic dural sheath forms the encephalic layer of the orbital compartment of the extra dural axis compartment which is an anatomic concept applied from the coccyx to the orbit.

References

1. Bonnet P (1955) La loge caverneuse et les syndromes de la loge caverneuse. Arch Ophtalmol 15: 332–57
2. Destrieux C, Kakou MK, Velut S, Lefrancq T, Jan M (1998) Microanatomy of the hypophyseal fossa boundaries. J Neurosurg 88: 743–52
3. Destrieux C, Velut S, Kakou MK, Lefrancq T, Arbeille B, Santini JJ (1997) A new concept in Dorello's canal microanatomy: the petroclival venous confluence. J Neurosurg 87: 67–72
4. Harris FS, Rhoton AL (1976) Anatomy of the cavernous sinus. A microsurgical study. J Neurosurg 45: 169–80
5. Hashimoto K, Nozaki K, Hashimoto N (2006) Optic strut as a radiographic landmark in evaluating neck location of a paraclinoid aneurysm. Neurosurgery 59: 880–87
6. Morard M, Tcherekayev V, de Tribolet N (1994) The superior orbital fissure: a microanatomical study. Neurosurgery 35: 1087–93
7. Mukherji SK, Tart RP, Fitzsimmons J, Belden C, McGorray S, Guy J (1994) Fat-suppressed MR of the orbit and cavernous sinus: comparison of fast spin-echo and conventional spin-echo. Am J Neuroradiol 15: 1707–14
8. Parkinson D (1965) A surgical approach to the cavernous portion of the carotid artery. Anatomical studies and case report. J Neurosurg 23: 474–83
9. Parkinson D (1991) Human spinal arachnoid septa, trabeculae, and "rogue strands". Am J Anat 1992: 498–509
10. Parkinson D (2000) Extradural neural axis compartment. J Neurosurg 92: 585–88
11. Parkinson D (2000) History of the extradural neural axis compartment. Surg Neurol 54: 422–31
12. Patouillard P, Vanneuville G (1972) The walls of the cavernous sinus. Neurochirurgie 18: 551–60
13. Rhoton AL, Natori Y (1996) Surgical approaches. In: Rhoton Al, Natori Y (eds) The orbit and sellar region: microsurgical anatomy and operative approaches. Thieme Medical publishers, New York
14. Ridley (1695) The anatomy of the brain, vol. 39. London
15. Seoane JR, Rhoton AL, de Oliveira EP (1998) Microsurgical anatomy of the dural collar (carotid collar) and rings around the clinoid segment of the internal carotid artery. Neurosurgery 42: 869–86
16. Taptas JN (1949) La loge du sinus caverneux sa constitution et les rapports des éléments vasculaires et nerveux qui la traversent. Sem Hop 40: 1719–22
17. Tsutsumi S, Rhoton AL (2006) Microsurgical anatomy of the central retinal artery. Neurosurgery 59: 870–79
18. Umansky F, Nathan H (1982) The lateral wall of the cavernous sinus. With special reference to the nerves related to it. J Neurosurg 56: 228–34
19. Weninger WJ, Streicher J, Muller GB (1997) Anatomical compartments of the parasellar region: adipose tissue bodies represent intracranial continuations of extracranial spaces. J Anat 191: 269–75
20. Winslow JB (1732) Exposition anatomique de la structure du corps humain, vol. 31. London
21. Yang Y, Wang H, Shao Y, Wei Z, Zhu S, Wang J (2006) Extradural anterior clinoidectomy as an alternative approach for optic nerve decompression: Anatomic study and clinical experience. Neurosurgery 59: 253–62

Surgical indications and techniques for failed coiled aneurysms

C. Raftopoulos; with the collaboration of G. Vaz

Department of Neurosurgery, University Hospital St-Luc, Université Catholique de Louvain (UCL), Brussels, Belgium

With 11 Figures and 8 Tables

Contents

Abstract 199
Introduction 200
Experience of our group 202
    Our population and illustrative cases 208
    Our classification of FCA and its lessons 213
Experiences of other teams 217
Conclusions 222
References 222

Abstract

For two decades, endovascular coiling has revolutionized the treatment of intracranial aneurysms. However, as with all techniques, it has limitations and endovascular radiologists and neurosurgeons are regularly confronted by what we call "failed" coiled aneurysms. Failed coiled aneurysms can occur in different situations: a) presence of a significant remnant at the end of an endovascular procedure; b) recanalization of an initially satisfactory occlusion; and c) coil extrusion deemed too thrombogenic or threatening the blood flow in the parent vessel. We and other teams around the world have developed strategies to manage these difficult cases. Here, we compare our own experience with other reports in the literature.

Keywords: Clipping; coil embolization; coiling; complications; endovascular therapy; intracranial aneurysm; recanalization; residual aneurysm; subarachnoid haemorrhage; surgery postembolization.

Introduction

Since 1991, endovascular coiling (EVC) with Guglielmi detachable coils (GDC, Boston Scientific, Fremont, CA, USA) has progressively become an additional, effective treatment for intracranial aneurysms (ICA), in particular for those of the posterior circulation and those that have ruptured [13, 28, 29]. However, as with all techniques, EVC has several limitations (Table 1). First, up to 69% of patients undergoing EVC have thromboembolic events demonstrated using diffusion-weighted MR imaging, with 27% experiencing clinical deterioration [30, 40, 45]; other teams report a 9% rate of clinical ischaemic events [17, 49], with 3% having haemorrhagic complications [17] and 5% persistent deficits [30]. Second, the technique requires considerable irradiation, with around 530 chest X-ray doses for an EVC procedure plus doses related to the control angiography and possible second EVC [3, 21, 24, 32, 42], which occurs in about 10% of all ICA treated by EVC [10]. Third, there is an aneurysm

Table 1. EVC presents a high rate of

TEE → PPMby	≤69% → 7.1%
Irradiation	530[1]
Residue	43.2% (81%)[2]
Recanalization	17.2% (2.4–71.4%)[3]
Cost at 1 year[4]	$45.493

EVC endovascular coiling; PPMby permanent procedural morbidity; TEE thromboembolic event observed by diffusion weighted magnetic resonance imaging.
[1]About 530 chest X-ray doses for an EVC procedure [32].
[2]Evaluation with time-of-flight magnetic resonance angiography [16].
[3]Depends on the aneurysm size [29].
[4]EVC is most costly at 1 year than surgical clipping [25].

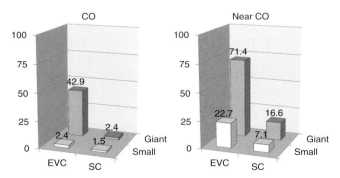

Fig. 1. Recanalization % varies depending on: Co complete occlusion; EVC endovascular coiling; SC surgical clipping

remnant in up to 43.2% of cases [15, 29], or even more if analyzed using time-of-flight resonance magnetic angiography [16]. Fourth, EVC shows a high rate of recanalization averaging about 17.2%, but varying between 2.4 and 71.4%, depending on the degree of aneurysm occlusion and its size (Fig. 1) [15, 29, 38]. It has been demonstrated that aneurysm recanalization occurs significantly more often after EVC than after surgical clipping (SC) [7, 29, 47]. When complete occlusion is achieved with EVC, the rate of recanalization varies between 2.4 and 42.9% [29], depending on the aneurysm size, while after SC this rate is 1.5 to 2.4% [7, 47]. This rate of recanalization is even higher in cases of near complete occlusion (residue of 5% or less; grade I or II of Sindou [44]), with 22.7 to 71.4% being recanalized after EVC compared to 7.1 to 16.6% after SC [7, 29, 47]. Fifth and finally, in the United States, EVC appears to be more costly at one year than SC although direct comparison of both treatment arms in the International Subarachnoid Aneurysm Trial (ISAT) showed similar costs for the two therapies at 24-month follow-up [25, 51].

Table 2. *Three types of failed coiled aneurysms (FCA)*

A	Attempts *no coil left in the aneurysm*
B	≥2 mm high aneurysmal residue *at ≥6 months post EVC*
C	Complication *Coil extrusion/compression*

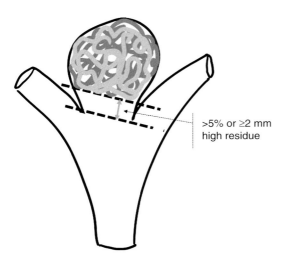

Fig. 2. Failed coiled aneurysm of group B

Table 3. *Rerupture % within 2 years after EVC [19]*

CO	1.1
Near CO *(Residue < 10%)*	2.9
Partial O	23.5

Median time to rerupture was 3 days (range 1 day to 1.1 year) and 58% died. *CARAT* Cerebral Aneurysm Rerupture After Treatment; *CO* complete occlusion; *EVC* endovascular coiling.

When an ICA is not completely or nearly completely occluded by EVC at a six month follow-up, it is labelled a failed coiled aneurysm (FCA; grade III to V of Sindou [44]) and can be one of three types (Table 2) [14]: type A, when an EVC attempt was carried out but no coil is left in the aneurysm; type B (Fig. 2), when there is an aneurysm residue of more than 5% or at least 2 mm between the aneurysm neck and the coil mass base at six months or later after EVC; and type C, when a complication related to EVC requires an urgent open surgical procedure (coil extrusion or nerve compression by the coil package).

Another problem associated with EVC is the risk of re-rupture (Table 3). In 2008, one study [19] reported that the re-rupture percentage following EVC was 1.1% after complete occlusion, 2.9% after near complete occlusion (residue < 10%), and as high as 23.5% after partial occlusion. It must be stressed that the median time to re-rupture was three days and 58% of the patients who re-ruptured died. Therefore, patients who have a marked aneurysm residue or recanalization after EVC always require strict follow-up, with an additional obliteration procedure when there is a treatable aneurysm residue.

Experience of our group

In February 1996, we instituted our department of Neurosurgery and our neurovascular group at the Saint-Luc University Hospital, Brussels. Since then, endovascular coiling (EVC) has been considered as the first-line treatment option for ruptured and unruptured intracranial aneurysms, notably in the following situations: first, no compressive haematoma requiring urgent evacuation; second, aneurysm located on the posterior circulation; third, patients with a poor medical condition or more than 65 years old; fourth, ruptured aneurysm, especially if not a middle cerebral artery aneurysm; and fifth, aneurysms with a fundus-neck ratio greater than or equal to 2.5, neck diameter less than 4 mm, not giant, and with no thrombus inside the aneurysm.

From February 1996 to August 2009, a consecutive series of 819 aneurysms, with significantly more cases in the last few years, was assessed by our group; 80% were treated while the other 20% were monitored (Fig. 3; Table 4). Of the aneurysms that were treated, 275 (42%) were recommended for an EVC procedure and 380 (58%) underwent SC. The EVC procedure performed

Surgical indications and techniques

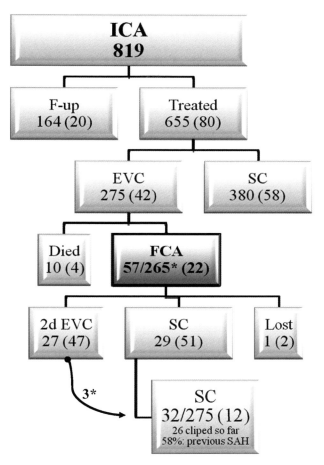

Fig. 3. Flowchart of our general ICA population from February 1996* to August 2009 with the management of our FCA (%). *EVC* endovascular coiling; February 1996*, creation of our department; *FCA* failed coiled aneurysm; *F-up* follow-up; *ICA* intracranial aneurysm; *SAH* subarachnoid hemorrhage; *SC* surgical clipping. 265*, = 275 ICA submitted to an EVC minus the 10 patients who died within one month post EVC 3*, three patients after a 2nd ineffective EVC procedure went for open surgery

by our team has already been reported in previous papers [35, 36]. EVC was essentially performed by one endovascular radiologist (P. Goffette) who used Guglielmi electrolitically detachable coils (GDC, Boston Scientific, Fremont, CA, USA) in all cases, associated regularly in recent years with a balloon-assist technique or stent deployment (Neuroform II, Boston Scientific).

EVC was associated with complete occlusion of the aneurysm in 62.4% of cases, near complete occlusion in 24%, partial occlusion in 5.6%, and attempted occlusion in 8% (Table 5). SC achieved complete occlusion in 90.5% of cases (95% if unruptured aneurysms [1]), near complete occlusion

Table 4. *Population with one or more ICA entered in our department between its opening in February 1996 to August 2009 and our management strategies (%)*

	Σ	Management strategies			
		Follow-up	Treatment		
			Σ	EVC	SC
Patients number	651	122 (19)	529 (81)	249 (47)	280 (53)
Sex					
F/M	2.1	2.2	2.1	2.1	2
Average age (min–max), mo					
F	51 (21–89)	58 (21–86)	50 (21–89)	50 (21–84)	51 (28–89)
M	52 (21–77)	60 (21–76)	49 (1.8–77)	50 (1.8–73)	49 (33–77)
Patient with multiple ICA	275 (42)	66 (24)	209 (76)	92 (44)	117 (56)
ICA number	819	164 (20)	655 (80)	275 (42)	380 (58)

EVC Endovascular coiling; *F* female; *ICA* intracranial aneurysm; *M* male; *mo* months; *SC* surgical clipping.

Table 5. *Occlusion rates obtained by EVC or SC in 655 consecutive ICA (%)*

	Treatment		
	Σ	EVC	SC
Aneurysm number	655	275 (42)	380 (58)
Occlusion rate			
CO	515 (79)	171 (62.4)	344 (90.5*)
Near CO	88 (13)	66 (24)	22 (6)
Partial O	19 (3)	15 (5.6)	4 (1)
Attempt	24 (4)	23[a] (8)	2[b] (0.5)
No postop angiography	8 (1)	–	8 (2)

CO complete occlusion; *EVC* endovascular coiling; *F* female; *ICA* intracranial aneurysm; *M* male; *Postop* postoperative; *SC* surgical clipping.
(90.5*), becomes 95% in case of unruptured aneurysms [1].
23[a], three patients had more than one EVC attempt.
2[b], 1 wrapping and one surgical approach impossible because of cerebral oedema.

in 6%, partial occlusion in 1%, and attempted occlusion in 0.5%. At the end of August 2009 and at least 6 months post-EVC, there were 57 (31 + 26) FCA, representing 22% of the cases that underwent an EVC procedure (Table 6; Fig. 3). These 57 cases comprised 69% of the partially occluded, and, of course, all aneurysms in which EVC had been attempted but failed.

Table 6. *Occlusion follow-up of ICA treated first by EVC and according to their initial occlusion rates (%) and 2nd treatment*

EVC	ICA	Death	Spont CO	Spont near CO	Stable occlusion rate	Rec	Res	2nd treatment				Lost
								2nd EVC		SC		
								Done	Pending	Done	Pending	
Σ	275	10 (3.6)	29 (11)	1	178 (67)	31 (12)	26 (10)	21*	6	26	6	1
CO	171	0	0	0	159 (93)	12 (7)		4	1	6	1	0
Near CO	66	2 (3)*	26 (41)	–	19 (30)	19 (29)		9	2	8	–	0
Partial O	15	2 (13)*	3 (23)	1 (7)	0		9 (69)	1	3	5	–	0
Attempt	23 (8)*	6 (26)*	–	–	–		17	4	–	7	5	1

CO complete occlusion; *EVC* endovascular coiling; *ICA* intracranial aneurysm; *Rec/Res* recanalization or residue with a ≥ 2 mm high neck remnant; *SC* surgical clipping; *Spont* spontaneous.

23 (8)*, three patients had more than one EVC attempt.

2 (3)*, one patient rebleeded post EVC; the second developed a L hemisph ischemic stroke post EVC.

2 (13)*, 2 pts with ruptured ICA and poor clinical condition.

6 (26)*, 3 pts showed an initial poor clinical condition (WFNS = 4 and 5); 2 pts experienced a subarachnoid hemorrhage during EVC followed by vasospasm; 1 pt died unexpectedly a few days later of possible new rebleeding.

21*, 3 patients recanalized after the 2nd EVC and went for SC.

Other percentages were calculated excluding the deaths.

Table 7. Summary of our 26 consecutive Failed Coiled Aneurysms treated by open surgery and distributed in three groups A, B and C

Patient no.	Age (yr)/ sex	SAH	Aneurysm				EVC			OS		
			Location	LA (mm)	Neck (mm)	F/N	1st/2nd	Rec (m/m)	GOS	Type	CO	GOS
Group A (attempted EVC, no coil inside the aneurysm)												
1	53/F	–	Ba Tr	10	4	2.5	Attempt	7	5	A	+	=
2	39/F	+	L-MCA	4	2	1	Attempt	–	5	A	+	=
3	37/F	–	L-PerCal	12	6	1	Attempt	1	5	A	+	=
4	56/F	–	L-MCA	5	2	2	Attempt	–	3	A	+	=
5	66/F	+	R-MCA	3	1	2	Attempt	–	4	A	+	=
6	40/M	–	ACoA	2	1	1.5	Attempt	–	5	A	+	=
7	54/M	–	ACoA	11	4	2	Attempt	2	5	A	+	=
Group B (coils inside the aneurysm, ≥2 mm high aneurysm residue)												
1	37/F	+	R-ICA Tip	12	3	4	P	12	4	B3	+	=
2*	53/M	–	R-MCA	34	8	4	P/P	1/64	5	B3	+	=
3	63/M	+	L-PCoA	21	4	2	P	24	4	B1	+	=
4	60/M	+	ACoA	5	2	2.5	CO	20	5	B1	+	=
5	61/M	–	ACoA	15	1.5	2	Near CO	8	5	B1	+	=
6	59/M	+	R-PCoA	5	2	2.5	Near CO	7	5	B1	+	=
7	48/F	+	R-Pcl (Oph)	25	7	4	Near CO	24	5	B2	+	=
8	53/M	–	L-MCA	22	8	3	Near CO	24	5	B3	+	=
9	65/F	+	ACoA	4	2	2	CO	11	5	B1	+	=
10	41/F	–	ACoA	5	2	2.5	Near CO	24	5	B1	+	=
11*	61/F	+	L-Pcl (Po)	20	8	2.5	CO/P*	7/72	5	B1	+	=***

12	55/F	–	L-PCoA	6	2	3	Near CO	24	5	B1	+	=
13	54/F	+	ACoA	4	2	2	Near CO	36	3	B1	+	5
14	44/M	+	L-PerCal	6	2.5	2.5	CO	17	4	B4	+	5
15	56/M	+	L-PICA	8	4.5	1	CO/Near CO*	8/12*	5	B2	Near	=
16	42/M	+	ACoA	4	3.5	1.1	P	5	5	B1	+	=
17	46/M	+	ACoA	6	3	2	CO	111	5	B1	+	4**

Group C (EVC complication: coil extrusion)

1	39/F	+	ACoA	4	1.5	2.5	Coil extrus	–	4	C1 (U)	+	5***
2	63/M	–	R-MCA	7	3	2.5	Coil extrus	–	5	C2 (U)	+	=

ACoA anterior communicating artery; *Bl* neck residue enough for direct plic application; *B2* neck residue with coil but direct clip application possible; *B3* Fundus coil resection en bloc followed by clipping of the residual neck; *B4* fundus coil resection followed by suture of the residual neck; *Cl* coil extraction through parent vessel; *C2* coil extraction through fundus followed by dipping; *CO* complete occlusion demonstrated by angiography; *EVC* endovascular coiling, one or two procedures; *Coil extru* coil extrusion Followed by an urgent (U) surgical procedure; *CO/Near CO** first EVC was complete, second EVC was near complete despite the use of a stent (Neuroform II, Boston Scientific); *CO/P** the first EVC was interrupted by a thrombosis of the internal carotid artery in the neck, the treatment by EVC was fully completed 13 days later with complete occlusion and a 3rd procedure was performed 72 months later after recanalisation and reached only partial occlusion which again slowly recanalized; *F* female; *F/N* fund/neck ratio; *GOS* Glasgow Outcome Scale (=means stable GOS); *ICA* internal carotid artery; *L* left; *M* male; *m* months; *LA* longest axis; *MCA* middle cerebral artery; *OS* open surgery classified accordingly to the type of surgical procedure performed; *Oph* ophtalmic aneurysm; *P* partial occlusion, residue > 5%; *Pcl* paraclinoid aneurysm; *PCoA* posterior communicating artery; *PerCal* pericallosal artery; *Po* posterior variety aneurysm; *PICA* posterior inferior cerebellar artery; *R* right; *Rec (m/m)* recanalisation or residue increase demonstrated by angiography performed a certain number of months (m) after each EVC (m/m); (U) OS in emergency; *yr* year.

2*, 11* these two patients were embolized before 1996; 8/12* during the 12 months after the 2nd EVC procedure, the patient underwent three angiographies and one angio-CT scan to monitor the progressive recanalisation 4** slight cognitives troubles; *** transient slight motor deficit.

In these 57 FCA, 27 (47%) underwent a second EVC procedure (Table 6; Fig. 3), 29 (10.5% of all the aneurysms initially treated by EVC) were selected for a surgical procedure, and one patient was lost. In three of the patients who had a second EVC procedure, the aneurysm recanalized and SC was performed. Of the 32 FCA (11.6%) that were selected for surgical occlusion, 26 had already undergone surgery by the end of August 2009, and 6 patients are scheduled for upcoming surgery. Among the 26 FCA who have already had the open surgical procedure, 58% had had a previous subarachnoid haemorrhage (Fig. 3).

For the FCA undergoing SC, since one year, the procedure is first performed virtually using the Dextroscope (Volumes Interactions, Bracco, Singapore) before going to the operating room. The Dextroscope allows the user to see a 3D virtual reality multimodal patient's head with its intracranial vessels and helps the neurosurgeon to familiarize him/her self to the forthcoming surgery. The SC procedure was performed under mild hypothermia (33°C) and electroencephalographic burst suppression [32, 33, 35–37]. Temporary clipping and evoked potentials were used when required. The most frequent surgical approach was a pterional approach. In all cases, clips designed by Perneczky were used (Zeppelin GbmH, Pullack, Germany and later Peter Lazic GbmH, Tuttlingen, Germany) [31]. This type of clip offers two fundamental advantages: (1) A larger operative field vision during the clipping process because the applying forceps hold the clip inside its ends; and (2) the possibility of removing these clips over a wide range of angles with a removing forceps fitting between the clip's ends. These clips can, thus, be easily removed allowing more clipping trials to obtain complete aneurysm occlusion. All the procedures were performed by the first author (CR) assisted by the co-author (GV). Intermittent temporary occlusion of the parent vessel was used in 54% of the 26 FCA, and was always less than ten minutes except in one case without clinical consequence (Table 7, group B, patient 14). If a longer temporary occlusion was required, we stopped the occlusion after ten minutes to allow reflow for at least five minutes before restarting temporary occlusion. All patients had post-operative cerebral angiography by femoral catheterisation.

Our population and illustrative cases

Group A (Table 7), with seven cases of attempted EVC, represents the standard procedure for the neurosurgeon, but these were difficult cases. Indeed, all these cases either had an unfavourable morphology (wide aneurysm neck, fundus-neck ratio <2.5, or arterial branch at the aneurysm neck) for stabilizing the coil inside the aneurysm or showed particularities, such as access vessel tortuosity, atheromatosis or fibromuscular dysplasia, which prevented the endovascular radiologist from navigating the endovascular catheter to the an-

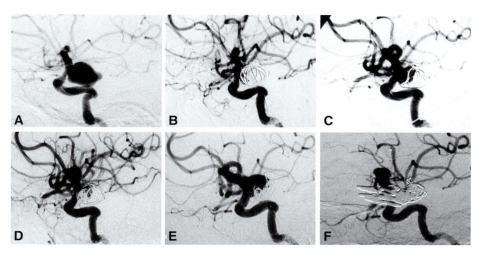

Fig. 4a. Large left paraclinoid aneurysm (posterior variant) (Table 7, group B, patient 11). (A) Before endovascular coiling (EVC); (B) after the first EVC with near complete occlusion (CO) but poor coil packing, this first EVC was interrupted by thrombus formation in the internal carotid artery at the neck that was removed surgically; the endovascular procedure was completed 13 days later; (C) recanalization; (D) second EVC with partial occlusion; (E) second recanalization; (F) complete occlusion by surgical clipping

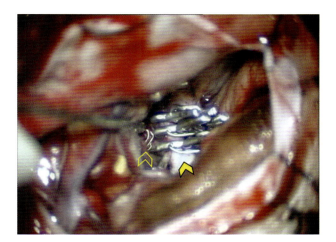

Fig. 4b. Intraoperative photograph showing, through a left pterional approach, the reconstruction of the internal carotid artery (*solid arrow head*) with three short slightly curved fenestrated clips. On the left (*open arrow head*), three coil loops are visible outside the aneurysm wall probably after a slow migration through the fundus wall itself

eurysm neck. EVC was attempted in these cases either because the endovascular radiologist thought he could succeed or because the patient was in a poor clinical condition and we agreed to try to at least occlude the fundus.

For FCA with coils inside the aneurysm (group B; Table 7), there were several specific situations. The less difficult case was when the recanalization was large enough to allow direct application of one or multiple clips (Table 7, patient 11) (Figs. 4a, 4b). Another situation was when the recanalization occurred with coils partly present in the aneurysm neck (Table 7, patient 7,

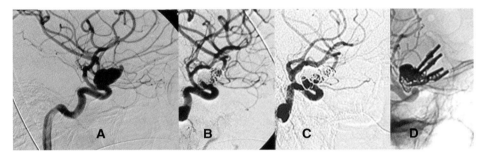

Fig. 5. Large right paraclinoid aneurysm (Table 7, group B, patient 7). (A) Just before the EVC; (B) at the end of EVC with near complete occlusion but poorly packed coils in the fundus and partly migrated in the parent vessel; (C) recanalization at 24 months; (D) surgical complete occlusion with the migrated coil incorporated in the neck and parent vessel walls

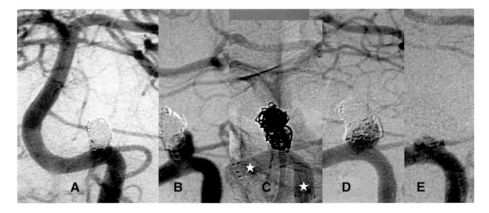

Fig. 6a. Small left PICA aneurysm (Table 7, group B, patient 15). (A) first complete endovascular coiling (EVC); (B) first recanalization; (C) second EVC with a stent (the two stars indicate the stent extremity markers, Neuroform II, Boston Scientific); (D) second recanalization; E, nearly complete occlusion after direct clip application (the only case considered not completely occluded after surgical clipping)

Surgical indications and techniques 211

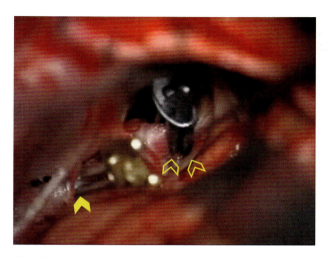

Fig. 6b. Intraoperative photograph showing, through a left retrosigmoid approach (the left ear is located at the upper left), two clips (*two open arrow heads*) on the part of the aneurysm neck which was not filled with coils. A temporary clip on the left vertebral artery through the left mixed nerves is also visible (*solid arrow head*).

Fig. 5 and patient 15, Figs. 6a, 6b) and, in one case, with a stent in the parent vessel (patient 15, Figs. 6a, 6b). In these situations, we had to dissect and precisely place the clips on the part of the aneurysm neck that was free of coil. In the case with the stent present in the parent vessel (Fig. 6a). we could temporarily clip the parent vessel, the left vertebral artery (Fig. 6b), with no difficulty probably because the stent was already integrated into the vessel wall. In three cases (Table 7, group B, patients 1, 2 and 8), although we thought there was enough aneurysm residue for direct clip application, we unfortunately experienced a parent vessel stenosis by the clip being pushed onto the parent vessel by the coil mass. We therefore resected the aneurysm fundus with the coil mass either in an en block (patient 8, Figs. 7a, 7b) or a piecemeal fashion. Once the fundus with the coil mass had been resected, we were able to streamline the clip application onto the aneurysm neck, avoiding any parent vessel stenosis. In another case (Table 7, group B, patient 14) (Figs. 8a, 8b), after piecemeal resection of the fundus with the coils, there was not enough neck remnant for clip application without parent vessel stenosis. In this case, we were obliged to perform a suture with 3 stitches of an 8.0 thread plus application of a microclip on a residual leak.

In group C cases (Table 7, group C), there were two different situations: In the first (Fig. 9a). an anterior communicating artery aneurysm was initially completely occluded by EVC, but then presented a coil extrusion into the parent vessel, up to the left Sylvian bifurcation. Because of the significant length of the extruded coil and the potential thromboembolic risk, we decided

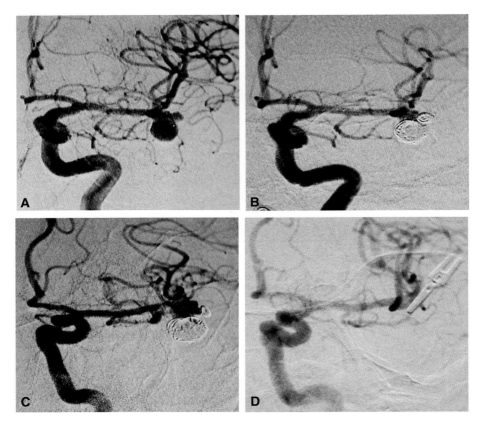

Fig. 7a. Small left middle cerebral artery aneurysm (Table 7, group B, patient 8). (A) Before endovascular coiling (EVC); (B) after near complete occlusion by EVC; (C) recanalization; (D) complete occlusion by surgical clipping after en bloc resection of the aneurysm fundus filled with coils.

to extract it as an emergency (Fig. 9b). A report of this case has previously been published in full [34]. It was a straightforward procedure consisting essentially of temporary clipping of both the left and right A1 segments and, with the help of a hook, anchoring the coil and extracting it (Fig. 9b). The post-operative evolution was uneventful. The second case (Fig. 10a) occurred after complete occlusion of a right small middle cerebral artery aneurysm by EVC when multiple coil loops extruded into the left mild cerebral artery bifurcation. The surgical procedure was also performed as an emergency and involved extracting the entire coil mass and the extruded coils through the fundus (Fig. 10b). During this procedure, we observed that already only two hours after the EVC, the coil mass was already very adherent to the aneurysm wall, but not enough to preclude its extraction. Regarding our entire series of 26

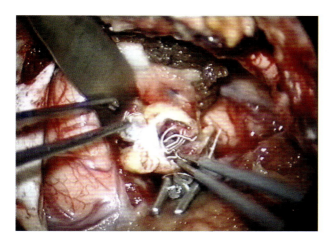

Fig. 7b. Intraoperative picture showing, through a left pterional approach, the "en bloc" resected fundus full of coils. The coils appear clearly imbedded into a dense intraaneurysmal fibrosis precluding all coil extraction. One straight clip is placed on the remaining aneurysm neck without any parent vessel stenosis. On the upper left, a blade is used to retract the left temporal lobe. No retractor on the left frontal lobe

consecutive FCA, complete occlusion was performed in 25 cases (96%), only one patient deteriorated slightly after surgery (patient 17 in group B; Table 7) and no mortality was observed.

Our classification of FCA and its lessons

Our experience has led us to subdivide group B into four subgroups (Fig. 11): Subgroup B1, in which there was enough remnant to allow direct clip application on the entire aneurysm neck without any coil manipulation ($n = 11$); subgroup B2, in which presence of coil in the neck obliged us to precisely locate the occluding clip on the free-of-coil aneurysm neck ($n = 2$); subgroup B3, in which we had to perform a fundus coil resection followed by clip application on the neck remnant ($n = 3$); and subgroup B4, in which after fundus and coil resection there was not enough neck remnant to allow a direct clip application so that a suture was required ($n = 1$). For group C FCA, we subdivided it into two subgroups: Subgroup C1, when the extruded coil could be extracted through a small opening at the aneurysm base on the parent vessel followed by closure of the opening with a single stitch ($n = 1$); and subgroup C2, when the coil mass with the extruded coil could be extracted through the aneurysm fundus ($n = 1$).

Among this population of 26 FCA that have been clipped so far, 23 (88%) were on the anterior circulation; 7 cases were in group A, 11 in B1, 2 in B2, 3 in B3, 1 in B4, 1 in C1 and 1 in C2 (Table 7; Fig. 11). The time between EVC and

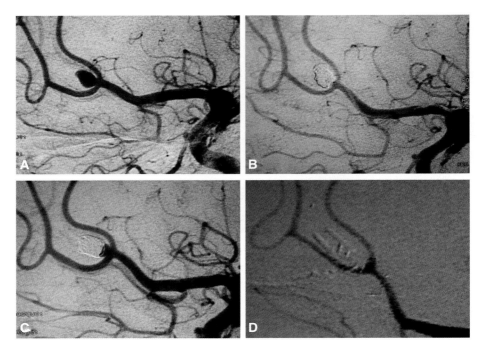

Fig. 8a. Small left pericallosal artery aneurysm seen from a right approach (Table 7, group B, patient 14). (A) Before endovascular coiling (EVC); (B) after complete occlusion by EVC; (C) recanalization; (D) complete occlusion by neck suture and one micro clip after piecemeal resection of the aneurysm fundus full of coils

SC of FCA of group B was on average 29 months, the median being at 24 months.

Our classification of FCA (Fig. 11), represents a modification of the Gurian classification [14], with group B subdivided into four subgroups of increasing difficulty, and group C into two subgroups of increasing difficulty. The cases in group A and subgroup B1 represent situations similar to our standard neurovascular practice but often on morphologically complex aneurysms. The cases in the other subgroups are different in terms of difficulty and risk. Subgroup C2, followed by subgroups B3 and B4, present difficulties of increasing magnitude. Situations such as those found in subgroup B4 should be carefully avoided, with regular radiological monitoring of the aneurysm to wait for a larger recanalization. The surgical danger in this subgroup clearly outweighs the risk of waiting for a larger neck remnant. Indeed, the only case we had in this group B4 (Table 7, patient 14) was also the only case where we had to temporarily clip the parent vessel for more than 10 minutes, fortunately without morbidity. Considering cases of type B3, the application on the aneurysm neck stenosing the parent vessel helps to guide the surgeon in his/her resection of

Surgical indications and techniques

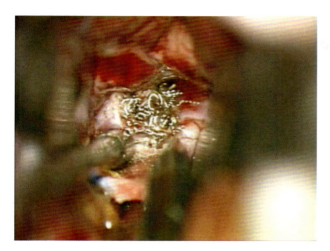

Fig. 8b. Intraoperative image showing, via a right interhemispheric approach, the opened aneurysm fundus full of incorporated coil which was piecemeal resected to access the aneurysm neck; unfortunately the residual aneurysm neck was too small to allow direct clip application and a difficult suture using three stitches with a 8.0 thread plus a microclip was required. Left: a blade slightly retracts the sagittal falx; right: another blade slightly retracts the right hemisphere

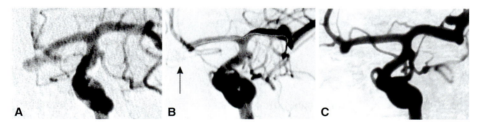

Fig. 9a. Small anterior communicant artery aneurysm (Table 7, group C, patient 1). (A) Before endovascular coiling; (B) after complete occlusion and unravelling of the last coil up to the left Sylvian artery bifurcation; (C) after complete removal of the floating extruded coil

the aneurysm fundus with the coil mass inside, maintaining sufficient neck for repositioning of a direct clip. For patients in subgroup C1, physicians must weigh the thromboembolic risks associated with extruded coils of different lengths and spatial volumes into the parent vessels [2, 40, 46], as recently reported in a case of delayed coil migration [12], against the risks of a few days or weeks of anticoagulant and antiaggregant treatment. Considering all types of FCA (Fig. 11), the lowest risk is associated with types A, B1 and B2. Types B3 and B4 should be left for a period of careful follow-up until the aneurysm neck is large enough for direct clip application. For group C, these

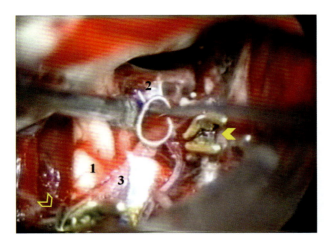

Fig. 9b. Intraoperative photograph showing, through a left pterional approach, the unravelled coiled on a hook used for its extraction through the parent vessel. (1) Left optic nerve; (2) aneurysm sac; (3) left A1; open head arrow temporary clip on left A1; solid head arrow temporary clip on right A1

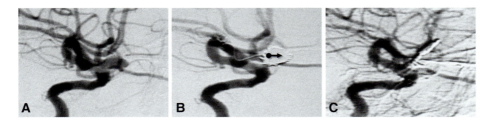

Fig. 10a. Small right middle cerebral artery aneurysm (Table 7, group C, patient 2). (A) Before endovascular coiling (EVC); (B) after complete occlusion but at the end of the EVC massive coil migration into the parent vessel and unravelling of a coil; (C) complete occlusion by one clip after transaneurysmal coil extraction

cases should remain rare with the development of better endoluminar tools and implants like protective stents or pipeline devices [23, 41, 43]. However, deployment of a stent increases the complication rate [11, 17, 27, 43] and the long-term stability of these new devices needs to be demonstrated [39].

In the majority of our 26 FCA treated with an open surgical procedure, temporary clipping was used either to reduce the pressure inside the aneurysm or to allow the resection en bloc or piecemeal of the aneurysm sac with its coils or to extract the coils through the aneurysm fundus. We have never had to use extra-intracranial (EC-IC) bypass, or a trapping or wrapping procedure to control the FCA. In order to avoid potentially very dangerous surgical procedures, as with FCA types B3 and B4, we now wait for a residue height of at

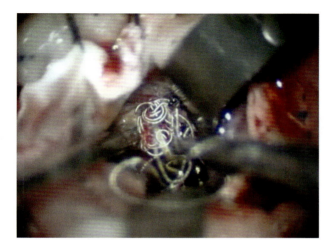

Fig. 10b. Intraoperative picture showing, through a right pterional approach, the coil mass extracted through the incised aneurysm fundus within two hours after the endovascular procedure complicated by coil migration into the parent vessel. Upper right, a blade slightly retracts the right temporal lobe

least 3 mm when the aneurysm neck width is 3 mm or more. A residue of this size should enable the aneurysm neck wall to be sufficiently large for direct clip application without causing parent vessel stenosis.

Experiences of other teams

Table 8 summarises the publications that have reported different surgical managements of FCA [4–6, 8, 9, 14, 18, 20, 22, 26, 37, 46, 48, 50, 52, 53]. Analysis of this table shows that FCA are predominantly anterior circulation aneurysms, the proportion varying between 65 and 100%. The majority of publications focused only on FCA of type B or C. In our experience, 50% of FCA (13/26) were distributed in subgroups B1 or B2 (direct clip application) while this percentage varies between 18 and 90% in the literature (Table 8). There is no other reported case of coil extraction through the parent vessel, probably indicating that physicians prefer to use an anticoagulant-antiaggregant treatment in most cases even though a coil that migrates into the parent vessel can induce severe permanent ischaemic stroke [12]. Considering coil extraction through an aneurysm fundus, in our classification subgroup C2 (Fig. 11), the largest series was reported by Thornton *et al.* in 2000 with 9 cases in a series of 11 FCA [46]. However, the majority of authors prefer to avoid such a procedure which is only relatively safe within hours after EVC before the development of strong coil adhesion to the aneurysm fundus. Complete occlusion of FCA was possible in 25 of our 26 cases (96%), while in the literature this rate

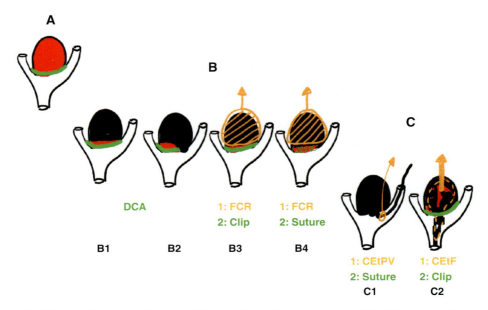

Fig. 11. Modified classification of Failed Coiled Aneurysms ($n = 26$), *Three main types according to Gurian et al.,* (A) attempted endovascular coiling without coil left in the aneurysm ($n = 7$); (B) at least 6 months after endovascular coiling, coils inside the aneurysm and a ≥ 2 mm high aneurysm residue ($n = 17$); (C) endovascular coiling complication, coil extrusion into the parent vessel ($n = 2$). *Six subtypes.* B1: enough residue along the aneurysm neck for direct clip application (DCA) ($n = 11$); B2: coil into the aneurysm neck but residue large enough for direct clip application ($n = 2$); B3: first fundus coil resection (FCR), in bloc or piecemeal, followed by clip application ($n = 3$); B4: first FCR followed by suture ($n = 1$); C1: coil extraction through parent vessel (CEtPV) followed by a single stitch of the small parent vessel opening ($n = 1$); C2: first coil extraction through fundus (CEtF) followed by clip application ($n = 1$); a subtype C3: corresponding to a coil mass compressing a neural structure could be imagined, however as we have never met such a situation we have not included this type in this classification ($n = 0$). *Red* aneurysm lumen or residue; *black* coils; *green* clip or suture; *orange* coil extraction within or outside the aneurysm fundus. *DCA* direct clip application; *FCR* fundus with coil resection; *CEtPV* coil extraction through parent vessel; *CEtF* coil extraction through fundus

varies between 50%, reported by Thornton *et al.* [46], and 98%, reported by Zhang *et al.* in 2003 using intraoperative angiography control [53].

Our morbidity percentage was 4% consisting in slight cognitive troubles in a small FCA of subgroup B1 (patient 17, Table 7); in the literature this rate varies between 0 and 10%. The highest percentage was reported by Lejeune *et al.* with 10% [22], a rate similar to the 9% reported by the International Subarachnoid Aneurysm Trial [4]. Reported mortality rates, absent in our

Surgical indications and techniques

group, vary between 0 and 14%. Gurian *et al.* in 1995 reported the highest mortality rate of 14% [14]; the majority of their perioperative deaths were in complex cases, either because of the aneurysm size, difficult location (posterior circulation) or due to the initial poor clinical condition of the patient.

If we consider only the series of at least 10 cases, each report has its own particularities. Gurian *et al.* reported a series of 21 FCA [14]; this team was the first to present a classification of the FCA into three groups, A, B and C, a classification which is now widely used in the literature. Four cases in their series were treated before GDC was available. This series showed the same rate of SC for FCA as we did, around 11% of all aneurysms submitted to an EVC (Fig. 3). These authors used 8 EC-IC bypasses and intraoperative angiography. They reported the highest mortality rate of 14%, but in two cases this was related to difficulties occurring during the EVC procedure.

Thornton *et al.* presented a series of 11 cases [46]. Nine of these 11 cases involved a coil extraction through the aneurysm fundus (subgroup C2, Fig. 11). These authors reported the lowest complete occlusion rate after surgery (50%).

Zhang *et al.*, reported a series of 40 cases [53] with 3 bypasses, 3 wrapping, 3 hypothermic circulatory arrests, intraoperative angiography in all cases, the highest complete occlusion rate (98%), and two perioperative deaths (5%).

Veznedaroglu *et al.*, in their 18 cases [48], reported 15 clippings with complete occlusion and 3 wrappings, with no morbidity and no mortality. These authors recommended that the height of the aneurysmal remnant should be at least twice that of the neck to avoid stenosing the parent vessel with the clips. They used intraoperative angiography.

In the small case series of König *et al.*, all 10 cases were located on the anterior circulation and had direct clip application with in one case coils extraction; no morbidity and no mortality was reported [20].

The series reported by Campi *et al.* was not focused on the surgical management of FCA [4]. If we consider their FCA operated late (more than 3 months after EVC; 25 cases) as being FCA of type group B, we observed a morbidity of 9%.

Lejeune *et al.* [22] reported 21 cases with only two cases of type A; all FCA were clipped; two coil extractions were reported; 19 FCA (90%) were completely occluded; two patients (9.5%) developed moderate disability.

The largest series of 43 cases was reported by Waldron *et al.* [50] and was characterised by an increasing trend in FCA occurrence and a 23% rate of unclippable FCA with 42% of cases being large or giant aneurysms and no coil extraction reported. Seven by-passes were performed. These authors presented a ratio of coil width to compaction height as potentially predictive of clippability. A perioperative mortality rate of 7% was reported.

Regarding our surgical experience with 26 FCA, there is a decreasing trend in FCA during recent years, in contrast to the findings of Waldron's group; three

Table 8. *Surgical clipping (SC) of Failed Coiled Aneurysms (FCA) distributed in three groups A, B and C. Literature Review and our experience (%)*

First author	Year	Surgery post EVC (%)	Ant circ nb (%)	Initial SAH (%)	A (attempt) No coil (%)	B (recanalization or residue)			C (coil extrusion or compression)			CO (%)	Outcome	
						DCA (%)	Fundus coil resection	Other	Coil extraction through		Other		Mby (%)	Mty (%)
									PV	Fundus				
Litofsky	1994	1	1	—	—	—	—	—	—	1 trap[a]	—	1	0	0
Gurian	1995	21 (11)	20 (95)	(61.9)	5 (24)	10 (48)	—	—	—	3 (1 balloon)	2 bp 1 ref	?	1 (5)	3 (14)[b]
Civit	1996	8	8 (100)	(100)	—	6	—	1 stop	—	1	—	7 (88)	3	1
Mizoi	1996	1	1	—	—	—	1	—	—	—	—	1	1	0
Horowitz	1999	5	3	3	—	3	—	—	—	2	—	5	0	0
Thornton	2000	11	10 (91)		—	2 (18)	—	—	—	9	—	4 (50)[c]	4	0
Boet	2001	7	7		—	7	—	—	—	—	—	6	1	0
Conrad	2002	7	7	(100)	—	4	—	3 lig	—	—	—	6	0	1[d]
Zhang	2003	40[e] NR	26 (65)	(60)	12 (30)	15 (37)	1	1 bp 2 trap 1 wrap 2 hca	—	6	2 bp 1 trap	39 (98)	1 (2)	3 (7)[f]
Deinsberger	2003	7	7		—	3	—	—	—	4	—	?	1	1[g]
Veznedaroglu	2004	18 (1.9)	15 (83)	(5.5)	—	15 (83)	—	3 wrap	—	—	—	15 (83)	0	0
Yoshida	2005	1	—	1	—	—	1[h]	—	—	—	—	—	0	0
Raftopoulos	2006	17	16 (94)		—	14 (82)	1	—	1	1	—	17 (94)	1 (6)	0
Deshmukh	2006	2	2		—	1	1	—	—	—	—	2	0	0
Minh	2006	7	7		2	3	—	—	—	—	2 encc	7	1	0
König	2007	10	10 (100)	(60)	—	9 (90)	1	—	—	—	—	8 (80)[i]	0	0
Campi	2007	25 (2.2)[j]	?	25 (100)	—	?	?	?	—	—	—	?	2 (9)[k]	0

Lejeune	2008	21 (2.2)	18 (86)	(95.2)	–	19 (90)	–	2 wrap	–	2	–	19 (90)	2 (10)	0
Waldron	2009	43 (?)	32 (74)	(88)	–	33 (77)	–	4 cmob 5 bp 1 wrap	–	–	2 bp 2 wrap	38 (88)	1 (2)	3 (7)[l]
Raftopoulos	2010	26 (9.4)	23 (88)	(58)	7 (27)	13 (50)	4	–	1	1	–	24 (92)	1 (4)	0
min–max %		1.9–11	65–100	5.5–100	0–30	18–90						50–98	0–10	0–14

Ant circ Anterior circulation; *Bp* by-pass; *CO* complete occlusion; *cmob* coil mobilization; *DCA* direct clip application; *encc* encircling clip of Sundt-Kees; *EVC* endovascular coiling; *hca* hypothermic circulatory arrest; *lig* ligature; *Mby* permanent morbidity; *Mty* mortality; *NR* not reported; *Other* other surgical procedure; *PV* parent vessel; *ref* one old patient refused surgery; *trap* trapping; *wrap* wrapping.

[a] one giant ophthalmic ICA nearly completely embolized in two steps but further visual loss required a surgical trapping after coil extraction.

[b] 3 died, one related to perioperative thalamic infarct and the two others related to complications occurred during the endovascular procedure (group C).

[c] only 8 patients had a postoperative angiography with four showing a complete occlusion.

[d] one patient died from a left MCA ischaemia related to the parent vessel stenosis post-clipping.

[e] 40 failed coiled aneurysms in 38 patients.

[f] 3 patients died, two as a result of the surgery (one with a hca) and one from subarachnoid hemorrhage induced myocardial infarction.

[g] despite early dipping after rerupture post coiling.

[h] only partial removal of the coils was possible.

[i] two patients refused the postoperative angiography.

[j] 103 FCA were send for SC but 75.7% of them were treated within 3months of the EVC (early retreatment).

[k] regarding the 25 cases with a late SC treatment.

[l] 3 died, two related to the endovascular procedure and one to a vasospasm post subarachnoid hemorrhage.

fundus coil mass resections and two coils extractions were performed; complete occlusion was possible in 92% of our series without any deaths and our experience led us to describe a modified Gurian classification with, in particular, four subgroups in group B and two subgroups in group C (Fig. 11). The increasing trend for FCA requiring a second, open surgical procedure that was recently reported by Waldron *et al.* [50] was related by the authors to a wider access to endovascular procedures, less experienced newly trained endovascular practitioners, and the preference of patients for minimally invasive procedures. We believe that our opposite observation of a decreasing trend in FCA, is related to that fact that since the start of our program, in February 1996, the same neurovascular team has been in charge of the neurovascular pathology in our University and each case is discussed by this team to ensure careful selection of the best technique for each aneurysm with 58% of the ICA being initially selected for SC (Fig. 3). The increased experience of our team during this time period, the considerable experience of our endovascular radiologist, and improvements in endovascular techniques and devices, such as new stents, represent other likely reasons for the reduced rate of FCA.

Conclusions

All FCA can be categorised into the different groups and subgroups of our modified classification, allowing the neurosurgeon to better appreciate the difficulties and potential risks associated with each type. This modified classification encourages the neurosurgeon to wait until an aneurysm residue is large enough for direct clip application. With better collaboration between endovascular radiologists and vascular neurosurgeons, increased experience of endovascular radiologists, and better endovascular tools and devices, the rate of occurrence of FCA should stabilise or even decrease. However, the most effective strategy to reduce the rate of FCA remains a pluridisciplinary approach to identify the best technique with the lowest risk and the highest probability of stable complete occlusion for each aneurysm. Even if endovascular techniques continue to improve, they will still have the inherent disadvantage of their endoluminal approach, including thromboembolic risks and difficulty to ensure a permanent stable complete or near complete occlusion of the aneurysm.

References

1. Aghakhani N, Vaz G, David P, Parker F, Goffette P, Ozan A, Raftopoulos C (2008) Surgical management of unruptured intracranial aneurysms that are inappropriate for endovascular treatment: experience based on two academic centers. Neurosurgery 62: 1227–34
2. Aviv RI, O'Neill R, Patel MC, Colquhoun IR (2005) Abciximab in patients with ruptured intracranial aneurysms. Am J Neuroradiol 26: 1744–50

Surgical indications and techniques

3. Bushong SC (1994) Hazards evaluation of neuroangiographic procedures. Am J Neuroradiol 15: 1813–16

4. Campi A, Ramzi N, Molyneux AJ, Summers PE, Kerr RS, Sneade M, Yarnold JA, Rischmiller J, Byrne JV (2007) Retreatment of ruptured cerebral aneurysms in patients randomized by coiling or clipping in the International Subarachnoid Aneurysm Trial (ISAT). Stroke 38: 1538–44

5. Civit T, Auque J, Marchal JC, Bracard S, Picard L, Hepner H (1996) Aneurysm clipping after endovascular treatment with coils: a report of eight patients. Neurosurgery 38: 955–60

6. Conrad MD, Pelissou-Guyotat I, Morel C, Madarassy G, Schonauer C, Deruty R (2002) Regrowth of residual ruptured aneurysms treated by Guglielmi's Detachable Coils which demanded further treatment by surgical clipping: report of 7 cases and review of the literature. Acta Neurochir (Wien) 144: 419–26

7. David CA, Vishteh AG, Spetzler RF, Lemole M, Lawton MT, Partovi S (1999) Late angiographic follow-up review of surgically treated aneurysms. J Neurosurg 91: 396–401

8. Deinsberger W, Mewes H, Traupe H, Boeker DK (2003) Surgical management of previously coiled intracranial aneurysms. Br J Neurosurg 17: 149–54

9. Deshmukh VR, Hott JS, Dumont T, Nakaji P, Spetzler RF (2006) Treatment of recurrent previously coiled anterior circulation aneurysm with minimally invasive keyhole craniotomy: report of two cases. Minim Invasive Neurosurg 49: 70–73

10. Ferns SP, Sprengers ME, van Rooij WJ, Rinkel GJ, van Rijn JC, Bipat S, Sluzewski M, Majoie CB (2009) Coiling of intracranial aneurysms: a systematic review on initial occlusion and reopening and retreatment rates. Stroke 40: e523–29

11. Fiorella D, Albuquerque FC, Deshmukh VR, McDougall CG (2004) In-stent stenosis as a delayed complication of neuroform stent-supported coil embolization of an incidental carotid terminus aneurysm. Am J Neuroradiol 25: 1764–67

12. Fiorella D, Kelly ME, Moskowitz S, Masaryk TJ (2009) Delayed symptomatic coil migration after initially successful balloon-assisted aneurysm coiling: technical case report. Neurosurgery 64: E391–92

13. Guglielmi G, Vinuela F, Sepetka I, Macellari V (1991) Electrothrombosis of saccular aneurysms via endovascular approach. Part 1: Electrochemical basis, technique, and experimental results. J Neurosurg 75: 1–7

14. Gurian JH, Martin NA, King WA, Duckwiler GR, Guglielmi G, Vinuela F (1995) Neurosurgical management of cerebral aneurysms following unsuccessful or incomplete endovascular embolization. J Neurosurg 83: 843–53

15. Hayakawa M, Murayama Y, Duckwiler GR, Gobin YP, Guglielmi G, Vinuela F (2000) Natural history of the neck remnant of a cerebral aneurysm treated with the Guglielmi detachable coil system. J Neurosurg 93: 561–68

16. Hayashi K, Kitagawa N, Morikawa M, Horie N, Kawakubo J, Hiu T, Tsutsumi K, Nagata I (2009) Long-term follow-up of endovascular coil embolization for cerebral aneurysms using three-dimensional time-of-flight magnetic resonance angiography. Neurol Res 31: 674–80

17. Henkes H, Fischer S, Weber W, Miloslavski E, Felber S, Brew S, Kuehne D (2004) Endovascular coil occlusion of 1811 intracranial aneurysms: early angiographic and clinical results. Neurosurgery 54: 268–80

18. Horowitz M, Purdy P, Kopitnik T, Dutton K, Samson D (1999) Aneurysm retreatment after Guglielmi detachable coil and nondetachable coil embolization: report of nine cases and review of the literature. Neurosurgery 44: 712–19

19. Johnston SC, Dowd CF, Higashida RT, Lawton MT, Duckwiler GR, Gress DR (2008) Predictors of rehemorrhage after treatment of ruptured intracranial aneurysms: the Cerebral Aneurysm Rerupture After Treatment (CARAT) study. Stroke 39: 120–25
20. Konig RW, Kretschmer T, Antoniadis G, Seitz K, Braun V, Richter HP, Perez de LM, Scheller C, Borm W (2007) Neurosurgical management of previously coiled recurrent intracranial aneurysms. Zentralbl Neurochir 68: 8–13
21. Kuwayama N, Takaku A, Endo S, Nishijima M, Kamei T (1994) Radiation exposure in endovascular surgery of the head and neck. Am J Neuroradiol 15: 1801–08
22. Lejeune JP, Thines L, Taschner C, Bourgeois P, Henon H, Leclerc X (2008) Neurosurgical treatment for aneurysm remnants or recurrences after coil occlusion. Neurosurgery 63: 684–91
23. Lylyk P, Miranda C, Ceratto R, Ferrario A, Scrivano E, Luna HR, Berez AL, Tran Q, Nelson PK, Fiorella D (2009) Curative endovascular reconstruction of cerebral aneurysms with the pipeline embolization device: the Buenos Aires experience. Neurosurgery 64: 632–42
24. Marshall NW, Noble J, Faulkner K (1995) Patient and staff dosimetry in neuroradiological procedures. Br J Radiol 68: 495–501
25. Maud A, Lakshminarayan K, Suri MF, Vazquez G, Lanzino G, Qureshi AI (2009) Cost-effectiveness analysis of endovascular versus neurosurgical treatment for ruptured intracranial aneurysms in the United States. J Neurosurg 110: 880–86
26. Mizoi K, Yoshimoto T, Takahashi A, Nagamine Y (1996) A pitfall in the surgery of a recurrent aneurysm after coil embolization and its histological observation: technical case report. Neurosurgery 39: 165–68
27. Mocco J, Snyder KV, Albuquerque FC, Bendok BR, Alan SB, Carpenter JS, Fiorella DJ, Hoh BL, Howington JU, Jankowitz BT, Liebman KM, Rai AT, Rodriguez-Mercado R, Siddiqui AH, Veznedaroglu E, Hopkins LN, Levy EI (2009) Treatment of intracranial aneurysms with the Enterprise stent: a multicenter registry. J Neurosurg 110: 35–39
28. Molyneux AJ, Kerr RS, Yu LM, Clarke M, Sneade M, Yarnold JA, Sandercock P (2005) International subarachnoid aneurysm trial (ISAT) of neurosurgical clipping versus endovascular coiling in 2143 patients with ruptured intracranial aneurysms: a randomised comparison of effects on survival, dependency, seizures, rebleeding, subgroups, and aneurysm occlusion. Lancet 366: 809–17
29. Murayama Y, Nien YL, Duckwiler G, Gobin YP, Jahan R, Frazee J, Martin N, Vinuela F (2003) Guglielmi detachable coil embolization of cerebral aneurysms: 11 years' experience. J Neurosurg 98: 959–66
30. Pelz DM, Lownie SP, Fox AJ (1998) Thromboembolic events associated with the treatment of cerebral aneurysms with Guglielmi detachable coils. Am J Neuroradiol 19: 1541–47
31. Perneczky A, Fries G (1995) Use of a new aneurysm clip with an inverted-spring mechanism to facilitate visual control during clip application. Technical note. J Neurosurg 82: 898–99
32. Raftopoulos C (2005) Is surgical clipping becoming underused? Acta Neurochir (Wien) 147: 117–23
33. Raftopoulos C (2009) Surgical management of intracranial aneurysms of the anterior circulation, In: Sindou M (ed) Practical handbook of neurosurgery from leading neurosurgeons. Springer, Wien New York, Vol. 1, pp 257–69
34. Raftopoulos C, Goffette P, Billa RF, Mathurin P (2002) Transvascular coil hooking procedure to retrieve an unraveled Guglielmi detachable coil: technical note. Neurosurgery 50: 912–14

Surgical indications and techniques

35. Raftopoulos C, Goffette P, Vaz G, Ramzi N, Scholtes JL, Wittebole X, Mathurin P (2003) Surgical clipping may lead to better results than coil embolization: results from a series of 101 consecutive unruptured intracranial aneurysms. Neurosurgery 52: 1280–87
36. Raftopoulos C, Mathurin P, Boscherini D, Billa RF, Van Boven M, Hantson P (2000) Prospective analysis of aneurysm treatment in a series of 103 consecutive patients when endovascular embolization is considered the first option. J Neurosurg 93: 175–82
37. Raftopoulos C, Vaz G, Docquier M, Goffette P (2007) Neurosurgical management of inadequately embolized intracranial aneurysms: a series of 17 consecutive cases. Acta Neurochir (Wien) 149: 11–19
38. Raymond J, Guilbert F, Weill A, Georganos SA, Juravsky L, Lambert A, Lamoureux J, Chagnon M, Roy D (2003) Long-term angiographic recurrences after selective endovascular treatment of aneurysms with detachable coils. Stroke 34: 1398–403
39. Raymond J, Guilbert F, Weill A, Roy D, LeBlanc P, Gevry G, Chagnon M, Collet JP (2004) Safety, science, and sales: a request for valid clinical trials to assess new devices for endovascular treatment of intracranial aneurysms. Am J Neuroradiol 25: 1128–130
40. Rordorf G, Bellon RJ, Budzik RE Jr., Farkas J, Reinking GF, Pergolizzi RS, Ezzeddine M, Norbash AM, Gonzalez RG, Putman CM (2001) Silent thromboembolic events associated with the treatment of unruptured cerebral aneurysms by use of Guglielmi detachable coils: prospective study applying diffusion-weighted imaging. Am J Neuro-radiol 22: 5–10
41. Sedat J, Chau Y, Mondot L, Vargas J, Szapiro J, Lonjon M (2009) Endovascular occlusion of intracranial wide-necked aneurysms with stenting (Neuroform) and coiling: mid-term and long-term results. Neuroradiology 51: 401–09
42. Shiralkar S, Rennie A, Snow M, Galland RB, Lewis MH, Gower-Thomas K (2003) Doctors' knowledge of radiation exposure: questionnaire study. BMJ 327: 371–72
43. Siddiqui MA, Bhattacharya J, Lindsay KW, Jenkins S (2009) Horizontal stent-assisted coil embolisation of wide-necked intracranial aneurysms with the Enterprise stent – a case series with early angiographic follow-up. Neuroradiology 51: 411–18
44. Sindou M, Acevedo JC, Turjman F (1998) Aneurysmal remnants after microsurgical clipping: classification and results from a prospective angiographic study (in a consecutive series of 305 operated intracranial aneurysms). Acta Neurochir (Wien) 140: 1153–59
45. Soeda A, Sakai N, Murao K, Sakai H, Ihara K, Yamada N, Imakita S, Nagata I (2003) Thromboembolic events associated with Guglielmi detachable coil embolization with use of diffusion-weighted MR imaging. Part II. Detection of the microemboli proximal to cerebral aneurysm. Am J Neuroradiol 24: 2035–38
46. Thornton J, Dovey Z, Alazzaz A, Misra M, Aletich VA, Debrun GM, Ausman JI, Charbel FT (2000) Surgery following endovascular coiling of intracranial aneurysms. Surg Neurol 54: 352–60
47. Tsutsumi K, Ueki K, Morita A, Usui M, Kirino T (2001) Risk of aneurysm recurrence in patients with clipped cerebral aneurysms: results of long-term follow-up angiography. Stroke 32: 1191–94
48. Veznedaroglu E, Benitez RP, Rosenwasser RH (2004) Surgically treated aneurysms previously coiled: lessons learned. Neurosurgery 54: 300–03
49. Vinuela F, Duckwiler G, Mawad M (1997) Guglielmi detachable coil embolization of acute intracranial aneurysm: perioperative anatomical and clinical outcome in 403 patients. J Neurosurg 86: 475–82

50. Waldron JS, Halbach VV, Lawton MT (2009) Microsurgical management of incompletely coiled and recurrent aneurysms: trends, techniques, and observations on coil extrusion. Neurosurgery 64: 301–15
51. Wolstenholme J, Rivero-Arias O, Gray A, Molyneux AJ, Kerr RS, Yarnold JA, Sneade M (2008) Treatment pathways, resource use, and costs of endovascular coiling versus surgical clipping after aSAH. Stroke 39: 111–19
52. Yoshida K, Wataya T, Hojo M, Doi D, Yamagata S (2005) Surgical clipping of a recurrent small saccular aneurysm after repeated coil embolization. Neurol Med Chir (Tokyo) 45: 356–59
53. Zhang YJ, Barrow DL, Cawley CM, Dion JE (2003) Neurosurgical management of intracranial aneurysms previously treated with endovascular therapy. Neurosurgery 52: 283–93

Author index volume 1–36

Advances and Technical Standards in Neurosurgery

Adamson TE, see Yaşargil MG, Vol. 18
Aebischer P, see Hottinger AF, Vol. 25
Agnati LF, Zini I, Zoli M, Fuxe K, Merlo Pich E, Grimaldi R, Toffano G, Goldstein M. Regeneration in the central nervous system: Concepts and Facts. Vol. 16
Alafuzoff I, see Immonen A, Vol. 29
Alafuzoff I, see Jutila L, Vol. 27
Ancri D, see Pertuiset B, Vol. 10
Ancri D, see Pertuiset B, Vol. 8
Ancri D, see Philippon J, Vol. 1
Andre MJ, see Resche F, Vol. 20
Auque J, see Sindou M, Vol. 26
Axon P, see Macfarlane R, Vol. 28

Backlund E-O. Stereotactic radiosurgery in intracranial tumours and vascular malformations. Vol. 6
Balagura S, see Derome PJ, Vol. 6
Basset JY, see Pertuiset B, Vol. 10
Bastide R, see Lazorthes Y, Vol. 18
Baumert BG, Stupp R. Is there a place for radiotherapy in low-grade gliomas? Vol. 35
Bello L, Fava E, Carrabba G, Papagno C, Gaini SM. Present day's standards in microsurgery of low-grade gliomas. Vol. 35
Benabid AL, Hoffmann D, Lavallee S, Cinquin P, Demongeot J, Le Bas JF, Danel F. Is there any future for robots in neurosurgery? Vol. 18
Benabid AL, see Caparros-Lefebvre D, Vol. 25

Benabid AL, see Torres N, Vol. 36
Bentivoglio P, see Symon L, Vol. 14
Berkelbach van der Sprenkel JW, Knufman NMJ, van Rijen PC, Luyten PR, den Hollander JA, Tulleken CAF. Proton spectroscopic imaging in cerebral ischaemia: where we stand and what can be expected. Vol. 19
Besser M, see Owler BK, Vol. 30
Bewernick BH, see Schlapfer TE, Vol. 34
Bitar A, see Fohanno D, Vol. 14
Blaauw G, Muhlig RS, Vredeveld JW. Management of brachial plexus injuries. Vol. 33
Blond S, see Caparros-Lefebvre D, Vol. 25
Boniface S, see Kett-White R, Vol. 27
Boon P, see Vonck K, Vol. 34
Borgesen SE, see Gjerris F, Vol. 19
Braakman R. Cervical spondylotic myelopathy. Vol. 6
Bret P, see Lapras C, Vol. 11
Bricolo A, see Sala F, Vol. 29
Bricolo A, Turazzi S. Surgery for gliomas and other mass lesions of the brainstem. Vol. 22
Brihaye J, Ectors P, Lemort M, van Houtte P. The management of spinal epidural metastases. Vol. 16
Brihaye J, see Klastersky J, Vol. 6
Brihaye J. Neurosurgical approaches to orbital tumours. Vol. 3
Brihaye J, see Hildebrand J, Vol. 5

Bull JWD, see Gawler J, Vol. 2
Bydder GM. Nuclear magnetic resonance imaging of the central nervous system. Vol. 11

Caemaert J, see Cosyns P, Vol. 21
Cahana A, see Mavrocordatos P, Vol. 31
Campiche R, see Zander E, Vol. 1
Caparros-Lefebvre D, Blond S, N'Guyen JP, Pollak P, Benabid AL. Chronic deep brain stimulation for movement disorders. Vol. 25
Cappabianca P, see de Divitiis, Vol. 27
Cappabianca P, Cavallo LM, Esposito F, de Divitiis O, Messina A, de Divitiis E. Extended endoscopic endonasal approach to the midline skull base: the evolving role of transsphenoidal surgery. Vol. 33
Caron JP, see Debrun G, Vol. 4
Carrabba G, see Bello L, Vol. 35
Caspar W, see Loew F, Vol. 5
Castel JP. Aspects of the medical management in aneurysmal subarachnoid hemorrhage. Vol. 18
Catenoix H, see Guénot M, Vol. 36
Cavallo LM, see Cappabianca P, Vol. 33
Ceha J, see Cosyns P, Vol. 21
Chabardès S, see Torres N, Vol. 36
Chaumier EE, see Loew F, Vol. 11
Chauvin M, see Pertuiset B, Vol. 10
Chazal J, see Chirossel JP, Vol. 22
Chiaretti A, Langer A. Prevention and treatment of postoperative pain with particular reference to children. Vol. 30
Chirossel JP, see Passagia JG, Vol. 25
Chirossel JP, Vanneuville G, Passagia JG, Chazal J, Coillard Ch, Favre JJ, Garcier JM, Tonetti J, Guillot M. Biomechanics and classification of traumatic lesions of the spine. Vol. 22
Choux M, Lena G, Genitori L, Foroutan M. The surgery of occult spinal dysraphism. Vol. 21

Cianciulli E, see di Rocco C, Vol. 31
Cinalli G, see di Rocco C, Vol. 31
Cinquin P, see Benabid AL, Vol. 18
Ciricillo SF, Rosenblum ML. AIDS and the Neurosurgeon – an update. Vol. 21
Civit T, see Marchal JC, Vol. 31
Cohadon F, see Loiseau H, Vol. 26
Cohadon F. Brain protection, Vol. 21
Cohadon F. Indications for surgery in the management of gliomas. Vol. 17
Coillard Ch, see Chirossel JP, Vol. 22
Coleman MR, Pickard JD. Detecting residual cognitive function in disorders of consciousness. Vol. 36
Cooper PR, see Lieberman A, Vol. 17
Cophignon J, see Rey A, Vol. 2
Costa e Silva IE, see Symon L, Vol. 14
Cosyns P, Caemaert J, Haaijman W, van Veelen C, Gybels J, van Manen J, Ceha J. Functional stereotactic neurosurgery for psychiatric disorders: an experience in Belgium and The Netherlands. Vol. 21
Crockard HA, Ransford AO. Surgical techniques in the management of colloid cysts of the third ventricle: stabilization of the spine. Vol. 17
Cuny E, see Loiseau H, Vol. 26
Curcic M, see Yaşargil MG, Vol. 7
Czosnyka M, see Kett-White R, Vol. 27

Danel F, see Benabid AL, Vol. 18
Dardis R, see Strong AJ, Vol. 30
Daspit CP, see Lawton MT, Vol. 23
Daumas-Duport C. Histoprognosis of gliomas. Vol. 21
de Divitiis O, see Cappabianca P, Vol. 33
de Divitiis E, Cappabianca P. Endoscopic endonasal transsphenoidal surgery. Vol. 27
de Divitiis E, Spaziante R, Stella L. Empty sella and benign intrasellar cysts. Vol. 8

de Divitiis E, see Cappabianca P, Vol. 33

de Kersaint-Gilly A, see Resche F, Vol. 20

de Seze M, see Vignes JR, Vol. 30

de Tribolet N, see Porchet F, Vol. 23

de Tribolet N, see Sawamura Y, Vol. 17

de Tribolet N, see Sawamura Y, Vol. 25

de Tribolet N, see Sawamura Y, Vol. 27

de Vries J, see DeJongste MJL, Vol. 32

de Herdt V, see Vonck K, Vol. 34

Debrun G, Lacour P, Caron JP. Balloon arterial catheter techniques in the treatment of arterial intracranial diseases. Vol. 4

DeJongste MJL, de Vries J, Spincemaille G, Staal MJ. Spinal cord stimulation for ischaemic heart disease and peripheral vascular disease. Vol. 32

Delalande O, see Villemure J-G, Vol. 26

Delliere V, see Fournier HD, Vol. 31

Delsanti C, see Pellet W, Vol. 28

Demongeot J, see Benabid AL, Vol. 18

den Hollander JA, see Berkelbach van der Sprenkel JW, Vol. 19

Derlon JM. The in vivo metabolic investigation of brain gliomas with positron emission tomography. Vol. 24

Derome P, see Guiot G, Vol. 3

Derome PJ, Guiot G in co-operation with Georges B, Porta M, Visot A, Balagura S. Surgical approaches to the sphenoidal and clival areas. Vol. 6

Deruty R, see Lapras C, Vol. 11

Detwiler PW, Porter RW, Han PP, Karahalios DG, Masferrer R, Sonntag VKH. Surgical treatment of lumbar spondylolisthesis. Vol. 26

DeWitte O, see Lefranc F, Vol. 34

Dhellemmes P, see Vinchon M, Vol. 32

Diaz FG, see Zamorano L, Vol. 24

Dietz, H. Organisation of the primary transportation of head injuries and other emergencies in the Federal Republic of Germany. Vol. 18

di Rocco C, Cinalli G, Massimi L, Spennato P, Cianciulli E, Tamburrini G. Endoscopic third ventriculostomy in the treatment of hydrocephalus in paediatric patients. Vol. 31

Dobremez E, see Vignes JR, Vol. 30

Dolenc VV. Hypothalamic gliomas. Vol. 25

Drake CG, see Peerless SJ, Vol. 15

du Boulay G, see Gawler J, Vol. 2

Duffau H. Brain plasticity and tumors. Vol. 33

Ebeling U, Reulen H-J. Space-occupying lesions of the sensori-motor region. Vol. 22

Ectors P, see Brihaye J, Vol. 16

Editorial Board. Controversial views of Editorial Board on the intraoperative management of ruptured saccular aneurysms. Vol. 14

Editorial Board. Controversial views of the Editorial Board regarding the management on non-traumatic intracerebral haematomas. Vol. 15

Epstein F. Spinal cord astrocytomas of childhood. Vol. 13

Esposito F, see Cappabianca P, Vol. 33

Fahlbusch R, see Nimsky C, Vol. 29

Fankhauser H, see Porchet F, Vol. 23

Faulhauer K. The overdrained hydrocephalus: Clinical manifestations and management. Vol. 9

Fava E, see Bello L, Vol. 35

Favre JJ, see Chirossel JP, Vol. 22

Favre JJ, see Passagia JG, Vol. 25

Fisch U, see Kumar A, Vol. 10

Fisch U. Management of intratemporal facial palsy. Vol. 7

Fohanno D, Bitar A. Sphenoidal ridge meningioma. Vol. 14

Fohanno D, see Pertuiset B, Vol. 5

Foroutan M, see Choux M, Vol. 21

Fournier H-D, see Hayek C, Vol. 31

Fournier H-D, Delliere V, Gourraud JB, Mercier Ph. Surgical anatomy of calvarial skin and bones with particular reference to neurosurgical approaches. Vol. 31

Fournier H-D, Mercier P, Roche P-H. Surgical anatomy of the petrous apex and petroclival region. Vol. 32

Fournier H-D, see Roche P-H, Vol. 33

Fox JP, see Yaşargil MG, Vol. 2

Frackowiak RSJ, see Wise RJS, Vol. 10

Francois P, Lescanne E, Velut S. The dural sheath of the optic nerve: descriptive anatomy and surgical applications. Vol. 36

Franke I, see Madea B, Vol. 36

Fries G, Perneczky A. Intracranial endoscopy. Vol. 25

Fuxe K, see Agnati LF, Vol. 16

Gaini SM, see Bello L, Vol. 35

Ganslandt O, see Nimsky C, Vol. 29

Garcier JM, see Chirossel JP, Vol. 22

Gardeur D, see Pertuiset B, Vol. 10

Gasser JC, see Yaşargil MG, Vol. 4

Gawler J, Bull JWD, du Boulay G, Marshall J. Computerised axial tomography with the EMI-scanner. Vol. 2

Genitori L, see Choux M, Vol. 21

Gentili F, Schwartz M, TerBrugge K, Wallace MC, Willinsky R, Young C. A multidisciplinary approach to the treatment of brain vascular malformations. Vol. 19

George B. Extracranial vertebral artery anatomy and surgery. Vol. 27

Georges B, see Derome PJ, Vol. 6

Gimbert E, see Sindou M, Vol. 34

Gjerris F, Borgesen SE. Current concepts of measurement of cerebrospinal fluid absorption and biomechanics of hydrocephalus. Vol. 19

Go KG. The normal and pathological physiology of brain water. Vol. 23

Goldstein M, see Agnati LF, Vol. 16

Gourraud JB, see Fournier HD, Vol. 31

Goutelle A, see Sindou M, Vol. 10

Griebel RW, see Hoffman HJ, Vol. 14

Griffith HB. Endoneurosurgery: Endoscopic intracranial surgery. Vol. 14

Grimaldi R, see Agnati LF, Vol. 16

Gros C. Spasticity-clinical classification and surgical treatment. Vol. 6

Guénot M, Isnard J, Catenoix H, Mauguière F, Sindou M. SEEG-guided RF-thermocoagulation of epileptic foci: A therapeutic alternative for drug-resistant non-operable partial epilepsies. Vol. 36

Guenot M, Isnard J, Sindou M. Surgical anatomy of the insula. Vol. 29

Guenot M, see Sindou M, Vol. 28

Guerin J, see Vignes JR, Vol. 30

Guglielmi, G. The interventional neuroradiological treatment of intracranial aneurysms. Vol. 24

Guidetti B, Spallone A. Benign extramedullary tumours of the foramen magnum. Vol. 16

Guidetti B. Removal of extramedullary benign spinal cord tumors. Vol. 1

Guillot M, see Chirossel JP, Vol. 22

Guilly M, see Pertuiset B, Vol. 10

Guimaraes-Ferreira J, Miguéns J, Lauritzen C. Advances in craniosynostosis research and management. Vol. 29

Guiot G, Derome P. Surgical problems of pituitary adenomas. Vol. 3

Guiot G, see Derome PJ, Vol. 6

Gullotta F. Morphological and biological basis for the classification of brain tumors. With a comment on the WHO-classification 1979. Vol. 8

Gur D, see Yonas H, Vol. 15

Gybels J, see Cosyns P, Vol. 21

Gybels J, van Roost D. Spinal cord stimulation for spasticity. Vol. 15

Haaijman W, see Cosyns P, Vol. 21

Halmagyi GM, see Owler BK, Vol. 30

Hame O, see Robert R, Vol. 32

Han PP, see Detwiler PW, Vol. 26

Hankinson J. The surgical treatment of syringomyelia. Vol. 5

Harding AE. Clinical and molecular neurogenetics in neurosurgery. Vol. 20

Harris P, Jackson IT, McGregor JC. Reconstructive surgery of the head. Vol. 8

Haase J. Carpal tunnel syndrome – a comprehensive review. Vol. 32

Hayek C, Mercier Ph, Fournier HD. Anatomy of the orbit and its surgical approach. Vol. 31

Hendrick EB, see Hoffman HJ, Vol. 14

Herrlinger U, see Kurzwelly D, Vol. 35

Higgins JN, see Owler BK, Vol. 30

Hildebrand J, Brihaye J. Chemotherapy of brain tumours. Vol. 5

Hirsch J-F, Hoppe-Hirsch E. Medulloblastoma. Vol. 20

Hirsch J-F, Hoppe-Hirsch E. Shunts and shunt problems in childhood. Vol. 16

Hoffman HJ, Griebel RW, Hendrick EB. Congenital spinal cord tumors in children. Vol. 14

Hoffmann D, see Benabid AL, Vol. 18

Hood T, see Siegfried J, Vol. 10

Hoppe-Hirsch E, see Hirsch J-F, Vol. 16

Hoppe-Hirsch E, see Hirsch J-F, Vol. 20

Hottinger AF, Aebischer P. Treatment of diseases of the central nervous system using encapsulated cells. Vol. 25

Houtteville JP. The surgery of cavernomas both supra-tentorial and infra-tentorial. Vol. 22

Huber G, Piepgras U. Update and trends in venous (VDSA) and arterial (ADSA) digital subtraction angiography in neuroradiology. Vol. 11

Hummel Th, see Landis BN, Vol. 30

Hurskainen H, see Immonen A, Vol. 29

Hutchinson PJ, see Kett-White R, Vol. 27

Iannotti F. Functional imaging of blood brain barrier permeability by single photon emission computerised tomography and Positron Emission Tomography. Vol. 19

Immonen A, Jutila L, Kalviainen R, Mervaala E, Partanen K, Partanen J, Vanninen R, Ylinen A, Alafuzoff I, Paljarvi L, Hurskainen H, Rinne J, Puranen M, Vapalahti M. Preoperative clinical evaluation, outline of surgical technique and outcome in temporal lobe epilepsy. Vol. 29

Immonen A, see Jutila L, Vol. 27

Ingvar DH, see Lassen NA, Vol. 4

Isamat F. Tumours of the posterior part of the third ventricle: Neurosurgical criteria. Vol. 6

Isnard J, see Guenot M, Vol. 29

Isnard J, see Guénot M, Vol. 36

Jackson IT, see Harris P, Vol. 8

Jaksche H, see Loew F, Vol. 11

Jennett B, Pickard J. Economic aspects of neurosurgery. Vol. 19

Jewkes D. Neuroanaesthesia: the present position. Vol. 15

Jiang Z, see Zamorano L, Vol. 24

Johnston IH, see Owler BK, Vol. 30

Joseph PA, see Vignes JR, Vol. 30

Jutila L, Immonen A, Partanen K, Partanen J, Mervalla E, Ylinen A, Alafuzoff I, Paljarvi L, Karkola K, Vapalahti M, Pitanen A. Neurobiology of epileptogenesis in the temporal lobe. Vol. 27

Jutila L, see Immonen A, Vol. 29

Kahan-Coppens L, see Klastersky J, Vol. 6

Kalviainen R, see Immonen A, Vol. 29

Kanpolat Y. Percutaneous destructive pain procedures on the upper spinal cord and brain stem in cancer pain – CT-guided techniques, indications and results. Vol. 32

Karahalios DG, see Detwiler PW, Vol. 26

Karkola K, see Jutila L, Vol. 27

Kelly PJ. Surgical planning and computer-assisted resection of intracranial lesions: Methods and results. Vol. 17

Kett-White R, Hutchinson PJ, Czosnyka M, Boniface S, Pickard JD, Kirkpatrick PJ. Multi-modal monitoring of acute brain injury. Vol. 27

Khalfallah M, see Robert R, Vol. 32

Kirkpatrick PJ, see Kett-White R, Vol. 27

Kirkpatrick PJ, see Patel HC, Vol. 34

Kiss R, see Lefranc F, Vol. 34

Kjällquist Å, see Lundberg N, Vol. 1

Klastersky J, Kahan-Coppens L, Brihaye J. Infection in neurosurgery. Vol. 6

Klein M. Health-related quality of life aspects in patients with low-grade glioma. Vol. 35

Knufman NMJ, see Berkelbach van der Sprenkel JW, Vol. 19

Konovalov AN. Operative management of cranio-pharyngiomas. Vol. 8

Kovacs K, see Thapar K, Vol. 22

Kreth FW, Thon N, Sieffert A, Tonn JC. The place of interstitial brachytherapy and radiosurgery for low-grade gliomas. Vol. 35

Krischek B, Tatagiba M. The influence of genetics on intracranial aneurysm formation and rupture: current knowledge and its possible impact on future treatment. Vol. 33

Kullberg G, see Lundberg N, Vol. 1

Kumar A, Fisch U. The infratemporal fossa approach for lesions of the skull base. Vol. 10

Kurzwelly D, Herrlinger U, Simon M. Seizures in patients with low-grade gliomas – incidence, pathogenesis, surgical management and pharmacotherapy. Vol. 35

Labat JJ, see Robert R, Vol. 32

Lacour P, see Debrun G, Vol. 4

Lacroix J-S, see Landis BN, Vol. 30

Landis BN, Hummel Th, Lacroix J-S. Basic and clinical aspects of olfaction. Vol. 30

Landolt AM, Strebel P. Technique of transsphenoidal operation for pituitary adenomas. Vol. 7

Landolt AM. Progress in pituitary adenoma biology. Results of research and clinical applications. Vol. 5

Langer A, see Chiaretti A, Vol. 30

Lanteri P, see Sala F, Vol. 29

Lantos PL, see Pilkington GJ, Vol. 21

Lapras C, Deruty R, Bret P. Tumours of the lateral ventricles. Vol. 11

Lassen NA, Ingvar DH. Clinical relevance of cerebral blood flow measurements. Vol. 4

Author index

Latchaw R, see Yonas H, Vol. 15

Lauritzen C, see Guimaraes-Ferreira J, Vol. 29

Lavallee S, see Benabid AL, Vol. 18

Laws ER, see Thapar K, Vol. 22

Lawton MT, Daspit CP, Spetzler RF. Presigmoid approaches to skull base lesions. Vol. 23

Lazorthes Y, Sallerin-Caute B, Verdie JC, Bastide R. Advances in drug delivery systems and applications in neurosurgery. Vol. 18

Le Bas JF, see Benabid AL, Vol. 18

Le Gars D, Lejeune JP, Peltier J. Surgical anatomy and surgical approaches to the lateral ventricles. Vol. 34

Lefranc F, Rynkowski M, DeWitte O, Kiss R. Present and potential future adjuvant issues in high-grade astrocytic glioma treatment. Vol. 34

Lejeune JP, see Le Gars D. Vol. 34

Lemort M, see Brihaye J, Vol. 16

Lena G, see Choux M, Vol. 21

Lenzi GL, see Wise RJS, Vol. 10

Lescanne E, see Francois P, Vol. 36

Lieberman A, Cooper PR, Ransohoff J. Adrenal medullary transplants as a treatment for advanced Parkinson's disease. Vol. 17

Lienhart A, see Pertuiset B, Vol. 8

Lindegaard K-F, Sorteberg W, Nornes H. Transcranial Doppler in neurosurgery. Vol. 20

Lindquist C, see Steiner L, Vol. 19

Livraghi S, Melancia JP, Lobo Antunes J. The management of brain abscesses. Vol. 28

Lobato RD. Post-traumatic brain swelling. Vol. 20

Lobo Antunes J, see Monteiro Trindade A, Vol. 23

Lobo Antunes J, see Livraghi S, Vol. 28

Lobo Antunes J. Conflict of interest in medical practice. Vol. 32

Loew F, Caspar W. Surgical approach to lumbar disc herniations. Vol. 5

Loew F, Papavero L. The intra-arterial route of drug delivery in the chemotherapy of malignant brain tumours. Vol. 16

Loew F, Pertuiset B, Chaumier EE, Jaksche H. Traumatic spontaneous and postoperative CSF rhinorrhea. Vol. 11

Loew F. Management of chronic subdural haematomas and hygromas. Vol. 9

Logue V. Parasagittal meningiomas. Vol. 2

Loiseau H, Cuny E, Vital A, Cohadon F. Central nervous system lymphomas. Vol. 26

Lopes da Silva FH. What is magnetocencephalography and why it is relevant to neurosurgery? Vol. 30

Lorenz R. Methods of percutaneous spino-thalamic tract section. Vol. 3

Lumley JSP, see Taylor GW, Vol. 4

Lundberg N, Kjällquist Å, Kullberg G, Pontén U, Sundbärg G. Non-operative management of intracranial hypertension. Vol. 1

Luyendijk W. The operative approach to the posterior fossa. Vol. 3

Luyten PR, see Berkelbach van der Sprenkel JW, Vol. 19

Lyon-Caen O, see Pertuiset B, Vol. 5

Macfarlane R, Axon P, Moffat D. Invited commentary: Respective indications for radiosurgery in neuro-otology for acoustic schwannoma by Pellet et al. Vol. 28

Madea B, Noeker M, Franke I. Child abuse – some aspects for neurosurgeons. Vol. 36

Manegalli-Boggelli D, see Resche F, Vol. 20

Mansveld Beck HJ, see Streefkerk HJ, Vol. 28

Mantoura J, see Resche F, Vol. 20

Marchal JC, Civit T. Neurosurgical concepts and approaches for orbital tumours. Vol. 31

Marshall J, see Gawler J, Vol. 2

Masferrer R, see Detwiler PW, Vol. 26

Massimi L, see di Rocco C, Vol. 31

Matthies C, see Samii M, Vol. 22

Mauguière F, see Guénot M, Vol. 36

Mavrocordatos P, Cahana A. Minimally invasive procedures for the treatment of failed back surgery syndrome. Vol. 31

McGregor JC, see Harris P, Vol. 8

Medele RJ, see Schmid-Elsaesser R, Vol. 26

Melancia JP, see Livraghi S, Vol. 28

Mercier Ph, see Hayek C, Vol. 31

Mercier Ph, see Fournier H-D, Vol. 31

Mercier P, see Fournier H-D, Vol. 32

Mercier P, see Roche P-H, Vol. 33

Merlo Pich E, see Agnati LF, Vol. 16

Mervaala E, see Immonen A, Vol. 29

Mervalla E, see Jutila L, Vol. 27

Messina A, see Cappabianca P, Vol. 33

Metzger J, see Pertuiset B, Vol. 10

Meyer B, see Stoffel M, Vol. 36

Michel CM, see Momjian S, Vol. 28

Miguéns J, see Guimaraes-Ferreira J, Vol. 29

Millesi H. Surgical treatment of facial nerve paralysis: Longterm results: Extratemporal surgery of the facial nerve – Palliative surgery. Vol. 7

Mingrino S. Intracranial surgical repair of the facial nerve. Vol. 7

Mingrino S. Supratentorial arteriovenous malformations of the brain. Vol. 5

Moffet D, see Macfarlane R, Vol. 28

Moisan JP, see Resche F, Vol. 20

Momjian S, Seghier M, Seeck M, Michel CM. Mapping of the neuronal networks of human cortical brain functions. Vol. 28

Momma F, see Symon L, Vol. 14

Monteiro Trindade A, Lobo Antunes J. Anterior approaches to non-traumatic lesions of the thoracic spine. Vol. 23

Mortara RW, see Yaşargil MG, Vol. 7

Muhlig RS, see Blaauw G, Vol. 33

Müller U, see von Cramon DY, Vol. 24

N'Guyen JP, see Caparros-Lefebvre D, Vol. 25

Nemoto S, see Peerless SJ, Vol. 15

Nicolelis MAL, see Oliveira-Maia AJ, Vol. 36

Nimsky C, Ganslandt O, Fahlbusch R. Functional neuronavigation and intraoperative MRI. Vol. 29

Noeker M, see Madea B, Vol. 36

Nornes H, see Lindegaard K-F, Vol. 20

Oliveira-Maia AJ, Roberts CD, Simon SA, Nicolelis MAL. Gustatory and reward brain circuits in the control of food intake. Vol. 36

Ostenfeld T, see Rosser AE, Vol. 26

Ostenfeld T, Svendsen CN. Recent advances in stem cell neurobiology. Vol. 28

Owler BK, Parker G, Halmagyi GM, Johnston IH, Besser M, Pickard JD, Higgins JN. Cranial venous outflow obstruction and pseudotumor cerebri syndrome. Vol. 30

Ozduman K, see Pamir MN, Vol. 33

Paljarvi L, see Immonen A, Vol. 29

Paljarvi L, see Jutila L, Vol. 27

Pamir MN, Ozduman K. Tumor-biology and current treatment of skull base chordomas. Vol. 33

Papagno C, see Bello L, Vol. 35

Papavero L, see Loew F, Vol. 16

Parker G, see Owler BK, Vol. 30

Partanen J, see Immonen A, Vol. 29

Partanen J, see Jutila L, Vol. 27

Partanen K, see Immonen A, Vol. 29

Partanen K, see Jutila L, Vol. 27

Passagia JG, Chirossel JP, Favre JJ. Surgical approaches of the anterior fossa and preservation of olfaction. Vol. 25

Passagia JG, see Chirossel JP, Vol. 22

Pasztor E. Surgical treatment of spondylotic vertebral artery compression. Vol. 8

Pasztor E. Transoral approach for epidural craniocervical pathological processes. Vol. 12

Patel HC, Kirkpatrick PJ. High flow extracranial to intracranial vascular bypass procedure for giant aneurysms: indications, surgical technique, complications and outcome. Vol. 34

Peerless SJ, Nemoto S, Drake CG. Acute surgery for ruptured posterior circulation aneurysms. Vol. 15

Pellet W, Regis J, Roche P-H, Delsanti C. Respective indications for radiosurgery in neuro-otology for acoustic schwannoma. Vol. 28

Peltier J, see Le Gars D, Vol. 34

Perneczky A, see Fries G, Vol. 25

Perrin-Resche I, see Resche F, Vol. 20

Pertuiset B, Ancri D, Lienhart A. Profound arterial hypotension (MAP £ 50 mmHg) induced with neuroleptanalgesia and sodium nitroprusside (series of 531 cases). Reference to vascular auto-regulation mechanism and surgery of vascular malformations of the brain. Vol. 8

Pertuiset B, Ancri D, Sichez JP, Chauvin M, Guilly M, Metzger J, Gardeur D, Basset JY. Radical surgery in cerebral AVM – Tactical procedures based upon hemodynamic factors. Vol. 10

Pertuiset B, Fohanno D, Lyon-Caen O. Recurrent instability of the cervical spine with neurological implications – treatment by anterior spinal fusion. Vol. 5

Pertuiset B, see Loew F, Vol. 11

Pertuiset B. Supratentorial craniotomy. Vol. 1

Philippon J, Ancri D. Chronic adult hydrocephalus. Vol. 1

Pickard JD, see Coleman MR, Vol. 36

Pickard J, see Jennett B, Vol. 19

Pickard JD, see Kett-White R, Vol. 27

Pickard JD, see Sussman JD, Vol. 24

Pickard JD, see Walker V, Vol. 12

Pickard JD, see Owler BK, Vol. 30

Piepgras U, see Huber G, Vol. 11

Pilkington GJ, Lantos PL. Biological markers for tumours of the brain. Vol. 21

Pitanen A, see Jutila L, Vol. 27

Poca MA, see Sahuquillo J, Vol. 27

Polkey CE. Multiple subpial transection. Vol. 26

Pollak P, see Caparros-Lefebvre D, Vol. 25

Pontén U, see Lundberg N, Vol. 1

Porchet F, Fankhauser H, de Tribolet N. The far lateral approach to lumbar disc herniations. Vol. 23

Porta M, see Derome PJ, Vol. 6

Porter RW, see Detwiler PW, Vol. 26

Powiertowski H. Surgery of craniostenosis in advanced cases. A method of extensive subperiosteal resection of the vault and base of the skull followed by bone regeneration. Vol. 1

Price SJ. Advances in imaging low-grade gliomas. Vol. 35

Puranen M, see Immonen A, Vol. 29

Raftopoulos C; with the collaboration of Vaz G. Surgical indications and techniques for failed coiled aneurysms. Vol. 36

Ransford AO, see Crockard HA, Vol. 17

Ransohoff J, see Lieberman A, Vol. 17

Ratial B, Sampaio C. Prophylactic antibiotics and anticonvulsants in neurosurgery. Vol. 36

Ray MW, see Yaşargil MG, Vol. 2

Regis J, see Pellet W, Vol. 28

Rehncrona S. A critical review of the current status and possible developments in brain transplantation. Vol. 23

Reifenberger G, see Riemenschneider MJ, Vol. 35

Resche F, Moisan JP, Mantoura J, de Kersaint-Gilly A, Andre MJ, Perrin-Resche I, Menegalli-Boggelli D, Richard Y. Lajat. Haemangioblastoma, haemangioblastomatosis and von Hippel-Lindau disease. Vol. 20

Rétif J. Intrathecal injection of neurolytic solution for the relief of intractable pain. Vol. 4

Reulen H-J, see Ebeling U, Vol. 22

Rey A, Cophignon J, Thurel C, Thiebaut JB. Treatment of traumatic cavernous fistulas. Vol. 2

Riant T, see Robert R, Vol. 32

Richard Y. Lajat, see Resche F, Vol. 20

Riemenschneider MJ, Reifenberger G. Molecular neuropathology of low-grade gliomas and its clinical impact. Vol. 35

Ringel F, see Stoffel M, Vol. 36

Rinne J, see Immonen A, Vol. 29

Roberts CD, see Oliveira-Maia AJ, Vol. 36

Robert R, Labat JJ, Riant T, Khalfahhah M, Hame O. Neurosurgical treatment of perineal neuralgias. Vol. 32

Roche P-H, see Pellet W, Vol. 28

Roche P-H, see Fournier H-D, Vol. 32

Roche P-H, Mercier P, Sameshima T, Fournier H-D. Surgical Anatomy of the jugular foramen. Vol. 33

Romodanov AP, Shcheglov VI. Intravascular occlusion of saccular aneurysms of the cerebral arteries by means of a detachable balloon catheter. Vol. 9

Rosenblum ML, see Ciricillo SF, Vol. 21

Rosser AE, Ostenfeld T, Svendsen CN. Invited commentary: Treatment of diseases of the central nervous system using encapsulated cells, by AF Hottinger and P. Aebischer. Vol. 25

Roth P, see Yaşargil MG, Vol. 12

Roth P, see Yaşargil MG, Vol. 18

Rynkowski M, see Lefranc F, Vol. 34

Sahuquillo J, Poca MA. Diffuse axonal injury after head trauma. A review. Vol. 27

Sala F, Lanteri P, Bricolo A. Motor evoked potential monitoring for spinal cord and brain stem surgery. Vol. 29

Sallerin-Caute B, see Lazorthes Y, Vol. 18

Sameshima T, see Roche P-H, Vol. 33

Samii M, Matthies C. Hearing preservation in acoustic tumour surgery. Vol. 22

Samii M. Modern aspects of peripheral and cranial nerve surgery. Vol. 2

Sampaio C, see Ratial B, Vol. 36

Sarkies N, see Sussman JD, Vol. 24

Sawamura Y, de Tribolet N. Immunobiology of brain tumours. Vol. 17

Sawamura Y, de Tribolet N. Neurosurgical management of pineal tumours. Vol. 27

Sawamura Y, Shirato H, de Tribolet N. Recent advances in the treatment of the central nervous system germ cell tumors. Vol. 25

Schlapfer TE, Bewernick BH. Deep brain stimulation for psychiatric disorders – state of the art. Vol. 34

Author index

Schmid-Elsaesser R, Medele RJ, Steiger H-J. Reconstructive surgery of the extracranial arteries. Vol. 26

Schwartz M, see Gentili F, Vol. 19

Schwerdtfeger K, see Symon L, Vol. 14

Seeck M, see Momjian S, Vol. 28

Seghier M, see Momjian S, Vol. 28

Shcheglov VI, see Romodanov AP, Vol. 9

Shirato H, see Sawamura Y, Vol. 25

Sichez JP, see Pertuiset B, Vol. 10

Siefert A, see Kreth FW, Vol. 35

Siegfried J, Hood T. Current status of functional neurosurgery. Vol. 10

Siegfried J, Vosmansky M. Technique of the controlled thermocoagulation of trigeminal ganglion and spinal roots. Vol. 2

Simon M, see Kurzwelly D, Vol. 35

Simon SA, see Oliveira-Maia AJ, Vol. 36

Sindou M, Auque J. The intracranial venous system as a neurosurgeon's perspective. Vol. 26

Sindou M, Goutelle A. Surgical posterior rhizotomies for the treatment of pain. Vol. 10

Sindou M, Guenot M. Surgical anatomy of the temporal lobe for epilepsy surgery. Vol. 28

Sindou M, see Guenot M, Vol. 29

Sindou M, see Guénot M, Vol. 36

Sindou M, Gimbert E. Decompression for Chiari Type I malformation (with or without syringomyelia) by extreme lateral foramen magnum opening and expansile duraplasty with arachnoid preservation: comparison with other technical modalities (literature review). Vol. 34

Smith RD, see Yaşargil MG, Vol. 4

Sonntag VKH, see Detwiler PW, Vol. 26

Sorteberg W, see Lindegaard K-F, Vol. 20

Spallone A, see Guidetti B, Vol. 16

Spaziante R, see de Divitiis E, Vol. 8

Spennato P, see di Rocco C, Vol. 31

Spetzler RF, see Lawton MT, Vol. 23

Spiess H. Advances in computerized tomography. Vol. 9

Spincemaille G, see DeJongste MJL, Vol. 32

Staal MJ, see DeJongste MJL, Vol. 32

Steiger H-J, see Schmid-Elsaesser R, Vol. 26

Steiner L, Lindquist C, Steiner M. Radiosurgery. Vol. 19

Steiner M, see Steiner L, Vol. 19

Stella L, see de Divitiis E, Vol. 8

Stoffel M, Stüer C, Ringel F, Meyer B. Treatment of infections of the spine. Vol. 36

Strebel P, see Landolt AM, Vol. 7

Streefkerk HJN, van der Zwan A, Verdaasdonk RM, Mansveld Beck HJ, Tulleken CAF. Cerebral revascularization. Vol. 28

Strong AJ, Dardis R. Depolarisation phenomena in traumatic and ischaemic brain injury. Vol. 30

Stüer C, see Stoffel M, Vol. 36

Stupp R, see Baumert BG, Vol. 35

Sundbärg G, see Lundberg N, Vol. 1

Sussman JD, Sarkies N, Pickard JD. Benign intracranial hypertension. Vol. 24

Svendsen CN, see Rosser AE, Vol. 26

Svendsen CN, see Ostenfeld T, Vol. 28

Symon L, Momma F, Schwerdtfeger K, Bentivoglio P, Costa e Silva IE, Wang A. Evoked potential monitoring in neurosurgical practice. Vol. 14

Symon L, see Yaşargil MG, Vol. 11

Symon L. Olfactory groove and suprasellar meningiomas. Vol. 4

Symon L. Surgical approaches to the tentorial hiatus. Vol. 9

Tamburrini G, see di Rocco C, Vol. 31

Tatagiba M, see Krischek B, Vol. 33

Taylor GW, Lumley JSP. Extra-cranial surgery for cerebrovascular disease. Vol. 4

Teddy PJ, see Yaşargil MG, Vol. 11

Teddy PJ, see Yaşargil MG, Vol. 12

TerBrugge K, see Gentili F, Vol. 19

Tew JM Jr, Tobler WD. Present status of lasers in neurosurgery. Vol. 13

Thapar K, Kovacs K, Laws ER. The classification and molecular biology of pituitary adenomas. Vol. 22

Thiebaut JB, see Rey A, Vol. 2

Thomas DGT. Dorsal root entry zone (DREZ) thermocoagulation. Vol. 15

Thon N, see Kreth FW, Vol. 35

Thurel C, see Rey A, Vol. 2

Tobler WD, see Tew JM Jr, Vol. 13

Toffano G, see Agnati LF, Vol. 16

Tonetti J, see Chirossel JP, Vol. 22

Tonn JC, see Kreth FW, Vol. 35

Torres N, Chabardès S, Benabid AL. Rationale for hypothalamus-deep brain stimulation in food intake disorders and obesity. Vol. 36

Tranmer BI, see Yaşargil MG, Vol. 18

Troupp H. The management of intracranial arterial aneurysms in the acute stage. Vol. 3

Tulleken CAF, see Berkelbach van der Sprenkel JW, Vol. 19

Tulleken CAF, see Streefkerk HJ, Vol. 28

Turazzi S, see Bricolo A, Vol. 22

Uttley D. Transfacial approaches to the skull base. Vol. 23

Valatx J-L. Disorders of consciousness: Anatomical and physiological mechanisms. Vol. 29

Valavanis A, Yaşargil MG. The endovascular treatment of brain arteriovenous malformations. Vol. 24

van der Zwan A, see Streefkerk HJ, Vol. 28

van Houtte P, see Brihaye J, Vol. 16

van Manen, see Cosyns P, Vol. 21

van Rijen PC, see Berkelbach van der Sprenkel JW, Vol. 19

van Roost D, see Gybels J, Vol. 15

van Veelen C, see Cosyns P, Vol. 21

Vanneuville G, see Chirossel JP, Vol. 22

Vanninen R, see Immonen A, Vol. 29

Vapalahti M, see Immonen A, Vol. 29

Vapalahti M, see Jutila L, Vol. 27

Vaz G, see Raftopoulos C, Vol. 36

Velut S, see Francois P, Vol. 36

Verdaasdonk RM, see Streefkerk HJ, Vol. 28

Verdie JC, see Lazorthes Y, Vol. 18

Vernet O, see Villemure J-G, Vol. 26

Vignes JR, de Seze M, Dobremez E, Joseph PA, Guerin J. Sacral neuromodulation in lower urinary tract dysfunction. Vol. 30

Villemure J-G, Vernet O, Delalande O. Hemispheric disconnection: Callosotomy and hemispherotomy

Vinas FC, see Zamorano L, Vol. 24

Vinchon M, Dhellemmes P. Transition from child to adult in neurosurgery. Vol. 32

Visot A, see Derome PJ, Vol. 6

Vital A, see Loiseau H, Vol. 26

von Cramon DY, Müller U. The septal region and memory. Vol. 24

von Werder K. The biological role of hypothalamic hypophysiotropic neuropeptides. Vol. 14

Vonck K, De Herdt V, Boon P. Vagal nerve stimulation – a 15-year survey of an established treatment modality in epilepsy surgery. Vol. 34

Vosmansky M, see Siegfried J, Vol. 2

Vredeveld JW, see Blaauw G, Vol. 33

Walker V, Pickard JD. Prostaglandins, thromboxane, leukotrienes and the cerebral circulation in health and disease. Vol. 12

Wallace MC, see Gentili F, Vol. 19

Wang A, see Symon L, Vol. 14

Whittle IR. What is the place of conservative management for adult supratentorial low-grade glioma? Vol. 35

Wieser HG. Selective amygdalohippocampectomy: Indications, investigative technique and results. Vol. 13

Williams B. Subdural empyema. Vol. 9

Williams B. Surgery for hindbrain related syringomyelia. Vol. 20

Willinsky R, see Gentili F, Vol. 19

Wirth T, Yla-Herttuala S. Gene technology based therapies. Vol. 31

Wise RJS, Lenzi GL, Frackowiak RSJ. Applications of Positron Emission Tomography to neurosurgery. Vol. 10

Wolfson SK Jr, see Yonas H, Vol. 15

Woolf CJ. Physiological, inflammatory and neuropathic pain. Vol. 15

Yaşargil MG, Fox JP, Ray MW. The operative approach to aneurysms of the anterior communicating artery. Vol. 2

Yaşargil MG, Mortara RW, Curcic M. Meningiomas of basal posterior cranial fossa. Vol. 7

Yaşargil MG, see Valavanis A, Vol. 24

Yaşargil MG, see Yonekawa Y, Vol. 3

Yaşargil MG, Smith RD, Gasser JC. Microsurgical approach to acoustic neurinomas. Vol. 4

Yaşargil MG, Symon L, Teddy PJ. Arteriovenous malformations of the spinal cord. Vol. 11

Yaşargil MG, Teddy PJ, Roth P. Selective amygdalohippocampectomy: Operative anatomy and surgical technique. Vol. 12

Yaşargil MG, Tranmer BI, Adamson TE, Roth P. Unilateral partial hemilaminectomy for the removal of extra- and intramedullary tumours and AVMs. Vol. 18

Yla-Herttuala S, see Wirth T, Vol. 31

Ylinen A, see Immonen A, Vol. 29

Ylinen A, see Jutila L, Vol. 27

Yonas H, Gur D, Latchaw R, Wolfson SK Jr. Stable xenon CI/CBF imaging: Laboratory and clinical experience. Vol. 15

Yonekawa Y, Yaşargil MG. Extra-Intracranial arterial anastomosis: Clinical and technical aspects. Results. Vol. 3

Young C, see Gentili F, Vol. 19

Zamorano L, Vinas FC, Jiang Z, Diaz FG. Use of surgical wands in neurosurgery. Vol. 24

Zander E, Campiche R. Extra-dural hematoma. Vol. 1

Zini I, see Agnati LF, Vol. 16

Zoli M, see Agnati LF, Vol. 16

Subject index volume 1–36

Advances and Technical Standards in Neurosurgery

Abscess
  brain, 2002, Vol. 28
Acoustic schwannoma
  hearing preservation, 1995,
    Vol. 22
  microsurgery, 1977, Vol. 4;
    2002, Vol. 28
  radiosurgery, 2002, Vol. 28
AIDS
  neurosurgery, 1994, Vol. 21
Alzheimer's disease
  gene therapy, 2005, Vol. 31
Amygdalohippocampectomy
  indications, investigations and
    results, 1986, Vol. 13
  operative anatomy and surgical
    technique, 1985, Vol. 12
Anatomy
  extended endoscopic endonasal,
    2008, Vol. 33
  insula, 2003, Vol. 29
  jugular foramen, 2008, Vol. 33
  lateral ventricles, 2008, Vol. 34
  optic nerve, 2010, Vol. 36
  orbit, 2005, Vol. 31
  petrous apex, 2007, Vol. 32
Aneurysms
  acute stage, 1976, Vol. 3
  acute surgery for ruptured
    posterior circulation, 1987,
    Vol. 15
  anterior communicating artery,
    1975, Vol. 2
  balloons, 1982, Vol. 9
  clipping, 2010, Vol. 36
  coiling, 2010, Vol. 36

controversies in their intraoperative
    management, 1986, Vol. 14
  embolisation, 2010, Vol 36
  genetics, 2008, Vol. 33
  giant, 2008, Vol. 34
  interventional neuroradiology,
    1982, Vol. 9; 1998, Vol. 24
  residual, 2010, Vol. 36
Anterior fossa
  preservation of olfaction, 1999,
    Vol. 25
Antibiotics (prophylactic), 2010,
    Vol. 36
Anticonvulsants (prophylactic), 2010,
    Vol. 36
Arteriovenous malformation, 1979,
    Vol. 6
  endovascular approaches, 1998,
    Vol. 24
  multidisciplinary approach to
    management, 1992, Vol. 19
  radical surgery, 1983, Vol. 10
  spinal cord, 1984, Vol. 11
  supratentorial, 1978, Vol. 5

Back pain, 2005, Vol. 31
Benign intracranial hypertension, 1998,
    Vol. 24; 2004, Vol. 30
Birth palsy (Brachial plexus), 2008,
    Vol. 33
Blood brain barrier
  permeability, 1992, Vol. 19
  single photon emission
    computerised tomography and
    positron emission tomography,
    1992, Vol. 19

Brachial plexus injuries, 2008, Vol. 33
Brain plasticity, 2008, Vol. 33
Brain protection, 1994, Vol. 21; 2004, Vol. 30
Brain swelling
  brain water, 1997, Vol. 23
  post traumatic, 1993, Vol. 20
Brain tumours
  biological markers, 1994, Vol. 21
  brain stem glioma, 1995, Vol. 22
  Central Nervous System lymphomas, 2000, Vol. 26
  chemotherapy, 1978, Vol. 5; 2008, Vol. 34
  childhood to adult, 2007, Vol. 32
  gene therapy, 2005, Vol. 31
  germ cell, 1999, Vol. 25
  gliomas, 1990, Vol. 17; 1994, Vol. 21; 1998, Vol. 24; 2008, Vol. 33; 2009, Vol. 35
  haemangioblastoma, 1993, Vol. 20
  histological prognosis, 1994, Vol. 21
  hypothalamic glioma, 1999, Vol. 25
  immunobiology, 1990, Vol. 17
  indications for surgery, 1990. Vol. 17
  low-grade gliomas, 2009, Vol. 35
    imaging
    molecular neuropathology
    conservative management
    seizure
    microsurgery
    radiotherapy
    interstitial brachytherapy
    quality of life
  medulloblastoma, 1993, Vol. 20
  petroclival, 2007, Vol. 32
  pineal: neurosurgical management, 2001, Vol. 27
  Positron Emission Tomography, 1998, Vol. 24
  prophylactic anticonvulsants, 2010, Vol. 36
  ventricular, 2008, Vol. 34

  von Hippel-Lindau disease, 1993, Vol. 20
  WHO classification, 1981, Vol. 8
Brain water
  normal and pathological physiology, 1997, Vol. 23

Cavernomas, 1995, Vol. 22
Cavernous fistulae
  traumatic, 1975, Vol. 2
Cerebral angiography
  digital subtraction, 1984, Vol. 11
Cerebral blood flow
  measurements, 1977, Vol. 4
  stable Xenon technique, 1987, Vol. 15
Cerebral ischaemia, 2004, Vol. 30
Cerebral revascularisation, 2002, Vol. 28
Cerebral vasospasm
  gene therapy, 2005, Vol. 31
  prostaglandins, 1985, Vol. 12
Cerebral venous system, 2000, Vol. 26; 2004, Vol. 30
Cerebrovascular autoregulation
  profound arterial hypotension, 1981, Vol. 8
Cerebrovascular disease
  balloon occlusion, 1977, Vol. 4
  extracranial arteries, 2000, Vol. 26
  extracranial surgery, 1977, Vol. 4
  extracranial vertebral artery anatomy and surgery, 2001, Vol. 27
  intracerebral haemorrhage (genetics), 2008, Vol. 33
Cervical spine
  anterior spinal fusion, 1978, Vol. 5
  instability, 1978, Vol. 5
Cervical spondylosis
  myelopathy, 1979, Vol. 6
Chiari malformation, 2008, Vol. 34
Child abuse, 2010, Vol. 36
Childhood transition to adult, 2007, Vol. 32

Subject index

Chordoma
  tumour biology, 2008, Vol. 33
  operative technique, 2008, Vol. 33
Chondrosarcoma
  tumour biology, 2008, Vol. 33
  operative technique, 2008, Vol. 33
Clinical Trials, 2008, Vol. 34
Clivus
  surgical approach, 1979, Vol. 6
Consciousness
  coma, 2003, Vol. 29
  neuropharmacology, 2003, Vol. 29
  vegetative state, 2010, Vol. 36
Cranial nerves
  jugular foramen, 2008, Vol. 33
  surgery, 1975, Vol. 2
Craniopharyngioma
  operative management, 1981,
    Vol. 8
Craniostenosis, 1974, Vol. 1
Craniosynostosis, 2003, Vol. 29
Craniotomy
  supratentorial, 1974, Vol. 1
CSF rhinorrhea, 1984, Vol. 11
CT Scanning, 1975, Vol. 2; 1982,
  Vol. 9

Deep Brain Stimulation, 2008, Vol. 34;
  2010, Vol. 36
Drug delivery
  advances, 1991, Vol. 18
  intra-arterial administration of
    chemotherapy, 1988, Vol. 16

Eating disorders, 2010, Vol. 36
Electrical stimulation mapping, 2008,
  Vol. 33
Endoscopy
  endonasal transsphenoidal surgery,
    2001, Vol. 27
  carpal tunnel syndrome, 2007,
    Vol. 32
  in neurosurgery, 1986, Vol. 14
  intracranial, 1999, Vol. 25
Epidemiology
  Child abuse, 2010, Vol. 36

Epilepsy
  hemispheric disconnection:
    callosotomy and
    hemispherotomy, 2000, Vol. 26
  low-grade gliomas, 2009, Vol. 35
  multiple subpial transection, 2000,
    Vol. 26
  neurobiology of epileptogenesis,
    2001, Vol. 27
  outcome, 2003, Vol. 29
  preoperative evaluation, 2003,
    Vol. 29
  SEEG-guided
    RF-Haemocoagulation, 2010,
    Vol. 36
  surgery, 2003, Vol. 29; 2008,
    Vol. 34; 2010, Vol. 36
  surgical anatomy of the temporal
    lobe, 2002, Vol. 28
  temporal lobe epilepsy, 2003,
    Vol. 29
  vagal nerve stimulation, 2008,
    Vol. 34
Ethics, 2008, Vol. 34
  conflict of interest, 2007, Vol. 32
Evoked potentials
  monitoring in neurosurgical
    practice, 1986, Vol. 14
Extradural haematoma, 1974, Vol. 1
Extra-intracranial arterial anastomosis,
  1976, Vol. 3; 2002, Vol. 28; 2008,
  Vol. 34

Facial nerve paralysis
  extra-temporal, 1980, Vol. 7
  intracranial repair, 1980, Vol. 7
  infratemporal, 1980, Vol. 7
  surgical treatment, 1980, Vol. 7
Feeding, 2010, Vol. 36
Foramen Magnum
  benign extramedullary tumours,
    1988, Vol. 16
  decompression, 2008, Vol. 34
Frameless stereotactic surgery
  neuronavigation, 2003, Vol. 29
  surgical wands, 1998, Vol. 24

Functional neurosurgery, 1983, Vol. 10
  brain plasticity, 2008, Vol. 33
  chronic deep brain stimulation,
    1999, Vol. 25
  functional neuronavigation, 2003,
    Vol. 29
  mapping of human cortical function
    2002, Vol. 28
  movement disorders, 1999, Vol. 25
  sacral neuromodulation, 2004,
    Vol. 30
  psychiatric disorders, 1994, Vol. 21;
    2008, Vol. 34

Gamma knife
  chondroma (chondrosarcoma),
    2008, Vol. 33
Gene therapy
  viral vectors, 2005, Vol. 31
Genetics
  cerebral aneurysms, 2008, Vol. 33
Glomus tumours, 2008, Vol. 33

Head injury
  child abuse, 2010, Vol. 36
  chronic subdural haematoma, 2010,
    Vol. 36
  diffuse external injury, 2001,
    Vol. 27
  multi-modal monitoring, 2001,
    Vol. 27
  Skull fracture (prophylaxis) 2010,
    Vol. 36
  transport, 1991, Vol. 18
  depolorisation phenomena, 2004,
    Vol. 30
Health economics of neurosurgery,
  1992, Vol. 19
Hydrocephalus
  adult, 1974, Vol. 1
  measurement of CSF absorption,
    1992, Vol. 19
  over drainage, 1982, Vol. 9
  prophylaxis, 2010, Vol. 36
  shunts and shunt problems in
    childhood, 1988, Vol. 16

  third ventriculostomy, 2005,
    Vol. 31
  transition from child to adult, 2007,
    Vol. 32
Hypothalamus
  neuropeptides, 1986, Vol. 14
  deep brain stimulation, 2010,
    Vol. 36

Infection
  brain abscess, 2002, Vol. 28
  neurosurgery, 1979, Vol. 6
  prophylactic antibodies, 2010,
    Vol. 36
  subdural empyema, 1982, Vol. 9
Intracranial pressure, 1974, Vol. 1.
Insula
  surgical anatomy, 2003, Vol. 29
Ischaemic heart disease, 2007, Vol. 32

Jugular foramen
  surgical anatomy, 2008, Vol. 33

Language
  brain plasticity, 2008, Vol. 33
Lasers in neurosurgery, 1986, Vol. 13
Lateral ventricles
  tumours, 1984, Vol. 11; 2008,
    Vol. 34
Lumbar spine
  discography, 2005, Vol. 31
  failed back syndrome, 2005, Vol. 31
  far lateral approach, 1997, Vol. 23
  prolapsed lumbar intravertebral
    disc, operative approach, 1978,
    Vol. 5
  prolapsed lumbar intravertebral
    disc, 1997, Vol. 23
  spondylolisthesis: surgical
    treatment, 2000, Vol. 26

Magnetic resonance imaging, 1984,
  Vol. 11
  carpal tunnel syndrome, 2007,
    Vol. 32
  brain plasticity, 2008, Vol. 33

Subject index

functional imaging, 2010, Vol. 36
intraoperative, 2003, Vol. 29
low-grade gliomas, 2009, Vol. 35
proton spectroscopy, 1992, Vol. 19
Magnetoencephalography, 2004,
Vol. 30
Memory
septal region, 1998, Vol. 24
Meningiomas
jugular foramen, 2008, Vol. 33
olfactory groove and suprasellar,
1977, Vol. 4
optic nerve sheath, 2005,
Vol. 31
parasagittal, 1975, Vol. 2
petroclival, 2007, Vol. 32
posterior fossa, 1980, Vol. 7
sphenoidal ridge, 1986, Vol. 14
Microsurgery
low-grade gliomas, 2009, Vol. 35
Minimally conscious state, 2010,
Vol. 36
Molecular neuropathology
low-grade gliomas, 2009, Vol. 35
Monitoring
brain stem surgery, 2003, Vol. 29
magnetoencephalography, 2004,
Vol. 30
motor evoked potentials, 2003,
Vol. 29
spinal cord surgery, 2003, Vol. 29
Myelomeningocoele, 2007, Vol. 32

Neuroanaesthesia, 1987, Vol. 15
Neurofibromatosis
orbital, 2005, Vol. 31
Neurogenetics in neurosurgery, 1993,
Vol. 20
Neuromodulation, 2007, Vol. 32;
2008, Vol. 34
Neurophysiology – carpal tunnel
syndrome, 2007, Vol. 32
Neuronavigation, 2003, Vol. 29

Obesity, 2010, Vol. 36
Olfaction, 2004, Vol. 30

Optic nerve, 2010, Vol. 36
Orbital tumours
operative approaches, 1976,
Vol. 3; 2005, Vol. 31
Outcome
age, 2007, Vol. 32

Paediatric neurosurgery
postoperative pain, 2004, Vol. 30
third ventriculostomy, 2005,
Vol. 31
Pain
intrathecal neurolysis, 1977, Vol. 4
nerve blocks, 2005, Vol. 31
percutaneous CT guided perineal,
2007, Vol. 32
physiological, inflammatory and
neuropathic, 1987, Vol. 15
postoperative, 2004, Vol. 30
radiofrequency lesions, 2005,
Vol. 31
spinal cord stimulation, 2005,
Vol. 31; 2007, Vol. 32
surgical posterior Rhizotomy, 1983,
Vol. 10
Parkinson's disease
gene therapy, 2005, Vol. 31
Peripheral nerves
carpal tunnel syndrome, 2007,
Vol. 32
pudendal nerve, 2007, Vol. 32
surgery, 1975, Vol. 2
Peripheral vascular disease, 2007,
Vol. 32
Pituitary adenomas
biology, 1978, Vol. 5
classification and molecular
biology, 1995, Vol. 22
endoscopic endonasal
transsphenoidal approaches,
2001, Vol. 27
extended endoscopic endonasal
approach, 2008, Vol. 33
surgery, 1976, Vol. 3
transphenoidal approach, 1980,
Vol. 7

Positron Emission Tomography, 1983,
Vol. 10; 1992, Vol. 19
blood brain barrier permeability,
1992, Vol. 19
in vivo metabolism of brain
gliomas, 1998, Vol. 24
low-grade gliomas, 2009, Vol. 35
Posterior fossa
operative approach, 1976, Vol. 3
Prophylaxis in Neurosurgery, 2010,
Vol. 36
Prostaglandins
cerebral circulation, 1985, Vol. 12
Pseudotumour cerebri, 1998, Vol. 24;
2004, Vol. 30
Psychiatry, 2008, Vol. 34

Quality of life
low-grade gliomas, 2009, Vol. 35

Radio frequency thermocoagulations,
2010, Vol. 36
Radiosurgery, 1992, Vol. 19
acoustic schwannoma, 2002,
Vol. 28
chondroma/chondrosarcoma, 2008,
Vol. 33
intracranial tumours, 1979, Vol. 6
low-grade gliomas, 2009, Vol. 35
Regeneration in the CNS, 1988,
Vol. 16
Robots in neurosurgery, 1991,
Vol. 18

Scalp flaps, 2005, Vol. 31
SEEG, 2010, Vol. 36
Sella
benign intrasellar cyst, 1981, Vol. 8
empty, 1981, Vol. 8
Sensori-motor region
space-occupying lesions, 1995,
Vol. 22
Skull base
chondroma/chondrosarcoma, 2008,
Vol. 33

skull base fracture, 2010, Vol. 36
skull base surgery, 2010, Vol. 36
extended endoscopic endonasal
approach to midline skull base,
2008, Vol. 33
infratemporal fossa approach, 1983,
Vol. 10
jugular foramen, 2008, Vol. 33
transfacial approaches, 1997,
Vol. 23
presigmoid approaches, 1997,
Vol. 23
scalp flaps, 2005, Vol. 31
Spasticity
clinical classification, 1979, Vol. 6
spinal cord stimulation, 1987,
Vol. 15
surgical treatment, 1979, Vol. 6
Sphenoid
surgical approach, 1979, Vol. 6
Spinal cord
extra-medullary, benign, 1974,
Vol. 1
stimulation, 2005, Vol. 31; 2007,
Vol. 32
Spinal cord tumours
astrocytomas of childhood, 1986,
Vol. 13
congenital in children, 1986,
Vol. 14
extra- and intramedullary tumours
and arteriovenous malformations,
1991, Vol. 18
unilateral partial hemilaminectomy,
1991, Vol. 18
Spinal dysraphism
surgery of occult, 1994, Vol. 21
Spinal epidural metastases
management, 1988, Vol. 16
Spinal stabilization, 1990, Vol. 17
Spinal trauma
biomechanics and classification,
1995, Vol. 22
Spino-thalamic tract
subcutaneous section, 1976,
Vol. 3

Subject index

Spontaneous intracranial haemorrhage
   controversies over management,
     1987, Vol. 15
Spreading depression
   cerebral blood flow, 2003, Vol. 29
   cerebral ischaemia, 2003, Vol. 29
   head injury, 2003, Vol. 29
Stem cells
   neurobiology 2002, Vol. 28
Stereotactic imaging, 1990, Vol. 17
Subarachnoid haemorrhage (see also
   aneurysms and AVM)
   clipping, 2010, Vol. 36
   medical management, 1991, Vol. 18
   endovascular therapy, 2010, Vol. 36
   genetics, 2008, Vol. 33
Subdural haematomas and hygromas
   chronic, 1982, Vol. 9
Syringomyelia
   hindbrain related, 1993, Vol. 20
   operative approaches, 1978, Vol. 5
   surgical approach, 1993, Vol. 20;
     2008, Vol. 34
Systematic review, 2010, Vol. 36
   prophylaxis in Neurosurgery, 2010,
     Vol. 36

Taste, 2010, Vol. 36
Tentorial hiatus
   surgical approaches, 1982, Vol. 9
Thermocoagulation, 1975, Vol. 2
   dorsal root entry zone (DREZ), 1987,
     Vol. 15
Third ventricle
   colloid cysts, 1990, Vol. 17

surgical techniques and
   management, 1990, Vol. 17
tumours of posterior part, 1979,
   Vol. 6
Thoracic spine
   anterior approaches to non-
     traumatic lesions, 1997, Vol. 23
Transcranial Doppler, 1993, Vol. 20
Trans-oral approaches
   epidural craniocervical pathology,
     1985, Vol. 12
Transphenoidal surgery
   extended endoscopic endonasal
     approach, 2008, Vol. 33
Transplantation
   brain, 1997, Vol. 23
   encapsulated cells, 1999, Vol. 25
   encapsulated cells: commentary,
     2000, Vol. 26
Transplants
   adrenal medullary for Parkinson's,
     1990, Vol. 17
Tumours
   brain plasticity, 2008, Vol. 33

Urinary tract, 2004, Vol. 30

Vagal nerve stimulation, 2008,
   Vol. 34
Ventricular shunt, 2010, Vol. 36
Vegetative state, 2010, Vol. 36
Vertebral artery
   spondylotic compression, 1981,
     Vol. 8

SpringerMedicine

J. Schramm (ed.)

Advances and Technical Standards in Neurosurgery, Vol. 35

Low-Grade Gliomas

2010. XIV, 256 p. 40 illus. in color.
Hardcover **EUR 139,95**
ISBN 978-3-211-99480-1

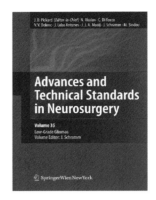

From the contents:
S. Price: Advances in imaging low-grade gliomas.- M. J. Riemenschneider, G. Riefenberger: Molecular neuropathology of low-grade gliomas and its clinical impact.- I. R. Whittle: What is the place of conservative management for adult supratentorial low-grade glioma.- D. Kurzwelly, U. Herrlinger, M. Simon: Seizures in patients with low-grade gliomas -- incidence, pathogenesis, surgical management, and pharmacotherapy.- L. Be lo et al: Present day's standards in microsurgery of low-grade gliomas.- B. Baumert and R. Stupp: Is there a place for radiotherapy in low-grade gliomas?.- F. W. Kreth et al: The place of interstitial brachytherapy and radiosurgery for low-grade gliomas.- M. Klein: Health-related quality of life aspects in patients with low-grade glioma.

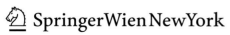

P.O. Box 89, Sachsenplatz 4–6, 1201 Vienna, Austria, Fax +43.1.330 24 26, books@springer.at, springer.at
Haberstraße 7, 69126 Heidelberg, Germany, Fax +49.6221.345-4229, SDC-bookorder@springer-sbm.com, springer.com
P.O. Box 2485, Secaucus, NJ 07096-2485, USA, Fax +1.201.348-4505, service@springer-ny.com, springer.com
All errors and omissions excepted. Recommended retail price. Net-price subject to local VAT.

SpringerNeurosurgery

Advances and Technical Standards in Neurosurgery

Volume 34

2009. XIV, 206 pages. 55 illus. in color.
Hardcover **EUR 134,95**
ISBN 978-3-211-78740-3

Advances: Present and potential future adjuvant issues in high-grade astrocytic glioma treatment (F. Lefranc et al.) • Deep Brain stimulation for psychiatric disorders – state of the art (T.E. Schlaepfer, B.H. Bewernick)

Technical Standards: High flow extracranial to intracranial vascular bypass procedure for giant aneurysm indications, surgical technique, complications and outcome (H.C. Patel, P.J. Kirkpatrick) • Decompression of Chiari Type I malformation ... (M. Sindou, E. Gimbert) • Vagal nerve stimulation – a 15-year survey of an established treatment modality in epilepsy surgery (K. Vonck, V. de Herdt, P. Boon) • Surgical anatomy of the lateral ventricles (D. Le Gars, J.P. Lejeune, J. Peltier)

Volume 33

2008. XIII, 282 pages. 74 figures, partly in colour.
Hardcover **EUR 134,95**
ISBN 978-3-211-72282-4

Advances: Brain plasticity and tumors (H. Duffau) • Tumor-biology and current treatment of skull-base chordomas (M.N. Pamir, K. Özduman) • The influence of genetics on intracranial aneurysm formation and rupture: current knowledge and its possible impact on future treatment. (B. Krischek, M. Tatagiba)

Technical Standards: Extended endoscopic endonasal approach to the midline skull base: the evolving role of transsphenoidal surgery (P. Cappabianca, L.M. Cavallo, F. Esposito, O. de Divitiis, A. Messina, E. de Divitiis) • Management of brachial plexus injuries (G. Blaauw, R.S. Muhlig, J.W. Vredeveld) • Surgical anatomy of the jugular foramen (P-H. Roche, P. Mercier, T. Sameshima, H-D. Fournier)

All prices are recommended retail prices
Net-prices subject to local VAT.

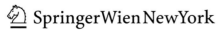

P.O. Box 89, Sachsenplatz 4–6, 1201 Vienna, Austria, Fax +43.1.330 24 26, books@springer.at, **springer.at**
Haberstraße 7, 69126 Heidelberg, Germany, Fax +49.6221.345-4229, SDC-bookorder@springer.com, springer.com
P.O. Box 2485, Secaucus, NJ 07096-2485, USA, Fax +1.201.348-4505, service@springer-ny.com, springer.com
All errors and omissions excepted.

SpringerNeurosurgery

Marc Sindou (ed.)

Practical Handbook of Neurosurgery

From Leading Neurosurgeons

3 volumes.
2009. XVIII, 1695 pages. 600 illus.
Hardcover **EUR 499.00**
ISBN 978-3-211-84819-7

The book invites the reader to an exciting journey through the vast fields of neurosurgery, accompanied by a large panel of leading neurosurgeons. At a time when neurosurgery has a tendency to segment in many subspecialties, the goal was to regroup practical lessons from experienced neurosurgeons. In addition, the book represents an anthology of ninety worldwide recognized neurosurgeons, with the main features of their curriculum and contributions. The book has three volumes which cover the following items: Volume 1: Techniques and cranial approaches; Vascular lesions; Cranial traumas; CSF/infectious diseases - Volume 2: Intracranial tumors; Intraoperative explorations; Pediatrics; - Volume 3: Spine; Functional neurosurgery; Peripheral nerves; Education.
The authors deliver their critical views and give useful guidelines.

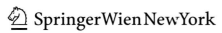

P.O. Box 89, Sachsenplatz 4–6, 1201 Vienna, Austria, Fax +43.1.330 24 26, books@springer.at, **springer.at**
Haberstraße 7, 69126 Heidelberg, Germany, Fax +49.6221.345-4229, SDC-bookorder@springer.com, springer.com
P.O. Box 2485, Secaucus, NJ 07096-2485, USA, Fax +1.201.348-4505, service@springer-ny.com, springer.com
Prices are subject to change without notice. All errors and omissions excepted.